HEALTH CARE SYSTEMS IN TRANSITION

HEALTH CARE SYSTEMS IN TRANSITION

An International Perspective

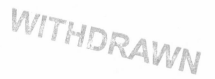

Francis D. Powell
Albert F. Wessen

Editors

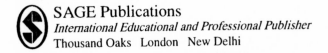

SAGE Publications
International Educational and Professional Publisher
Thousand Oaks   London   New Delhi

For information:

SAGE Publications, Inc.
2455 Teller Road
Thousand Oaks, California 91320
E-mail: order@sagepub.com

SAGE Publications Ltd.
6 Bonhill Street
London EC2A 4PU
United Kingdom

SAGE Publications India Pvt. Ltd.
M-32 Market
Greater Kailash I
New Delhi 110 048 India

Printed in the United States of America

Library of Congress Cataloging-in-Publication Data

Main entry under title:

Health care systems in transition: An international perspective /
   edited by Francis D. Powell and Albert F. Wessen.
      p.   cm.
   Includes bibliographical references and index.
      ISBN 0-7619-1081-6 (cloth: acid-free paper)
      ISBN 0-7619-1082-4 (pbk.: acid-free paper)
         1. Medical policy.   2. Medical care.   3. Health care reform.   4. Insurance,
Health.   I. Powell, Francis D. (De Sales), 1918-   II. Wessen, Albert F.
   RA393.H414 1998
   362.1—ddc21   98-19744

This book is printed on acid-free paper.

99   00   01   02   03   04   05   7   6   5   4   3   2   1

Acquiring Editor:	Dan Ruth
Editorial Assistant:	Anna Howland
Production Editor:	Sanford Robinson
Editorial Assistant:	Denise Santoyo
Copy Editor:	Elisabeth Magnus
Typesetter/Designer:	Lynn Miyata

Contents

Part III. *The Canadian Experience*

Part IV. *The Swedish Experience*

Part V. *The British Experience*

Part VI. *Health Care Reform: Toward a Synthesis*

Preface

The capacity of health care systems to alter their structures and functioning in response to new and challenging conditions is an outstanding—and perhaps underreported—feature of these systems. The experiences of the four countries analyzed in this volume provide striking examples of this ability to adapt to changing economic, political, and social circumstances. Thus, in the United Kingdom, the massive changes described by the term *internal market reforms* were a response to the perceived necessity for greater efficiency and "value for money" as well as for greater responsiveness to community needs. The Swedish health care system has progressively followed the path of decentralization, allowing local governments to find innovative ways of reconciling local desires with the framework of national health care goals. Sustained conditions of budgetary and economic restriction in Canada have stimulated the provinces to embark on a variety of management reforms aimed at cost containment and also to develop some innovative programs of primary care. Continuing budgetary problems, especially as a result of the unanticipated magnitude of the costs of national reunification, have compelled the historically autonomous corporatist structures of German national health insurance to accommodate to more centrally controlled systems of management.

Each of the selected countries has confronted, with more or less success, the problem of medical cost inflation. In two of the countries, Great Britain and Germany, reform has taken place primarily through policy changes initiated and carried through by the national government. In Canada and Sweden, however, experimentation has taken place at regional levels of government. Two of the countries, Great Britain and Sweden, have systems that are largely owned and operated by governmental agencies; in Germany and Canada, on the other hand, the delivery of both ambulatory and hospital care takes place primarily within the private/voluntary sector. In terms of the way in which policy decisions are made and implemented, Germany and Sweden lean toward a corporatist model, whereas Britain and Canada manifest the Anglo-Saxon liberal model of majoritarian rule. In short, in terms of some of the parameters differentiating the polities of nations, the selected countries offer a good range of differences.

The ability of these systems to respond to straitened economic conditions while maintaining universal coverage for health care is a manifestation of their vitality. This resiliency has probably been made possible in these countries by their underlying commitment to equitable access to services by their populations. The possibility for appropriate change is enhanced when there is assurance that, within broad limits, the needs of all segments of society will be considered when new health system problems are addressed.

For a nation such as the United States, which has not committed itself to guaranteed coverage for the whole population, the experience of these four countries offers a valuable fund of knowledge. In each of them, progress toward universal coverage was quite gradual, and each has continued to alter its structures and procedures to meet emerging circumstances. Their experience shows that the road to universally assured access to care is winding and often tortuous and that when this objective has been met, new and unforeseen obstacles appear. The journey of health care policy making is not made without struggle and is not marked by clear signposts. The development of an effective and equitable health care system is arduous and never finalized, but it is one that nations undertake out of fear of a greater failure.

Plan of the Book

Whereas many analyses of the health care systems of various countries have used a "broad-brush" approach, providing information on a number of countries, we have chosen to look at fewer countries in greater depth. By presenting the analyses of several experts, we have tried to examine each country's system from several perspectives.

This book stresses the unique ways in which each country has coped with the common problems facing all contemporary health care systems. We have been careful, therefore, to stress the historical context within which contemporary "reforms" have developed. But our authors have also emphasized what they believe to be innovative solutions that might be suggestive elsewhere.

Part I provides an introductory chapter offering conceptual materials designed to highlight major issues and to provide an analytic framework for their consideration. In addition to this introduction, two essays provide overall perspective: David Mechanic considers what might be learned by Americans from the experience of others, and Mark Field discusses the relationship between the universal and particularistic aspects of health care systems by reexamining the convergence hypothesis.

The three papers of Part II, on Germany, analyze two major issues: how Germany has coped with the increasingly onerous pressures of the cost of care and how it dealt with the socialist health care system of East Germany after the collapse of the German Democratic Republic. Thus, Christa Altenstetter's analysis of the institutional basis of Germany's system is complemented by Bradford Kirkman-Liff's analysis of its repeated efforts in recent years to attain cost containment and by Bradley Scharf's analysis of the consequences of unification for health care in the former East German states.

In Part III, on Canada, Catherine Charles and Robin Badgley analyze the evolution of national health insurance in Canada, emphasizing attempts to maintain universal access to high-quality care at a price the nation can afford to pay. Catherine Fooks elaborates on the problems of Canadian provinces in the area of cost control during the period from 1989 to 1992. François Béland describes how Quebec has sought to improve its system by addressing the issues of primary care and preventive medicine.

Part IV, on Sweden, focuses on the implications of Scandinavia's commitment to combine governmental provision of comprehensive services with a maximum of local initiative and control. Ellen Immergut's chapter on the historical and institutional foundations of the Swedish system emphasizes the importance of the nation's overall approach to policy making. Richard Saltman examines in detail the relations between national and local government in this decentralized system. And Casten von Otter analyzes Sweden's cost containment efforts, arguing that success in this area need not follow the prescriptions of neoclassical economists.

Part V, on Great Britain, concerns the reforms of the National Health Service announced by the Conservative government in 1989 and implemented beginning in 1991. Because many changes have taken place since 1991, the structure of the system has been in unprecedented flux. Patricia

Day and Rudolf Klein's article "Britain's Health Care Experiment," first published in 1991, provides background for and an early assessment of the reforms. John Appleby provides an evaluation 6 years later, and Donald Light considers some lessons that might be drawn from the experience of the National Health Service.

In conclusion, Part VI attempts to synthesize the foregoing analyses. Albert Wessen offers a topical and conceptual summary aimed at a better understanding of why health care reforms in the countries studied here have had different trajectories and outcomes. And Francis Powell uses one approach to describing social system differences to show that the underlying structures shaping the reforms made in our study countries may have analogues in various American states and in their health programs.

Acknowledgments

The original impetus for this book came from an International Conference on the theme "Can New England and the United States Learn From Other Health Care Systems?" held in Boston on October 21-23, 1993. Principal sponsors of the conference were the Massachusetts Institute for Social and Economic Research, the University of Massachusetts School of Public Health, and the New England Council of State Governments, and we appreciate their support.[1]

We thank *Health Affairs* for permission to reprint Patricia Day and Rudolf Klein's article on "Britain's Health Care Experiment," which originally appeared in Fall 1991 (Vol. 10, No. 3). We also appreciate permission from Cambridge University Press to include an abridged version of the chapter on Sweden from Ellen Immergut's *Health Politics: Interests and Institutions in Western Europe* (1992, Chapter 5).

We would like to acknowledge the assistance of the staff of the Department of Community Health at Brown University in support of our editorial endeavors. Special thanks go to Monelle Lawrence, who faithfully served as student assistant on this project and to Paul Wessen for preparing the index. Finally, the editors would like to thank the contributors for their patience and helpfulness throughout the process of developing this manuscript. In a real sense, it is indeed their book.

Note

1. Attention of the conferees was focused on possible lessons from Germany, Sweden, and Canada. We have taken account of more recent developments in our analyses and have added a fourth nation, Great Britain, because of the importance of the extensive reforms of its system.

PART I

Introduction

CHAPTER 1

The Comparative Study of Health Care Reform

ALBERT F. WESSEN

The surge of interest in health reform, which reached a peak in the 1992 election campaign and in the months leading to the introduction of the Clinton health plan, has subsided. With the failure of Congress to pass any health care reform in 1994 and the Republican triumph in the midterm elections of that year, many have despaired that they will see any meaningful American health care reform in their lifetimes. Because many people see the national government as unable to afford additional commitments or as unworthy of trust, health care reform at a governmental level may be left to the states, which have their own problems. Meanwhile, the payers, insurers, and providers in the private sector have tried both to control costs and to adapt to fast-changing conditions. In the process, they are radically changing the structure of health care in the United States.

Before the collapse of Clinton's legislative agenda for health care reform, there was widespread interest in the health care systems of other developed countries. Perhaps their experience could provide insights, or a model, in terms of which Americans could design their own reforms. Thus, for example, many advocated the adoption of a "single-payer" program, which would draw on the Canadian experience. Many others, however, concluded that what works in Canada would not work in the United States.

Cultural and ideological differences apparently place sharp limitations on the transferability of health policies from one country to another. If this is the case, are there any practical reasons for the analysis of other countries' health care systems?

Our answer is that there are. Despite the cultural and institutional differences among the nations, modern health care systems share many similarities. Not only do "Western" or cosmopolitan health care systems depend on contemporary biomedical science and its technology, but the liberal Western democracies, with their mature economies and high standards of living, also share many social and economic characteristics. In many respects, these countries have a common heritage, common goals for their health systems—which confront similar problems—and a number of common ideological and policy concerns. These commonalities provide a context for an analysis of their various and sometimes singular efforts to deal with similar issues.

It is frequently argued that over time there has been a tendency for convergence in the methods and organization of medical care.[1] As modern biomedical science has developed and achieved hegemony in developed countries, its technologies and ideology have set the standards for practice and the delivery of health care. Scientific communication has become worldwide in scope, and professional and organizational methods for achieving consensus on matters of health care and public health policy have become increasingly influential.[2] Insofar as health problems are seen as *technical* in nature, to be solved by the application of biomedical science, approaches to their solution are likely to be similar everywhere. Thus, for example, the content of the medical curriculum differs only slightly from country to country, and hospitals and clinics throughout the world have similar goals and attempt to practice similar methods of diagnosis and care.

Moreover, similarities among health care systems of Western countries stem from the fact that they share a set of similar goals for their health care systems, face broadly similar economic and social problems, and have been exposed to ideologies and "expert" policy prescriptions of worldwide currency. At the same time, the structures of their health care systems differ in a number of ways that stem in large part from differences in the polities of nations and in their several histories. These structural differences can be described in terms of a set of parameters along which variation is observed from country to country. The performance of various systems and the health care reforms that are occurring throughout the Western world can be studied in these terms.

Common Goals

The many similarities among modern societies are suggested by descriptive terms such as the *global economy* or metaphors such as the *global village*. At least at a general level, similar goals and problems are clearly apparent among national health care sectors. All nations share the goal of *maximizing the health of their population* (and of the individuals composing them). However, they might not fully agree about what "health" is. Is it the absence of disease? Or, as the World Health Organization (WHO) would have it, is it to be understood as "a state of complete physical, mental and social well-being and not merely the absence of disease or infirmity" (WHO, 1996, p. 1)? Though few would disagree that their health care system should have the goal of caring for the sick and disabled and curing them if possible, differences of opinion arise about the extent to which the socially handicapped are really "sick" or have a medical disability. There is also likely to be a lack of consensus concerning the relative priority of the goals of "caring" and "curing." Students of comparative health care systems would do well to consider whether differing interpretations of the goal of improving the nation's health help to account for differences in health system design and health policy. Such disagreements almost certainly reflect broader social and political values as well.

Moreover, it appears that most nations share the goal that their health care system should be *equitable*. That is to say, the system should be fair, just, and impartial in its treatment of those who need its services. To the extent that health care is perceived as inequitable, popular dissatisfaction is likely. But what is fair and just? Is a system that offers the opportunity for all to receive health care really equitable if all groups in the population seem unable, for one reason or other, to take advantage of it when they need it? Is health care a right or a privilege?[3] How these issues are treated in various countries will have much to do with the structure of their systems and how they change.

In connection with the National Health Planning and Resource Development Act of 1975, five goals (or criteria for evaluation) for local or regional health care systems were set out. Although this law has since been repealed, the five goals provide a useful framework for comparison of national health care systems:

1. *Availability.* Are resources available to provide the services needed by the population? Availability is most often thought of in geographic terms, and in the health care systems of developed countries it tends to be attained

reasonably well, although many rural areas chronically suffer from a dearth of available facilities. However, the assessment of availability depends on agreement on what services populations actually need. Here there is room for real difference of opinion, especially with respect to the availability of various technologies. Can a service or a technology be said to be truly available if substantial waiting lists for its use regularly occur?

2. *Accessibility.* Given that resources are available, can individuals (or groups) gain access to them? Are there barriers of cost, of time, or of discriminatory practices that prevent those in need from receiving timely care? In the United States, issues of accessibility are most often seen as economic. Thus, the large numbers of the population without health insurance are presumed to lack access to the system—and this is almost certainly the case in many situations. But problems of accessibility also surface in countries where health care is free at the point of service because facilities are inconvenient or because of delays or bureaucratic barriers to accessing service. Problems of accessibility are, of course, closely bound up with issues of equity.

3. *Acceptability.* Even accessible services may not be utilized by individuals or groups who find that, for one reason or another, a given service is unwelcome or unsatisfactory. Here issues of cultural expectations and the sensitivity of health service staff to patients' needs and expectations become important, as do the amenities (material or psychological) provided. Among minority groups, issues of acceptability frequently arise, especially when needs are perceived as not urgent, as in the case of many preventive services.

4. *Quality of care.* Though acceptability is a criterion that highlights the importance of patients' expectations and willingness to cooperate, the goal of quality of care refers more to the attainment of professional and community standards of good practice. What is "good medicine" anyway, and how can consensus on this point be developed? Given a normal range of differences in performance among providers, at what point is the judgment made that care is (or is not) of "good quality"? How can this be ensured? Should it be judged only (or largely) by professional criteria? Should it be measured by assessing the process or the outcome of care?

5. *Affordable cost.* Can the system provide accessible and acceptable services of high quality to a population at a price that the community can afford or is willing to pay? Because in all countries the cost of care continuously escalates, often at a faster rate than does income, the issue of cost containment is pervasive. It is clear that there must be trade-offs between affordable costs on the one hand and the availability and accessibility of high-quality care on the other. But countries differ in how they make these judgments and in the degree to which there is pressure for cost containment.

Though modern health care systems share these broad goals, there are many differences in how they specify and operationalize them. The cultural and political traditions of various nations may largely account for these differences. At the same time, however, broad agreement concerning the general goals of health care, as well as common belief in biomedical science and in the efficacy of its technologies, may result in convergence in the structure of health care systems. To the degree that nations have experienced similar socioeconomic and political conditions, this convergence is likely to be enhanced.

A Common Heritage

All of the developed countries have experienced powerful forces of demographic, cultural, and economic change that have shaped their health care systems. The industrial revolution and urbanization led both to unprecedented increases in the wealth of nations and to acute problems of poverty and discontent stemming from the constraints on self-sufficiency imposed on the "masses." The long-term result was the piecemeal development of the state interventions characteristic of the welfare state.[4] Improved living conditions, coupled with rapid scientific advances in biomedical science, led to the emergence of modern institutions of medical care during the second half of the 19th century. In all countries, medical practitioners united as a self-conscious and self-governing profession devoted to (and legitimized by) biomedical science. Application of modern medical knowledge resulted in an exponential increase in the range, intensity, and success of medical interventions. This transformed hospitals from "places for the poor to die" into "life-saving" centers for specialized treatment of the acutely ill. The needs of hospitals and their specialists have dominated 20th-century medical care.[5]

The combination of improved living conditions, ameliorative social legislation, and the burgeoning technical capabilities of medical science led to what Omran (1971) described as the "epidemiologic transition." This transition is characterized by marked reduction in mortality, especially of infants and young children, increasing life expectancy, a marked reduction in the burden of infectious diseases, and a concomitant increase in long-term illness and disability.[6]

Common Problems

This common heritage has led to several health system problems faced by all Western nations. The health care reforms of recent years constitute their various attempts at solutions—or adaptations—to changed conditions. Four common problems merit attention here.

Effects of Aging Populations

All Western nations are experiencing a marked aging of their populations, with the proportions over 65 having at least doubled since the beginning of World War II and with the "old old" (those 85 and over) becoming the most rapidly increasing age group in most countries. With the large cohort of postwar "baby boomers" approaching retirement age within a decade or two, gerontological problems may assume almost crisis proportions. From the perspective of the economy, the problem lies in the increased proportion of the population that is no longer economically productive and that may be expected to draw on transfers from the employed segment of the population for an ever-increasing span of years. In health system terms, this problem is greatly compounded by the greatly increasing need (and demand) for medical services in the last years of life. Because these needs involve both acute medical care and the provision of a variety of support and domiciliary services, care for the elderly is both a complex problem and one that transcends the traditional parameters of medical care.

Chronicity and Disability

Diseases such as heart disease, arthritis, AIDS, and mental illness are characterized both by their long duration and by the multiple needs they impose on their victims. The effects of serious accidents, substance abuse, and violence take their chronic toll as well. It is important to note that chronic problems are by no means restricted to the elderly. Because, in large part, chronic disease and disability cannot be reversed or cured, health services must focus on rehabilitation and maintenance of function instead. This entails multiple interventions, provision of services in the community, and a commitment to long-term support of the incapacitated. Clearly, chronicity and disability not only impose financial stress on health care systems but pose challenges to their structures, which have been focused on hospital-centered acute care.

Heightened Expectations and Demands

All Western countries are having to cope with demands for more and better services. The proliferation of new biomedical discoveries continues unabated. The media provide instant and extensive coverage of these developments. Both providers and patients then demand access to these "state-of-the-art" technologies. Despite efforts to develop rational means of technology assessment, only budget constraints that are unresponsive to these demands succeed in deferring or negating them. This, of course, reaps a harvest of dissatisfaction.

As educational levels have improved in most countries, so has the sophistication of the consumers of health care. Patients tend to be less respectful of providers and more assertive of their wishes. They have become less tolerant of unresponsive providers or shabby amenities. Often this has led to their willingness to move from provider to provider or even to take legal action against providers with whose service they are dissatisfied.[7] These enhanced demands for a responsive and effective health service have been associated with collective action on the part of specific interest groups, such as patients' rights groups, advocacy groups for those with particular problems, and the women's health movement.

Cost Escalation and Budgetary Pressures

The problems discussed thus far all lead to increased demands for health services. Responses to these escalating levels of demand have led to health services of increased complexity. The tendency is for different services to be provided more frequently, using more sophisticated—and expensive—inputs. So health care costs rise accordingly, often at a rate higher than that of overall inflation.[8]

At the same time, in recent years almost all countries have experienced economic difficulties that have led to sharp constraints on available resources. Slow economic growth, high unemployment, competitive weakness in the international economy, restructuring of business organizations to enhance profitability, deficit spending, increased resistance to taxation: Some or all of these have limited the ability of payers—public and private—to meet constantly increasing health care costs. Resulting cutbacks or budgetary ceilings may result in lessened accessibility and/or decreased quality of services. This, in turn, engenders political discontent.

Shared Ideological and Policy Concerns

Approaches to health care reform in various countries have in recent years also been conditioned by some common ideological and policy concerns. Though they have been more prominent in some countries than in others, these concerns have motivated debate in all of the developed nations. We shall briefly identify five of them.

The first has been *questioning of the value of the welfare state and of governmental interventions.* If the period between the end of World War II and the early 1970s represented the time of flowering of "welfare state" legislation in most countries, the "oil shock" and ensuing times of economic stringency led to questions about the sustainability of these initiatives. However, doubts were not limited to issues of affordability. A resurgent libertarian ideology denounced the substitution of governmental mandates for individual initiative and preached the superiority of the private sector. Although these "conservative" ideas were especially in evidence in Reagan's America and Thatcher's Britain, they everywhere put advocates of the welfare state on the defensive. Even in Britain and the United States, however, the scope of governmental social programs has been little affected (although their further growth has been circumscribed).

The second development has been an increasing *emphasis on the values of choice and the competitive discipline of the market.* Along with increasing skepticism concerning the role of government has come a strong reassertion of the superiority of the "free" market over all other forms of economic organization. Flexibility in adapting to changing conditions is thought to be maximized when the individuals (or groups) desiring a given product or service have the opportunity to choose among a number of alternative providers. The possibility of choice is thought to provide both greater satisfaction to consumers and greater responsiveness by providers. Thus, competition is thought to enhance efficiency, and the discipline of the market is believed to promote "the greatest good for the greatest number." This economic ideology offered a promising alternative to central planning for welfare and seemed to be justified by the decay of the socialist economies.

The third development has been an increasing *emphasis on outcome rather than process, on quality of life, and on prevention.* Another broadly accepted set of ideas has stressed the importance of evaluating the outcomes of health care programs: judging them by what they do for people rather than simply by the volume or scope of their activities. If a health care system exists to promote health, it should be evaluated in terms of its success in improving the health of populations, whether measured by declines in morbidity and mortality or by other means. Increasingly, desired health system outcomes include consumer satisfaction as well as more "objective" criteria of physiologic functioning. There is a strong emphasis on "quality of life" as a goal of health care. In turn, attainment of a high quality of life has been increasingly seen to depend on preventing unnecessary illness or disability. These emphases of the "new public health," of course, may sometimes be in conflict with antigovernment and strongly economistic ideologies.

A fourth development has been *the search for "painless cost control" and the quest for efficiency*. Given the incessant pressure of medical inflation, every nation has tried to achieve what Bodenheimer and Grumbach (1995, p. 89) have called "painless cost control": that is, minimizing reductions in service to consumers while striving to keep providers happy. Gains in productivity are seen as the key to "painless" cost control. Much attention has been given to operational objectives such as overcoming organizational slack, consolidating or redirecting the use of underutilized facilities, preventing unnecessary procedures or referrals, reducing inappropriate use of medical technology, and providing economic incentives to reward efficient behaviors. Such aims require better management. The restructuring of work has become a raison d'être of the "new managerialism" of recent years.

A final development has been *attacks on the dominance of specialist providers and hospital medicine*. All of these trends have led to attacks on the power of those thought to be the prime beneficiaries of the status quo. Specialist providers and the doyens of hospital medicine are thought by many to have undue influence in determining health policy. Just as "big government" is thought to be unresponsive to the needs of the society, so tertiary care hospitals and superspecialists are thought to be unresponsive to the needs of the majority of the population. Thus, stress on decentralization of power and stress on the priority of primary care have gone hand in hand in recent policy thinking. Reforms enhancing the roles of primary caregivers and local communities have been seen as essential to the achievement of "Health for All by the Year 2000."[9]

Thus, policy making for health care systems has been affected by changing doctrines and ideologies. Whether they originated in the wider world of political and social thought or in changing perceptions of health care priorities, these trends have provoked worldwide discussion and, to varying degrees, have influenced the policy trajectories of most societies.

Salient Differences in the Structure of Health Care Systems

Common goals and problems, a shared heritage, and the influence of powerful ideological concerns have combined with the thrust of modern medical science to foster convergence among contemporary health care systems. But although the tendency toward convergence has fostered similar approaches to health care, it has not established a standard, prescriptive structure within which to carry them out. The institutions of government and health care delivery in modern societies have evolved in the context of the unique histories of each. Accordingly, the structures of health care systems differ along numerous parameters; figuratively, they constitute a set of variations on the theme of "modern health care." We shall discuss two relevant characteristics of national polities that clearly lead to structural differences in health systems and also 11 structural "parameters" or "dimensions" along which the systems of various countries differ. Such differences are the result of policy decisions taken at various times. They may—sometimes in unanticipated ways—affect the effectiveness and efficiency of health care systems.

Degree of Market Orientation

Anderson (1989) saw the degree of market orientation, from "market minimization" to "market maximization," as a fundamental parameter of comparison.[10] He stressed that, in general terms, a nation's place on this "continuum" is the result of the historical evolution of its polity; thus, the market orientation of health care systems may change over time and is correlated with that of the economy as a whole. Moreover, the systems of all nations have at least some market-oriented characteristics and are constrained to some degree by collective (governmental) action. At least three factors determine the degree of market orientation in a system:

1. The degree to which resources are allocated through the bargaining of "free" agents

2. The extent of a plurality of providers and purchasers to participate in this bargaining

3. The degree to which collective or governmental action limits the nature and extent of bargaining through means such as direct regulation, modification of incentives through taxation and subsidy, or direct collective ownership of services

Of these, the latter distinction between governmentally owned and privately owned and controlled services has been especially consequential for the shape of health care systems.

Context of Decision Making: Corporatist Versus Pluralistic Interest Competition

A second parameter of interest derives from the way in which decisions are made—or not made—in various polities. Many European nations are characterized by what has been called a "corporatist" approach to decision making, in which many (or most) decisions are rationalized and harmonized by negotiations between aggregated functional interest groups, such as employers' associations and trade unions.[11] By contrast, in other countries, perhaps most markedly in the United States, decisions tend to be the majoritarian resultant of competition to set policy among a plurality of competing interest groups, each of which may be able to block the initiatives of others, if not to attain its own ends.[12] In no country are decisions made in the context of only one of these modes; some decisions may be corporatist in nature (as in the negotiation of health and other fringe benefits in labor-management bargaining in this country), whereas others may involve the full free-for-all of winner-take-all interest group politics. One might expect that where corporatist institutions are effective, the structure of institutions will be more stable than where political competition is untrammeled.

Structural Characteristics of Health Care Systems[13]

Health care is dispensed by various "hands-on" providers in hospitals or other institutional settings. Much of the structure of health care systems is concerned with the relationships of providers to one another and to the institutions in which they work. Whereas most providers are organized into professional collectives, hospitals and other health care institutions are bureaucratically organized. The ways in which hospitals and physicians are reimbursed typically differ. In short, the structure of health care is largely concerned with the arrangement of the "building blocks" of providers and institutions, and health policy is preoccupied with issues concerning physicians and hospitals.

In addition to the population that uses health care systems, principal types of actors include (a) providers of care, (b) those who pay for care (often employers), (c) insurers (or other agents) who mediate between the payers and the providers, and (d) the governmental authorities who in various ways monitor and regulate health care. The roles of these actors vary from system to system (and through time as well). These variations may be described in terms of a number of "parameters." We have selected 11 of these that may be expected to have consequences for system performance.

Degree of "Medical Dominance"

Systems differ in the degree to which providers of care, especially physicians, have organizational power and autonomy (see Freidson, 1970). Historically, physicians acted as autonomous providers who took individual responsibility for providing good care to patients who chose them freely. Responsibility for ensuring that physicians provided competent and ethical care was vested in the medical profession itself, which acted both to vouch for the competence of its members and to protect their technical and economic freedom. This ideal of the free "liberal" profession has been the platform of medical professions in all countries and has been implemented to varying degrees. However, with the increasing organizational complexity of medical care, institutions such as hospitals became necessary both to provide resources and to coordinate the activities of an increasingly diverse cadre of providers. The increasing complexity of the institutional environment in which medicine is practiced has tended to place limits on medical dominance in several respects:

- Limitations on the *clinical* autonomy of physicians within hospitals (and other medical care settings): the extent to which individual physicians' decisions must be shared—with other physicians, with other professionals, and/or with institutional managers
- The extent to which physician autonomy is constrained by the reimbursement system
- The extent to which the medical profession has been able to control decision making within health care institutions—with respect to developing norms for care, monitoring quality of care, and allocating resources
- The extent to which the medical profession has been able to exert influence and control over political decisions affecting the health care system

Role of Payers

To what extent are those who pay the bills for health care active in determining the ground rules and structure of the system? These payers—whether individual patients, employers contributing health insurance premiums, or governmental agencies—may be more or less active in negotiating both terms and conditions of payment and its amount. These negotiations affect the financial well-being of providers and patients and also may alter institutional cultures and the very structure of the health care system.[14] To the extent that payers are active rather than passive and are united enough to have real leverage on decision making, they may play major roles in altering health policy. When payers act in concert—or there is a "single-payer" situation—their decisions and negotiations can result in major changes in the health care system. When they act alone, they may attain their own ends to some degree, but providers are likely to find ways to circumvent the effects of their actions, as in the case of shifting costs from one payer to another.

Role of Insurers ("Third-Party Agents")

We distinguish those who actually provide the financing (the payers) from their agents, who administer this financing. Thus, in countries, such as the United States, where private health insurance is widespread, the health care plans offered by insurers play a major role in setting the conditions for care. Negotiations between payers and their "third-party agents" (or insurers) are consequential for determining the extent and price of coverage for various groups. These agents arrange with providers to offer care to their clients and thus are a major influence in determining the structure of health care. Competition among insurers is apt to complicate the structure of the reimbursement system. In countries with public or "statutory" health care insurance, there may be a "single payer" (usually a governmental unit, as in Canada). Alternatively, a plurality of "insurers," either quasi-public or private (as in Germany or France), may share these intermediary administrative tasks. In countries (such as Great Britain or New Zealand) where a governmental health system has experimented with "internal markets," the agencies that contract for services from providers become, in effect, third-party agents.

Role of Government

In all health care systems, government plays a significant role, although its extent varies across time and space. All governments take responsibility for setting the basic legal ground rules by which health care is delivered. However, the extent to which these ground rules define in detail the structure of medical care organization and financing is variable, as is the degree to which governments actively intervene in the process of care. But all governments are involved in regulation of the health care system.

All governments also provide at least some resources for the health care system. This may be limited largely to provision of "infrastructural" elements (such as financing of medical education or research) and to provision of capital resources. Or it may also involve financing the actual provision of care (with varying degrees of coverage of the population). Clearly, the more the government participates in providing resources for the system, the more it is able to determine its shape.

Finally, all governments participate to some degree in the delivery of health services. Activities directed to securing the public health are everywhere a governmental function. Facilities for at least some groups—for example, military hospitals or institutions for the mentally ill—are usually provided directly by government. The extreme case is, of course, the development of a national health service in which a government directly provides most of the care for most of the population.

The role and influence of government are key determinants of the character of health care. There is a tendency for health policy to be politicized rather than left to "individual initiative." In general, the influence of governments has been directed toward rationalizing the system.

Degree of Centralization

In modern large-scale societies, a pervasive issue is whether effectiveness and efficiency are better achieved through consolidation and coordination of activities across communities or by allowing local units maximal freedom. Economies of scale and the resources and power of large organizations must be weighed against the possibilities for greater responsiveness to local situations and for the enhanced individual commitment that may be elicited in smaller, more "face-to-face" settings. Is progress more likely to occur by fostering uniformity or diversity? These issues—perhaps ultimately philosophical—arise in both the public and private sectors. In the latter, issues of mergers of local units and of vertical or horizontal integration are fought out in the marketplace. In the public sector, the issue may most frequently be posed in terms of the level of government—local, regional, national—to which responsibility should be entrusted. In either case, the degree of consolidation and centralization of systemic activity is likely to have important consequences for system performance.[15]

Degree of Specialization: The Balance Between Primary, Secondary, and Tertiary Care

As medical knowledge and technology have multiplied, there has been an inexorable trend toward increased specialization. In the medical profession, specialization has led to the proliferation of recognized specialty and subspecialty groups, each with its own technical domain. It has also involved the increasing importance of a number of paraprofessional or technical occupational groupings attached to the "health care team." Such specialization of function complicates the problem of meeting consumers' needs. Not only must patients find the right type of specialist, but in the case of multiple needs, the activities of numerous specialists must be coordinated. Because institutions also specialize, the problem of finding the right hospital or service also arises. Specialization leads to increased need for communication among relevant personnel and hence to increased paperwork. This in turn leads to the emergence of new administrative or managerial cadres to coordinate work. Moreover, if the thrust of specialization is to divide responsibility for health problems according to functional (or anatomic) criteria, who is to be responsible for meeting the needs of the "whole patient"?

Such problems frame the issue of primary versus specialty health care, which is faced by all modern health care systems. What structures can best ensure the provision of comprehensive yet individually responsive care for persons who may have multiple needs? At what point should the competence of the generalist give place to that of the specialist? Given the intellectual and economic attractions of specialization, how can an adequate number of competent generalists be recruited? Because specialization involves competence in problems experienced by small fractions of the population, there is a natural tendency for specialists to concentrate in urban areas and in large institutions; this being so, how can access to care best be ensured for those who dwell on the periphery?

In most Western systems, these problems have focused on the status and role of the general practitioner (GP) or family physician. How can the GP be provided with adequate status in a profession that values specialized knowledge so highly? To what extent should GPs be "gatekeepers," controlling access to specialized services? Should the generalist have hospital privileges or work only in community ambulatory settings? The ways different countries deal with these questions have important consequences for the character of their health care systems.[16]

Extent of Pluralism in the System

Health care systems differ in the number of provider units available to serve a community of given size. Whether measured by the number of physicians (or nurses or hospital beds) or in terms of the number of health care institutions (or health plans), the number of available participants will affect the extent of choice—and hence the degree of competition. If there are qualitative differences among services and providers (e.g., choice among health plans offering different sorts of coverage), both individuals' range of choice and system complexity will increase. On the other hand, if only one practitioner or one hospital is accessible to a community, the benefits of competition will be withheld. Moreover, systems also differ in the extent to which choice by individual consumers is facilitated or impeded.

Sources of Financing

Four major sources of funds to pay for health care are used in modern health care systems. The simplest—and most "market-friendly"—method is, of course, *direct payment by the consumer of services.* But many consumers are unable to meet the costs of the services they need, and because providing health care to the suffering is a moral imperative in modern societies, three other sources of financing have evolved to allow care to be given to those who may need it.

Of these, the oldest is *charity.* Care for the sick has been seen as a religious duty or vocation, and various religious organizations have offered care to the needy at little or no charge. Physicians and other providers have also cared for the needy, either freely or on a "sliding scale," and philanthropic donors have established institutions to offer charitable care or to provide special services.[17] However, charity never has sufficed to meet all the needs of the indigent.

Governments, therefore, had to step in to provide necessary care for the most dependent and needy, whether by hiring town physicians on a retainer or by establishing public hospitals and kindred institutions.[18] However, not all the needy are indigent. The costs of sickness are unpredictable and can render those who are normally self-sufficient, and thus "respectable," unable to pay for necessary care.

This led to the development of *insurance,* by which individuals share the risks of illness through contributing to a common fund from which the costs of care are paid.[19] Although historically, insurance mechanisms were first developed by cooperative groups such as guilds or sick benefit societies, they later often became the commercial products of entrepreneurs who accepted the risk of contracting to meet specified needs for a term on payment of a set "premium."

These four sources of payment are used in varying degrees in most societies and have had different degrees of importance throughout history. In general, it may be said that as modern medicine has become more complex and expensive, both direct payment and charity have accounted for less and less of the overall cost of care. Reliance on insurance has thus increased, and voluntary types of insurance have often been supplanted by governmentally sponsored universal insurance programs or by direct governmental provision of care. As the institution with the power to command and direct the allocation of a society's resources, government becomes the agency that meets the needs that voluntary or market-based institutions do not—or cannot—satisfy. The result is that health care has increasingly become a major budgetary responsibility of governments and hence an ongoing political issue.

Methods of Financing Health Care

Certain alternative arrangements for the allocation of resources within health care systems are so important for system structure and performance that they are often taken as critical determinants of overall system performance. Among these are the methods of health care financing, modes of payment to health care providers, and mechanisms for cost control. Methods of health care financing differ in the extent of control that they give to the financing agency. Various methods, of course, can be either a public or a private responsibility.[20]

The simplest method of financing is, of course, *direct out-of-pocket payment* by consumers of service. It is found to at least some degree in all systems. Out-of-pocket payment is least problematic—and most commonly used—when costs are trivial or low. Perhaps the most common example of its use is the purchase of over-the-counter drugs. Under this method, prices are usually set by the provider/seller and are usually not negotiable. They tend also to be "unbundled"—that is, they are set for specific items or procedures rather than aggregated.

Because of the need for protection against unanticipated and/or very large expenditures for health care, three types of "insurance" financing have also evolved. They offer different degrees of control to the insurer; each method may be conducted under either public or private auspices.

1. *Direct-reimbursement models.* These involve the post hoc reimbursement of consumers of health care by insurers, usually according to specific reimbursement schedules and with or without co-participation by the user. Traditional indemnity insurance provided by commercial insurers is an example of a private direct-reimbursement model, and statutory health insurance for ambulatory medical care in countries such as France and Switzerland provides an example of the public direct-reimbursement model.

2. *"Contract" models.* These involve contractual arrangements whereby insurers agree to provide for care on behalf of their insurees and then contract with a set of providers to reimburse them for care covered under the terms of their insurance policies. Examples of private contract models in America include traditional service-benefit health insurance, independent practice association (IPA) or network-type HMOs, and preferred provider organizations. Examples of public contract models include HMO waiver arrangements under Medicare in the United States and contractual arrangements between sickness funds and medical associations in Germany.

3. *Integrated models.* In these models, the insurer directly provides services to the insured through facilities that the former owns or manages. An example of the private contract model is the American staff-model HMO. Public integrated models involve direct provision of medical care by a governmental agency—for example, the British National Health Service or the Veterans Administration health care system in the United States.

Control of medical care by the insurer is, in principle, least in the direct-reimbursement models and greatest in the integrated models.

Modes of Payment to Providers

A number of different forms of payment to providers for their services have been developed. Theoretically, they have different implications for system performance because they affect the incentives of providers. Modes of payment are usually different for professional providers than for medical care institutions such as hospitals. To begin with the latter, hospitals have historically wished to be paid, like other sellers, on the basis of *charges* for services developed by the hospitals themselves. But in many settings, negotiations have produced agreements that there should be *retrospective reimbursement* on the basis of actual costs (with or without allowance for a profit). In the United States, at least, the terms of cost-based reimbursement may vary as negotiated by various payers, and there is usually a substantial difference between costs and charges for the same service.[21] Finally, payment may be made on a *prospective* basis, either through a negotiated overall budget to which the hospital must conform or on the basis of an agreed-on schedule of payments (such as for patients falling in various diagnosis-related groups). These prospective payments may be adjusted to account for unusually difficult cases or for volume of services. Frequently, arrangements may be made for providers to keep all or part of any surplus that may result—and similar arrangements may exist in terms of sharing losses. Clearly, prospective reimbursement affords the insurer the greatest degree of cost control and payment of charges the least.

Traditionally, the three major modes of payment for physicians' services have been *fee for service, capitation,* and *salary.* Often, some combination of these methods is agreed on. Fee-for-service payments can be made only retrospectively and vary according to volume of service rendered. Capitation and salary payments are prospectively negotiated and in principle do not take account of the volume of services rendered. Primary care physicians are most often paid on a fee-for-service basis or by capitation or by some combination of these. On the other hand, hospital-based physicians are often salaried (except where hospital services are provided on a "private" basis by the provider, as is typically the case in American community hospitals).

In general, these modes of payment may be classified in terms of the degree to which they "lump" or "split" payments. Fee-for-service methods are the epitome of the "splitting" approach, and services are frequently "unbundled" to a great degree. On the other hand, salaries for professionals and overall or "global" budgets for institutions aggregate payment for services to a maximum degree. Clearly, payment methods emphasizing "splitting" allow more discretion to providers, who can increase or decrease their income by controlling the volume of services for which they bill. Prospective and "lumped" forms of payment tend to take away this flexibility and accordingly are thought to provide an incentive for providers to perform efficiently. However, they may also provide an incentive for undertreatment.

Rigor of Cost Control Methods

All health systems make at least some effort to control costs. At a minimum, claims for payment are audited, and buyers of services tend to utilize services on the basis of their price. Despite varying degrees of vigilance in auditing claims, substantial fraud is often encountered, especially in the case of fee-for-service payments. A second, more intrusive method of audit involves prospective or concurrent review mechanisms of utilization management (see Gray, 1991, Chapter 11). Thus, second opinions may be required before surgery, and lengths of hospital stay may be subject to external control by payers in an effort to ensure that services are used appropriately and provided efficiently. The price of care may also be subject to control through the use of voluntary targets, fee schedules, or prospective rate setting. Finally, costs may be controlled by the negotiation or imposition of overall budgets that may leave more or less room for modification in the face of changing conditions. Naturally, from the perspective of the system as a whole, the more cost control methods are uniform and extended to all elements of the system, the more rigorous they are likely to be. Thus, in theory, global budgets are probably the most rigorous form of cost control. When rigorous cost controls are instituted, accessibility of services is frequently limited, resulting in waiting lists or other forms of rationing.

Conclusion

In the preceding discussion, we have selected structural features of health care systems that are thought to have special relevance for the comparison of health care systems. Various combinations of these features have been incorporated by the health services of different nations. And recent attempts to reform the systems have involved planned changes of many of these features. Analysis of what has taken place in various countries should therefore prove instructive about what might work elsewhere. However, a major caveat must be that, however promising the results of a reform in another country might be, these results might not be transferable. A given change that works under one set of conditions might not work under others, or the organizational and political culture of one country might find what works elsewhere to be incompatible with its ethos and norms. The comparative analysis of health care systems may thus provide insight into what the effects of possible change *might* be. But given the present state of our knowledge, the engineering of health care systems is far from a prescriptive science.

Notes

1. For a recent analysis that emphasizes the importance of convergence among health care systems, see Mechanic and Rochefort (1996). See also the discussion in Chapter 3 of this volume.

2. Witness the role of the World Health Organization in promoting the development and application of this consensual knowledge throughout the world.

3. For a discussion of equity in various health care systems, see van Doorslaer, Wagstaff, and Rutten (1993). The chapter by Alan Williams in that volume (pp. 287-299) on the implications of different concepts of equity may be of special interest.

4. This process took place in most countries over a period extending roughly from the mid-19th century through the period of reconstruction after World War II. The impact of industrialization and urbanization differed in intensity and in timing among Western countries; this partly explains differences in the character of their social legislation. It is worth pointing out that among the earliest state interventions in the social conditions of most countries were sanitary and other public health measures. For historical perspective on the American case, see Wilensky and Lebeaux (1958).

5. This social history has been well documented for the United States by Starr (1982). A classic account of the historical development of hospitals in Great Britain is Abel-Smith (1964).

6. This transition developed unevenly among Western nations over the past two centuries. Since World War II, it has also begun to transform the health and demographic situation of developing nations as well. McKeown and others have argued that the most important causes of changes in the burden of disease are to be found in changing living conditions, especially improved nutrition. See McKeown (1979) and McKinlay and McKinlay (1977).

7. For discussion of this tendency to "consumerism" in the United States, see Haug and Lavin (1983). Popular discontent with waiting lists and lack of ability to choose providers have fueled policy changes in both Sweden and the United Kingdom.

8. Comparative data on health care costs are further discussed in Chapter 16 of this volume.

9. The Thirtieth World Health Assembly of WHO unanimously decided in 1977 that "Health for All by the Year 2000" should be the main objective both of the organization and of its member nations.

10. As Anderson (1989) put it,

> For purposes of international comparison, if the personal health services delivery systems of the United States did not exist, they would have to be invented. This country has become a convenient international reference point, not to be emulated, of the extreme of inequality and wasted resources. Likewise, . . . if the British National Health Service did not exist, it would also have to be invented. It has become a convenient international reference point of the opposite extreme, for relatively low cost, equity and fairness. (p. 3)

For Anderson, the United States represented an empirical extreme of a market-maximized system, whereas Great Britain (in 1989) represented a high degree of market minimization.

11. The concept of corporatism is discussed by Schmitter and Lehmbruch (1979) and by Cawson (1986). For examples of this approach to decision making in health care systems, see Chapters 4 and 11 of this volume.

12. One example is the effective use of lobbying by groups purporting to represent the interests of the elderly in securing the repeal of President Reagan's initiative to provide new benefits under Medicare (to be financed by increased taxes on Social Security payments). Another example might be the failure of Clinton's health care plan.

13. In the following paragraphs, we concentrate on the provision of clinical care, leaving aside those aspects that are concerned with public health activities or with infrastructural arrangements. Thus, for example, we do not discuss the pharmaceutical or medical appliance industries, even though they are important parts of every health care system.

14. For example, in the United States, many payers have demanded the institution of managed-care procedures. As cost containment measures, they may limit the incomes of providers by refusing payment for various procedures. They certainly have affected the culture of hospitals and, in some cases, have added a whole new type of organization—the utilization management organization—to the American health care system. For further discussion, see Gray (1991, especially Chapter 11).

15. For a discussion of issues relating to health system decentralization, see Mills, Vaughan, Smith, and Tabibzadeh (1990).

16. Starfield (1992) has analyzed the issues relating to primary care at length, including a comparison of primary care in 10 nations; see especially Chapter 15.

17. In Europe, medieval hospitals were regularly established and operated as religious foundations, and in the Anglo-Saxon countries most hospitals were established on a "voluntary" basis, either under church sponsorship or as nonprofit philanthropic foundations. Only during the 20th century were "private" patients regularly admitted and expected to pay the cost of their care. On the other hand, charitable hospitals always attempted to secure contributions from the larger community (and the government), as well as from patients who were able to meet some of the costs of their care.

18. Governmentally supported care for the indigent has commonly been of low quality because of the reluctance of society to spend more than the minimum to care for the poor, whom many regarded as "undeserving."

19. Intrinsic to the concept of insurance are both the notion of the individual's responsibility to "save for a rainy day" and the idea of solidarity between the well and those unfortunate enough to become ill. Insurance both carries the cachet of social responsibility and is often seen by individuals as an entitlement.

20. Here we follow the classification adopted by the Organization for Economic Cooperation and Development (OECD) and described by Hurst (1991). See also OECD (1992).

21. Insurers generally can negotiate cost-based reimbursement terms with providers, whereas out-of-pocket payers ordinarily are confronted with a provider's set charges.

References

Abel-Smith, B. (1964). *The hospitals, 1800-1948: A study in social administration in England and Wales.* Cambridge, MA: Harvard University Press.

Anderson, O. (1989). *The health services continuum in democratic states: An inquiry into solvable problems.* Ann Arbor, MI: Health Administration Press.

Bodenheimer, T., & Grumbach, K. (1995). *Understanding health policy: A clinical approach.* Norwalk, CT: Appleton & Lange.

Cawson, A. (1986). *Corporatism and political theory.* Oxford, UK: Basil Blackwell.

Freidson, E. (1970). *Professional dominance: The social structure of medical care.* New York: Atherton.

Gray, B. (1991). *The profit motive and patient care: The changing accountability of doctors and hospitals.* Cambridge, MA: Harvard University Press.

Haug, M., & Lavin, B. (1983). *Consumerism in medicine: Challenging physician authority.* Beverly Hills, CA: Sage.

Hurst, J. (1991). Reforming health care in seven European nations. *Health Affairs, 10*(3), 7-20.

McKeown, T. (1979). *The role of medicine: Dream, mirage or illusion.* Princeton, NJ: Princeton University Press.

McKinlay, J., & McKinlay, S. (1977). The questionable contribution of medical measures to the decline of mortality in the United States in the twentieth century. *Milbank Memorial Fund Quarterly, 55,* 405-428.

Mechanic, D., & Rochefort, D. (1996). Comparative medical systems. *Annual Review of Sociology, 22,* 239-270.

Mills, A., Vaughan, J. P., Smith, D. L., & Tabibzadeh, I. T. (1990). *Health system decentralization: Concepts, issues and country experience.* Geneva: World Health Organization.

Omran, A. (1971). The epidemiologic transition: A theory of the epidemiology of population change. *Milbank Memorial Fund Quarterly, 49,* 509-538.

Organization for Economic Cooperation and Development. (1992). *The reform of health care: A comparison of seven OECD countries.* Paris: Author.

Schmitter, P., & Lehmbruch, G. (1979). *Trends toward corporatist intermediation.* Beverly Hills, CA: Sage.

Starfield, B. (1992). *Primary care: Concept, evaluation, and policy.* New York: Oxford University Press.

Starr, P. (1982). *The social transformation of American medicine.* New York: Basic Books.

van Doorslaer, E., Wagstaff, A., & Rutten, F. (1993). *Equity in the finance and delivery of health care: An international perspective.* New York: Oxford University Press.

Wilensky, H., & Lebeaux, C. (1958). *Industrial society and social welfare: The impact of industrialization on the supply and organization of social welfare services in the United States.* New York: Russell Sage.

World Health Organization. (1996). *Basic documents* (43rd ed.). Geneva: Author.

CHAPTER 2

Lessons From Abroad
A Comparative Perspective

DAVID MECHANIC

Scientific medicine is part of an internationally shared culture, but the financing and organization of services are much less so. Nevertheless, Western countries—facing many of the same pressures of advancing technologies, changing demographics, and limited economic growth— look with great interest at service innovations in other countries, adapting some to their own social and political circumstances. Factors intrinsic to the advancement of medical knowledge and technology, economic constraints, and a variety of other factors have put health reform high on the agenda of most developed nations. Many of these nations, including the United Kingdom, the Netherlands, New Zealand, Sweden, Italy, Turkey, and many countries in eastern Europe and Asia, have been struggling in recent years with structural reforms that go well beyond evolutionary changes. Health reform in the United States, which was high on the agenda in 1993-94, is now in limbo. However, current and impending difficulties make it inevitable that reform issues will be revisited in the foreseeable future.

The particular formats of health services organization are never inevitable and depend a great deal on prior history, professional patterns, culture, and politics. But the development of a world culture and easily available information on events elsewhere affect what people want and

25

expect, and the tendency is for local politics to respond. A recent study of health care reform in 17 Organization for Economic Cooperation and Development (OECD) countries observed that "the most remarkable feature of the health care system reform among the seventeen countries is the degree of emerging convergence. Whether intentionally or not, the reforms follow in the general direction of those pioneered earlier in other countries" (OECD, 1994, p. 43). Moreover, developed countries—and developing countries as well—share the challenges of aging populations, reduced mortality and changing disease patterns, and a growing burden of chronic diseases, disabilities, and behavioral disorders, as well as increasing aspirations for sophisticated medical care.

Beyond medical inflation, growing medical care costs in all Western countries reflect the growing proportion of elderly people and the dramatic potentialities that arise from changing medical knowledge and technology. The medical product has changed substantially in recent years: Technological innovations and a higher intensity of care, especially in hospitals, have become characteristic. New technology is valued and aggressively marketed throughout the world. Though the United States is well beyond most in pursuing the technological imperative, all Western nations are struggling with the diffusion of new technologies and are searching for prudent ways to use and control them.

Moreover, changing disease profiles associated with the delay of mortality and the growing prevalence of chronic disabling disease pose a new set of challenges in long-term and community care. The long-term care challenge requires an appropriate blend of medical and social services designed to maintain function in home and community contexts. Long-term care may require a range of resources and interventions, including social security, housing, social services, rehabilitation, and medical care, that cross bureaucratic institutional cultures. Such welfare functions, to a much greater degree than acute medical care, are embedded in unique cultural and institutional systems that have their own priorities, bureaucratic arrangements, ideologies, and reward structures. They are susceptible to battles over control and tendencies toward cost shifting.

The challenges of keeping pace with technology and long-term care needs increasingly occur in a context of growing public expectations, encouraged by worldwide media that quickly bring news of new possibilities into the home A culture of rights is common throughout developed countries, and efforts to organize services take place within a growing concern about equity of access and sometimes even equity of outcomes. Perhaps nowhere are populations as demanding of immediate access and the latest innovations as in the United States, but in all countries growing expectations make heavy demands on existing medical systems.

Escalating costs have put rationing on the agenda of all developed nations, and there is continuing evidence of restructuring of organizational arrangements, reimbursement mechanisms, and regulatory devices designed to rein in medical costs. Countries differ in their willingness to discuss rationing openly. However, the nature of the rationing agenda and its evolution in various countries is revealed by the growing attention to prospective budgets, gatekeeper roles, waiting lists, technology controls, and insurance changes to shift risk to providers and to increase consumer cost sharing.

Given their varying histories, cultures, and political systems, how countries learn from one another is a disjointed process, but the willingness to consider elements seemingly foreign to one's existing system reflects the extent of perceived crisis in many settings and the degree to which a world culture is emerging on economic and technological issues. With the collapse of the socialist economies in eastern Europe and the former Soviet Union, national systems of care are giving way to more decentralized, pluralistic, entrepreneurial, and privatized approaches. Who, for example, could have anticipated the wide interest in American health maintenance organizations (HMOs) in many countries or the influence on the British National Health Service of the ideas of Alain Enthoven and the notion of "internal markets" within the government system?

Goals for Health Care Reform

Almost everyone agrees on the desirability of having a universal system of medical care that offers people security in case of serious illness, is reasonably comprehensive, and is portable from one geographic area to another. Despite spending far more on medical care than any system in the world, Americans debate health reform as if a universal system would tax our political ingenuity and economic capacities. Perhaps the most important lesson we should learn from experience around the world is that a comprehensive system of health care within economic limits is doable; indeed, such systems are almost universal. We all understand that millions of people depend on our health care system for their livelihoods and profits; hence the unwillingness of these interests to yield current advantages. But it should also be clear from our own past experience, and from the experience of other nations as well, that unless we are prepared to make choices, we cannot meet our aspirations at an acceptable cost.

Any rational solution obviously will involve losers as well as winners; thus, selling health care reform requires framing issues in a way that appeals to important shared values and is convincingly fair. An important goal underlying reform is that its resultant distributional effects will be fair. Fairness, however, is in the eye of the beholder, as the acrimonious debate over the small business mandate in the Clinton proposals made obvious. It is a reasonable contention, however, that burdens should have some clear relationship to the ability to pay and that resulting distributional effects should be responsive to existing disadvantage and growing inequalities in health. Most people accept this idea in principle, but in the noise of the health care debate it has been difficult to avoid distortion and confusion.

The debate about the Clinton health plan pragmatically focused on health insurance reform. At the periphery were those who argued that the debate should have focused less on sickness care and more on health itself and on the types of initiatives that could contribute to the prevention of illness and disability. It is inevitable that more immediate and tangible issues such as insurance coverage and financing take precedence, but in recent years many nations have been seriously considering what measures might be taken to promote health. See, for example, Canada's Lalonde Report (Lalonde, 1974), the Health of the Nation Initiative in the United Kingdom (Secretaries of State for Health, 1992), and the objectives for the year 2000 formulated by the U.S. Public Health Service (U.S. Department of Health and Human Services, 1991). A full-scale debate about the broad determinants of health and health inequalities is comfortable neither for powerful interests nor for governments that must adjudicate among them, but it is imperative that health promotion occupy a more central place in the constellation of issues considered.

Health care systems, however organized and financed, must be responsive to the realities of changing demography, emerging patterns of disease and disability, and new threats to health. Given the changing balance of importance between the diseases of childhood and infectious disease as opposed to chronic disorders and disabilities, medical care systems must accommodate to the needs for long-term treatment and the prevention of secondary impairments and disabilities. As medicine increasingly becomes a geriatric endeavor, the challenges are less to find the "silver bullet" and more to manage illness in a way that facilitates continuing function and the maintenance of a decent quality of life. The goals of acute and long-term care are not in conflict, and there is much specialized knowledge and technology that has had dramatic consequences for the functioning of elderly persons and those with serious chronic disease. Nevertheless, long-term treatment and care requires somewhat different caring arrangements and more complex connections with other sectors. Long-term care is an essential aspect of medical care arrangements, although many policy-makers would like to wish the financial and organizational issues away.

There is now an extensive and growing literature on how varying nations finance and organize services; how they approach new challenges associated with changing technology, demography, and patterns of disease; and how they attempt to do this within predetermined budgetary limits. None have been so successful as to be complacent, and throughout the world there is intense interest in the steps that other nations are taking to meet public and professional expectations within permissible financial limits. Some of the changes have been remarkable and surprising—for example, the abandonment of public systems of medical care in eastern Europe, efforts to establish quasi-markets within the public services in Britain and Sweden, and the establishment of general practitioner (GP) fund-holding in the United Kingdom as a way of bringing cost-consciousness into professional decision making. In the space remaining, I examine some lessons that the United States can learn from developments elsewhere as we consider alternative reforms in the years ahead.

Lessons From Abroad

Despite the impressive technical capabilities of the United States, experience around the world should teach us to seek a more reasonable balance between the epidemiology of need and the distribution of services. A key lesson is that although good access to care is essential, too much intervention is often the enemy of the good and can be harmful as well as costly. That the United States, despite its technical ingenuity, lags far behind many other nations in health outcomes does not support the contention that American health care is poor—a point that critics make through these comparisons—but it does reaffirm that the proliferation of technology is not the answer to promoting health.

Although our advanced technologies are admirable, they are often used inappropriately and wastefully and are commonly a source of iatrogenic injury. The sophistication of our screening and imaging technologies allows us to identify seeming pathologies whose significance is unknown and often exaggerated. As Black and Welch (1993) observed, "Many patients have been labeled with disease they do not really have, and many have been given therapy they do not really need" (p. 1242). It seems clear that many newer interventions such as coronary artery bypass surgery and coronary angioplasty are probably too infrequently used in some European countries that ration the availability of new technologies, but the extraordinarily high rates in the United States are difficult to justify. At the same time that we spend many billions on uncertain applications of technology, we fail to provide as widely as necessary many proven services such as appropriate primary care and such simple preventive modalities as immunizations. Experience elsewhere tells us that a better balance is not only desirable but also feasible.

A second lesson to be learned from examining experience abroad is that by using a variety of financing approaches, it is possible to hold cost at an agreed-on level without significantly damaging the population's health. However, all such approaches are crude and very imperfect in distinguishing between efficacious and ineffective care. Few parties in the debate in any nation readily acknowledge such real uncertainties. Many American policymakers believe they can reduce waste by making patients cost-conscious—for example, through increased cost sharing. As the RAND Health Insurance Experiment showed, however, cost sharing functions as a general barrier and has comparable effects on both efficacious and less worthwhile services (Newhouse & the Insurance Experiment Group, 1993).

Studies of waiting lists and practice variations suggest that planned systems, common abroad, also fail to achieve their promise of rationality. Though in theory physicians carefully give preference to those most in need of service, in reality many other factors intervene, including practice incentives, physician training and preferences, and poor judgment. Variations become exaggerated with increased uncertainty. Nevertheless, systems of triage function reasonably well, and practice guidelines, physician education, and improved information systems should help to get closer to the ideal.

In the United States, a core issue is whether managed care results in withholding useful and efficacious care. Whether considering prospective payment or utilization management, it seems inevitable that medical uncertainty and the nonspecificity of these approaches will result in the denial of some useful care as well as the curbing of wasteful practices. Experience elsewhere suggests the importance of a thoughtful perspective that acknowledges the dilemma but recognizes that despite errors, reasonable gatekeeping works in the interest of most of the population. The perfect can be the enemy of the good, and it is prudent to keep in mind iatrogenic injuries that accompany unnecessary aggressive interventions.

Provision of care within a budget—the dominant pattern around the world—offers the better option. Physicians may make errors, but they clearly are in a better position to make prudent judgments of medical need than are patients as consumers. Safeguards to assist judgment—such as practice guidelines, outcomes research, and vigorous peer review—are required. It is also necessary to control perverse incentives that seek to distort physicians' judgment—for example, by tying their incomes closely to utilization targets.

During the acrimonious debate over the Clinton plan, there was much heated rhetoric but little thoughtful discussion of the choice issue. Choice is important in medicine because it contributes to trust and increases the probability that patients will reveal important information to doctors, cooperate in treatment, adhere to appropriate medical regimens, and make meaningful efforts to change their behavior when required. The placebo effect in medicine has long been recognized as a powerful force; the practitioner's credibility is fundamental to the potency of therapeutic relationships and influence processes. Choice also allows dissatisfied people to shift their care easily, thus reducing disruptions and conflicts within therapeutic relationships and insurance plans, and it has some value in making providers of service more responsive to patients.

The drawback to excessive choice is that it encourages shopping among specialists and the unnecessary use of many services. Choice, however, remains one of the strengths of the American system. Providing patients incentives to join programs such as HMOs that offer point-of-service plans will encourage some restraint in use of services while maintaining opportunities for choice.

Among the weaknesses of many systems abroad are restraints on choice, lack of responsiveness to patients, and bureaucratic officiousness. One important function associated with the emergence of quasi-markets within nationalized systems is to facilitate patient choice as well as competition. In the United Kingdom, for example, the new reforms make changing GPs easier, and GP fundholding allows doctors to buy services for their patients at other facilities when waiting lists are long or when consultants are unresponsive. The challenge in the American context is to maintain the benefits of choice without fostering too much waste. This can be achieved by providing a great deal of choice of primary care physicians and by creating incentives that discourage self-referral to specialists.

Projections for the next century of an aging population and its effect on demand for medical care alarm many American policymakers about potential needs and costs of long-term care. Experience in countries that have a much larger proportion of elders in their populations (e.g., Sweden and Germany) shows that it is possible to provide a high level of care at lower investment of gross domestic product than we now spend. With the increasing medicalization of aging and social problems, the technologically aggressive traditional model of acute care characteristic of American medicine will not be sustainable without significant modification.

Changing disease patterns require that medical care give greater priority to broad interventions designed to maintain function. Current medical organization is poorly structured to provide the range of judgment and services needed to provide coherent and coordinated management of long-term care problems. We tend too frequently to substitute expensive technology for thoughtful assessment and for building collaborative relationships with patients and their families. These problems are exacerbated by poorly developed primary care services and the failure to effectively use other professional services that have much to contribute to effective functioning, such as physical therapy, nutritional services, and rehabilitation.

Medical systems that are insensitive to how people define their problems and use help tend to respond in a more technical fashion than is desirable. Throughout the world, a vast amount of help seeking is triggered by social and personal problems that contribute to physical and psychological distress. Psychological disorder is a major source of disability in everyday living and has more damaging effects on function than do most physical illnesses. No nation has successfully confronted the implications of psychological morbidity, and we have much to learn in this area. It is clear, however, that the frameworks for financing and organizing services will either enable or make impossible a meaningful response to these types of challenges.

Because it is common for psychological distress to be presented to doctors in the form of somatic symptoms, patients with psychosocial problems are commonly subjected to extensive and costly diagnostic workups that reinforce their sense of distress and illness behaviors while ignoring many salient and important aspects of their concerns. Monitoring patients without instituting premature and intrusive interventions requires a strong primary care system that maintains continuity and can make rapid responses as circumstances change. In many nations, primary care is better positioned to take on this task than is the case in the United States, although everywhere cost pressures and increasing expectations put great stress on primary care.

Primary care is best conceptualized as a set of functions that can be performed in alternative ways depending on the needs of the population served, the types of medical and nursing personnel available, the availability and capacity of specialized facilities, and the dispersion of population and supporting resources. There is no single best model of primary care, although all systems must work out some reasonable balance between the functions of the service of first contact and the more specialized secondary and tertiary care facilities. Varying models may fit different circumstances, but experience abroad shows the value of a strong primary care service not only in maintaining continuity of care but also in restraining demand for specialized services.

How varying levels of care are organized depends not only on the professionals and resources available in any system but also on how the system pays providers (Glaser, 1970, 1987). Payment shapes the behavior of professionals and institutions and indirectly determines the priorities of systems of care. Experience around the world provides ample evidence that each form of payment—whether capitation, fee for service, or case payment—has both advantages and disadvantages. Thus, no one form of payment is intrinsically preferable. Professionals appear to prefer the systems of payment to which they have become most accustomed.

Some lessons, however, seem fairly obvious from experience around the world. First, payment arrangements must be consistent with the priorities of the system because professionals respond to the incentives in such arrangements. The incentives, however, should be sufficiently complex to make reimbursement gamesmanship difficult, and mixed systems of reimbursement are more likely to achieve this. Second, we should be careful not to confuse how the population pays for health care with how professionals are reimbursed. Capitated systems often become more efficient and responsive when combined with appropriate fee-for-service incentives. We need more experimentation with mixed reimbursement schemes that combine a basic capitation with enhancements related to levels of skills, performance indicators, productivity, and patient satisfaction. Improved information and available information technology make feasible what would have been totally impractical a short time ago.

A final lesson that experience around the world teaches us is that there is no single, ideal model for financing and organizing services. Each system of care evolves from particular cultures, local circumstances, and patterns of preexisting professional groupings and infrastructures. Population expectations, political institutions and processes, and the personalities and political skills of reformers all play some part. There is much convergence in reform proposals around the world; this reflects common biomedical knowledge and technology as well as economic, demographic, and political pressures. Though such common factors narrow the options theoretically available, no particular approach is inevitable (Mechanic & Rochefort, 1996).

Health reform efforts can either cement in place long-standing patterns or strike out in innovative ways. Their effects at any point in time are not predictable, depending greatly on public attitudes, political institutions, advocacy skills, the vigor of important interest groups, and the types of coalitions and compromises that emerge. Health reform is rarely successful if it does not make allies of at least some important components of the professional community. Many systems, whatever their political orientation, find that regularizing negotiations with the medical profession often makes possible innovations that would otherwise be impossible.

Political processes may at any point thwart reform, but politics is a changing scene. In all Western countries, the pressures of health care costs, population expectations, demographic changes, and concerns about inequalities all ensure that health reform will remain on the agenda. Changes may come about either by small iterations or by larger transformations. As we seek new ways in the future, it is important that we examine alternatives in other countries. What we actually do, of course, will be responsive to our own culture and politics, but by learning from the experience of others we can expand our options and help limit our mistakes.

References

Black, W., & Welch, G. (1993). Advances in diagnostic imaging and overestimations of disease prevalence and the benefits of therapy. *New England Journal of Medicine, 328,* 1237-1243.

Glaser, W. (1970). *Paying the doctor: Systems of remuneration and their effects.* Baltimore: Johns Hopkins University Press.

Glaser, W. (1987). *Paying the hospital: The organization, dynamics and effects of differing financial arrangements.* San Francisco: Jossey-Bass.

Lalonde, M. (1974). *A new perspective on the health of Canadians: A working document.* Ottawa: Government of Canada.

Mechanic, D., & Rochefort, D. (1996). Comparative medical systems. *Annual Review of Sociology, 22,* 239-270.

Newhouse, J., & the Insurance Experiment Group. (1993). *Free for all? Lessons from the Rand Health Insurance Experiment.* Cambridge, MA: Harvard University Press.

Organization for Economic Cooperation and Development. (1994). *The reform of health care systems: A review of seventeen OECD countries* (Health Policy Studies No. 5). Paris: Author.

Secretaries of State for Health. (1992). *The health of the nation: A strategy for health for England.* London: HMSO, Command No. 1986.

U.S. Department of Health and Human Services. (1991). *Healthy people: National health promotion and disease prevention objectives* (DHHS Pub. No. [PHS] 91-50212). Washington, DC: Government Printing Office.

CHAPTER 3

Comparative Health Systems and the Convergence Hypothesis

The Dialectics of Universalism and Particularism

MARK G. FIELD

For about 200 years, the United States has had a system of "socialized" education. Although this system has a variety of problems, the general principles that undergird it have been accepted as part of the American way of life. It is universally available, financed from tax monies, with salaried teachers, and with facilities built by the community or the state. And it does not preclude, for those parents that want it and can afford it, privately financed schools. It is true that at the time of Jefferson and well into the 19th century, there were those who argued against universal education, saying that the children of the poor could not benefit from it and that it should be reserved for the middle and particularly the upper orders of society. But both Jefferson and, later, Horace Mann carried the day. They argued that an educated citizenry could only benefit the community and society. This included even those who did not have children, in terms of domestic tranquillity, through the teaching not only of the three R's but also of morality and codes of civil conduct. Moreover, it was held that in a society that was industrializing, the schools could contribute to the learning of the necessary traits of obedience, discipline, and punctuality. Moreover, education was seen as an important instrument in the absorption of immigrants, or their children, into American life and culture. The provision of personal health care, however, has followed a quite different path.

If education is meant to shape the capacity to act through socialization, then health or medical care is meant, among other objectives, to repair, enhance, and prolong the individual's capacity to act. And yet, until today, access to medical care has not been considered as a right, an essential component of the good life and the "pursuit of happiness," or as a boon to society. Rather, it has been seen first as a privilege of the well-to-do. Or it has been seen as a consumer good, a commodity that one can purchase if one can afford it. When need for care becomes pressing, one can insure for it, or eventually it may be made available as a charity. It was possible until quite recently for some to argue that personal medical care may be like a Cadillac: "If a person can afford one, so much the better, but society does not *owe* everyone a Cadillac."

In recent years, these attitudes have changed significantly. In most industrial societies, particularly after World War II, health care has been defined as a right of citizenship, guaranteed one way or another by the state. In the United States, we are still struggling and arguing about a universal guarantee for health care. Recent national events in this country involving proposed changes in the health care system are indicative of the politically and ideologically charged nature of the issue of universal access in the American context. Indeed, health security has become one of the most controversial issues of the moment, particularly in view of the fact that health care involves one seventh of the U.S. economy, so that the stakes are enormous.

This issue also brings into relief the question of equity because it is estimated that at any one time about 40 million Americans do not have health insurance or coverage. A study carried out between 1970 and 1987, using a sample of nearly 5,000, found that the uninsured were one and one quarter times more likely to die of the same conditions as those who were insured (Franks, Clancy, & Gold, 1993).

The public sector, particularly the federal government, has increasingly been concerned with the health situation. In the 19th century, health—particularly public health—was, by default, the responsibility of the states. This situation gave rise to a number of problems—for example, the stemming of epidemics and the imposition of quarantines affecting more than one state. Only in the 20th century, with the passage of the Social Security Act of 1935, were the welfare concerns of the federal government recognized as constitutional, though health care was not included. In fact, throughout American history, until perhaps the passage of Medicare and Medicaid, the separation of personal medicine from the state was almost as sacrosanct as that of church and state.

Now we have at last begun to embark on a process of debating health care as a universal right of citizenship. But the question that remains is how to decide on a program of health care for a population of over a quarter of a billion people. One alternative involves a move in the direction of universal national health insurance, which is in fact a financing mechanism more than a health care program but is compatible with American ideology. The second alternative involves the institution of a national health service in which the polity would dispense health care much as it does public education. The second alternative, so far, does not have much of a chance, for it would amount to socialized medicine, which, contrary to socialized education, still raises the hackles of Americans. This aversion is not only because of its association with communism, the traditional foe. There exists also a fear that a national health plan would give too great a role to the government, particularly the federal government, which, after the collapse of the Soviet Union has become, for many, the new enemy.

But the question will not go away: How can America extend the benefits of modern health care to all those who need it, not only to the insured and the affluent? The problem is complicated by the fact that no society can build a health care system completely *de novo*. It must accept the system that exists today, with its practitioners, institutions, and other characteristics, and attempt to change it or bend it in a different direction—a task made difficult by the multiplicity of vested interests that want their particular turf protected or even enhanced. The recent explosive growth of managed care seems an almost spontaneous development, propelled by the perceived need to control the escalation of costs. Managed care is a revolution that has not yet run its course. It has brought to the fore a surge of vexing questions, not the least of which is the downsizing of the medical profession's traditional autonomy.

So, for a perspective on these problems, the logical step would be to look around at other countries that have implemented their own programs and see what could be learned and avoided. This, then, is the genesis of comparative health systems. Comparison is at the heart of the scientific enterprise, as when we compare a control and an experimental group. It is a way to make judgments, to assess changes and progress. We do it all the time: Mothers compare their children; when we appoint someone to be a professor, comparison is the essential ingredient of evaluation. It is often only through comparison that the contours of a phenomenon become meaningful.

Comparison may be either synchronic or diachronic. In the first instance, we go horizontally, so to speak, to determine, for example, how much of the gross national product (GNP) each country spent on health in a given year. This is the cross-national approach. The diachronic measure is a historical or vertical one: We compare, for example, the infant mortality rate of 10 years ago with that of today. Discussions of health care reform mainly take the synchronic approach, though I feel that the historical and evolutionary approach also has a great deal to offer.

This led me to ask whether there might be some regularity in the evolution of health systems, as there is in the evolution of morbidity in the developing world, with its increasing burden of chronic illness. This evolution is associated with the demographic patterns of societies as they change from a pattern of high birth rates and high death rates to a pattern of high birth rates and low death rates, and finally to a pattern of low birth rates and low death rates. Is there some common dynamism and regularity in the organization of health services that would permit us to compare and learn? Would this regularity also allow us to some extent to predict changes in health systems, as we are able to predict an increase in heart disease and cancer in societies that are modernizing? This is the idea behind the general hypothesis of the *convergence* of modern societies all over the world (Form, 1979). There is a transition from an agricultural to an industrial and urbanized society, and this will in time lead to the emergence of social structures and personality traits dictated by the logic of this type of economic activity, typified, for instance, by the assembly line. This technological determinism, though different from the inexorable historical materialism of Marxism, does postulate certain consequences. As Inkeles and Smith (1974) explained, "Men from different cultures might nevertheless respond in basically the same way to certain of the relatively standard institutions and interpersonal relations introduced by economic developments and sociopolitical modernization" (p. 12). Among these elements one might note the importance of the time dimension, the use of clocks and watches, and the relevance of the punctuality and discipline that Horace Mann, and those who emulated him, sought to impart to the future industrial workers who sat as children in their classrooms.

It is not only the logic of industrialism that produces increasing convergence but also the principle of emulation and imitation, facilitated by instant global communication. Industrialism, like the proverbial wheel, does not have to be reinvented time and again. The convergence theory does not postulate that all societies are becoming like peas in a pod. It means that shared elements are increasing and that the differences and divergences are decreasing. Just stand at a busy intersection in any one of the major cities around the world, whether Paris, Tokyo, New York, or Boston, and you will recognize the resemblances.

If there is some validity to this idea, then why not postulate that it also operates for health systems, given that these systems are constantly being affected and transformed by research, science, and the new technologies—that is, the universal means of "medical production"? The use of antibiotics or of insulin, like the action of these drugs, knows no national or other boundaries.

Indeed, as we go around the world, we see many striking similarities in health care systems. These commonalities embrace a wide range of phenomena prevalent in the health systems of many countries, including some important problems and issues facing these systems. A recurrent feature in many countries involves the increasing portion of the GNP consumed by medical care. A constant pattern is the growing significance and the role played by the polity, with the public sector often assuming financial, organizational, managerial, and control functions in health care. Another recurring trend in most of these systems involves the constant introduction of medical technologies. These generally are both capital and labor intensive and are more and more expensive; they also contribute to the alienation of the patient from the therapist. This alienation is fostered by the unending process of internal differentiation associated with specialization and superspecialization. This trend toward the proliferation of specialties in turn gives rise to the perceived need, often unfulfilled, to integrate the increasingly narrow outputs of superspecialists.

A parallel set of new circumstances and problems is also confronted by the medical profession in many of these health care systems. Thus, a growing proportion of physicians are now renumerated on a salaried basis, and many are employed in bureaucratic organizations. This change in situation is associated with an increasing alarm on the part of doctors, who fear that their professional and particularly their clinical autonomy is being steadily eroded by the bureaucrats, the managers, the bean counters, and the cost reduction experts. Accompanying these changes is the widening cultural lag caused by advances in prolonging and maintaining life, with resulting legal, ethical, spiritual, and religious implications. These problematic trends, found in many countries, contribute to the prospects for introduction of formal rationing of health care.

Following the theory of convergence, the structures, arrangements, and institutions in which contemporary medical care is provided should be expected to be affected and shaped by these trends, modalities, and processes. For example, the very requirements of asepsis in the operating

•

room dictate not only what we might call "measures of security" against infection but also personal behavior patterns in hospitals that admit of little if any variability if available knowledge is to be applied effectively. Thus, one might expect that every hospital, particularly in the developed world, should resemble every other hospital. Yet observation and, in some cases, personal experience with American, French, Soviet, and German hospitals suggest that this is not precisely the case. A hospital is part of the community in which it exists and of the society and culture of which it partakes. The passage from that community into the hospital is not one regulated by pressure chambers and airtight doors. There is a constant flow from the community and society into and out of the hospital. Passing through its doors does not mean passing from one distinct world to another, from the community to a distinct medical and antiseptic world. The hospital is an amalgam of the two; the dialectic confrontation of two cultures, particularistic and universalistic, results in a synthesis that varies from society to society.

But this encounter is not limited to the hospital; it is part of the clinical picture and of medical practices themselves. One would assume, at first glance, that these practices should be similar, as doctors everywhere apply universal knowledge and the use of up-to-date equipment and technology. Not so: As Payer (1988) observed, there are amazing differences in the manner in which American, British, French, and German doctors practice, and "while medicine benefits from a certain amount of scientific input, culture intervenes every step of the way" (p. 26). For one, doctors from one country rarely read the literature of any country but their own. American doctors are characterized by their aggressiveness—the coronary bypass is performed many times more often than in most countries, even those that have the same rate of heart disease. The Americans are six times more likely to have a coronary bypass than the English. For the American doctor, the heart is just a pump, a machine, an organ fed by tubes that must be unclogged if necessary. For the German doctor, the heart is not just a pump but an organ with a life of its own that pulsates in response to different stimuli, including emotions, and that has metaphoric associations with love and affective feelings. On the other hand, German doctors prescribe six times as many heart drugs as the French and the English. And there is in Germany the diagnosis of *Herzinsuffizienz*, which we may translate, but not quite correctly, as either congestive heart failure or cardiac insufficiency. Lack of appetite is a much more serious symptom, and understandably so, for the French than for the English or the Swedes. There is a belief among the French, including many doctors, and not denied by their winegrowers, that moderate drinking protects from heart attack. This may be correct (not causally, of course, but as an observation). Though the French have the highest rate of cirrhosis in the world, they have a much lower incidence of heart attacks: 100 per 100,000 versus 240 for Germans, 300 for Americans, and 350 for the British (Payer, 1988, p. 56). The "liver crisis" has become a legendary French complaint. In 1970, there were 300 different drugs for the liver in France, together accounting for 5% of drug consumption. In 1976, a French study absolved the liver of responsibility for most ailments (cirrhosis excepted), and now the *crise de foie* has become less fashionable in the Gallic heartland (Payer, 1988, p. 59). On the other hand, the French are much more prone to accept parallel medicines, the *médecines douces,* than the more aggressive Americans. Thomas Hewes, who has long practiced internal medicine at the American Hospital of Paris, says:

> I came to Europe thinking medicine, as a science, was the same all over. I soon learned that it's not. . . . The French consider it more art than a science. . . . You'll get three different answers if you go to three different physicians. (quoted in Harris, 1995, p. 98)

American plastic surgeons have identified a disease that apparently affects millions of American women and which they have called *micromastia* (or "small breasts"), and the disease has been aggressively treated, as the brouhaha about silicone implants suggests.[1] The aggressiveness of American medicine can also be seen in the fact that an American woman has two or three times as much chance of having a hysterectomy as her French, British, or German sister. This also holds true to a similar extent for cesarean sections. Indeed, a British general practitioner has called Americans "Godsakers," as in "For God's sake, do something," thus expressing the obsessive-compulsive nature of American doctors and their patients, who think that "more is better" and who want it fast. This attitude makes it more difficult for Americans to accept chronic illnesses, where there is no easy formula for a possible cure.

The hospice movement is well developed in England, possibly because of the greater English acceptance of death and dying, whereas Americans regard dying as the ultimate failure. The British prefer lumpectomies to mastectomies. Economy indeed characterizes British medicine. The blood pressure is taken considerably less often in Great Britain than in the United States, and the threshold is likely to be considerably higher.

The upshot is, as Payer (1998) noted, that "the choice of diagnosis and treatment is *not* science. . . . The weighing of risks and benefits will always be made on a cultural scale" (p. 154). It is precisely that element of cultural diversity that makes meaningful comparisons of national health care systems a complicated and sometimes difficult if not frustrating task. All kinds of unjustified conclusions can be drawn from international statistics.

As a final note, Gaylin (1993) has suggested that the health crisis in America is so severe not only because America is preeminent in high technology culture but also

> because of the American character. . . . Americans refuse to believe there are limits to anything—let alone to life itself. . . . Consider the struggle to define such terms as "death with dignity" and growing old gracefully; the latter means living a long time without aging. Dying in one's sleep at 92 after having won three sets of tennis from one's 40 year old grandson . . . and having made love to one's wife twice that same evening—this is about the only scenario most American men [are] willing to accept as fulfilling their idea of death with dignity. (p. A27)

So as we leave aside for the time being the softly deterministic theory of convergence, we are left with the open question of the didactic value of the comparative approach. For example, in the United States, we are obsessed with the increasing costs of health care, and there has been a great deal of soul-searching and solution seeking in looking at other entities to see how they have managed this vexing problem. In the last few years, Canada has emerged as a possible model to emulate: It is, after all, a society with which the United States shares many features. And Canada, while assuring its population universal health care coverage, has been able to keep its costs at a manageable 9% to 10% of the GNP, whereas with our 14% of the GNP we still have close to 40 million people who have no health insurance and who must rely on welfare, charity, or nothing. And in the Canadian system, there is a partnership between the provinces and the central government, similar to that established in this country for Medicaid. But as William Glaser (1990) pointed out, the completely government-financed system of health care is "an irrelevant model" because of widely different political cultures in the very area of financing personal health services. Glaser suggested that the United States take a closer look at the highly relevant statutory health insurance systems of Europe.

The particularism of medical practice complicates the process of comparison and limits the didactic nature of the comparative exercise by narrowing the transferability of effective patterns and arrangements from one society to another. The universalism of medicine as applied science, in the sense of verifiable, tested knowledge, must always be tempered by the setting into which it is introduced and applied. Thus, each health system is a synthesis of the universal and the particular. It has been said that culture is destiny, a paraphrase of the famous dictum of Freud about anatomy. But anatomy and physiology are invariant, whereas culture, which I define as humanity's nongenetic inheritance, does evolve constantly. Thus, an editorial in the *Massachusetts General Hospital News* ("Editorial," 1993), commenting on recent political events concerning health care reform, expressed the view that

> the United States tends to swing wildly from one end of the spectrum to the other. Whether it is a new system of education, a new craze in music, or a new medical procedure, we seem to treat novel ideas with unrestrained enthusiasm, only to find out we have overreacted. (p. 2)

This, then, is a measured plea for levelheadedness in our use of the comparative approach. There is much to learn from other systems, but what we learn must be judiciously calibrated to fit into American culture and its particularities.

Note

1. We still have not heard of its counterpart, which would logically be called *macromastia*. Large breasts are considered not as a clinical problem in today's American culture but rather as an asset (as Mae West or Dolly Parton have made abundantly clear). But fashions change. In the 1920s, flat chests were considered by flappers to be chic!

References

Editorial. (1993, September). *Massachusetts General Hospital News*, p. 2.

Form, W. (1979). Comparative industrial sociology and the convergence hypothesis. *Annual Review of Sociology, 5*, 1-25.

Franks, P., Clancy, C., & Gold, M. B. (1993). Health insurance and mortality: Evidence from a national cohort. *Journal of the American Medical Association, 270,* 737-741.

Gaylin, W. (1993, September 15). The health plan misses the point. *New York Times,* p. A27.

Glaser, W. (1990). Comparative research methods. In French Ministry of Social Affairs, Research Section (MIRE) and International Social Security Association (Eds.), *The international comparison of social security policies and systems* (pp. 289-297). Paris: Editors.

Harris, J. (1995, June). Uncommon cures. *Condé Nast Traveler,* pp. 98-99.

Inkeles, A., & Smith, D. (1974). *Becoming modern: Individual change in six developing countries.* Cambridge, MA: Harvard University Press.

Payer, L. (1988). *Medicine and culture: Varieties of treatment in the United States, England, West Germany and France.* New York: Henry Holt.

PART II

The German Experience

CHAPTER 4

From Solidarity to Market Competition?

Values, Structure, and Strategy in German Health Policy, 1883-1997

CHRISTA ALTENSTETTER

In moving toward the 21st century, Germany is going its own way. Whereas many other nations have introduced some form of "internal markets" or "managed care" based on the superiority of market forces (Jérôme-Fourget, White, & Wiener, 1995; Organization for Economic Cooperation and Development [OECD], 1994, 1995), Germany has retained—though it has restructured—its 100-year-old national health insurance program. To understand why Germany continues on its estab-

AUTHOR'S NOTE: Portions of this chapter were written while I was in residence at the GSF National Research Center for Environment and Health, Ingolstädter Landstr.1, D-85764 Oberschleißheim, Germany, in July 1995 and January 1997. The opinions expressed here are my own and do not represent the position of the Institut für Medizinische Informatik und Systemforschung (MEDIS). The research for this chapter was completed in February 1997. I would like to thank Ellen J. Hammer in New York and Jürgen John, Andreas Mielck, and Walter Satzinger at MEDIS, the GSF National Research Center for Environment and Health. I wish to thank in particular Professor Dr. Wilhelm van Eimeren, director of MEDIS, for his continuing support.

lished path and how the German health insurance system functions within a federal structure, it is necessary to consider the values, ideas, and principles that have shaped health policy making in Germany over more than 100 years.

The Health Care Structural Reform Act became law in 1993 (Bundes-ministerium für Arbeit und Sozialordnung, 1993; "Gesetz zur Sicherung," 1992). Though some observers (Franco, 1992; Knox, 1993; U.S. General Accounting Office, 1993; numerous German authors as cited by Giaimo & Manow, 1997) have viewed it as a radical departure, it will be argued that it does not yet mark the end of the organizing principles of health care and statutory health insurance policy (Döhler, 1993; Döhler & Manow-Borgwardt, 1992, 1995). Rather, the 1993 Structural Reform Act builds on the existing regulatory and corporatist insti-tutional framework joining purchasers and providers. It fully reaffirms the principle of providing nearly universal access to medical care while mod-erately redefining solidarity (Giaimo & Manow, 1997).

However, the implementation of the 1993 reform has added much more organizational and procedural complexity to an already complex and fragmented regulatory regime. There is now a greater variety of contracts (collective, regional, selective, and individual), less homogeneity of rules, less transparency, more procedural differentiation, and less uniformity in the conditions under which providers work (Advisory Council, 1995, p. 33).

The 1993 Structural Reform Act imposed capped global and regional budgets, which between 1993 and 1997 were tied to the revenue base of statutory insurance. The implementation of this policy, led by the Health Minister, Mr. Seehofer, has wreaked havoc with the entire delivery system since mid-1996. Mr. Seehofer staged a most vigorous campaign against all providers, especially office-based physicians and dentists, and in 1997 he also stepped up his attacks on the sickness funds for alleged failure to maximize resources and increase efficiency. Although physicians are losing much political and, above all, economic ground, the Health Minister gave in to the pressures by the pharmaceutical industry, which in 1997 seems to be regaining influence that it lost in 1993.

According to a good many observers, these "third-phase reform poli-cies" are ruining a fairly well-functioning system that has been driven by a national policy of solidarity since 1883. Thus, for example, *Die Zeit* (Hoffmann, 1996) saw Mr. Seehofer as having earned his place in history already; it suggested that in the year 2050, a reader of *Brockhaus* (the German equivalent to *Webster's Dictionary*) would find this entry on Mr. Seehofer: "Christian Democratic Minister of Health known for having destroyed the Bismarckian system" (p. 27). On the other hand, the level of public support of the existing system continues to be high and a "culture of solidarity" prevails among the insured (Hinrichs, 1995, p. 653).

The key issue raised by this political controversy is: What is this system that is "being dismantled," and where is it going? Preexisting regulatory regimes and the values, norms, and rules embedded in them are known to generate long-lasting effects on contemporary health policy. It is therefore important to understand the history of health care policy in Germany in order to assess where it may be going in the future.

What follows is an attempt to provide a broad picture of the causal structure of forces at work in German health care reform. Six sections will examine the following issues:

1. A brief history of German health insurance from 1883 to the present
2. A description of the values and political goals binding policymakers and stakeholders, as well as the rules and procedures by which they agreed to play
3. A comparison of the main components of the delivery systems of the former Federal Republic of Germany and the former German Democratic Republic
4. An examination of the transfer of statutory health insurance, medical care policy, and institutional mechanisms from West Germany to former East Germany
5. A description of the complex federal framework for health policy development and implementation, including the role of state and intermediary nonstate decision-making bodies
6. A discussion of the most salient issues raised by the Health Care Structural Reform Act of 1993

Historical Background

Germany was the first country to institute nationwide insurance-based social and health programs. It adopted the Health Insurance Act in 1883, the Accident Insurance Law in 1884, and the Old Age and Invalidity Act in 1889. These acts, which were part of Bismarck's political strategy for undermining support for socialism, established the main principles that have guided the development of social and health policy in Germany up to the present day. They established close and contingent links between the financing of health care, social insurance-based programs, labor legislation, and the economy in both growth and decline.

Several fundamental characteristics of these acts should be noted:

1. Membership in insurance programs is mandated by law for covered workers earning under an income ceiling.
2. The administration of these programs is delegated to nonstate bodies governed by representatives of the insured and their employers.
3. Entitlement to benefits is linked to past contributions (rather than to other criteria such as need).
4. Benefits and contributions are primarily earnings related.
5. Financing is secured through wage taxes levied on the employer and the employee and, depending on the program, sometimes by additional financing by the state.
6. Until 1997, reimbursement for medical services was made directly to the provider (rather than to the consumer after deduction of copayments, as in France and other neighboring countries).

With the expansion of coverage to an ever-increasing proportion of the population, and the expansion of the scope of services now covered by health insurance, Characteristics 3 and 4 have been replaced by those of universality and health security. The right to health care has been socially defined and now is independent of keeping a job or the ability to make contributions. Because of the opposition of political forces opposed to centralized program structures under the control of the Bismarck regime (Alber, 1988, pp. 1-11; Altenstetter, 1986a), the administration of these insurance programs was not given to the state and, except during the Nazi period and in East Germany during the years between 1945 and 1990, has remained the province of nonstate organizations.

What is remarkable is that during most of this 100-year history, these policies and the principles of solidarity and income redistribution have remained immutable. Today they bind both private and public employers. They permeate the political arenas and all public health insurance-specific decision-making bodies.

In 1885, the Health Insurance Act provided medical protection for only 26% of the lower-paid blue-collar labor force (or for 10% of the population). In 1901, coverage was extended to transport and commercial (office) workers, in 1911 to agricultural and forestry workers and domestic servants, and in 1914 to civil servants. It was extended to the unemployed in 1918, to seamen in 1927, and to all dependents in 1930.[1] In 1941, legislation was passed allowing workers whose income had risen above the national ceiling for compulsory membership to continue their health insurance coverage on a voluntary basis. In the same year, coverage was extended to all retired Germans. Farm workers and sales people were covered in 1966, self-employed agricultural workers and their dependents in 1972, and students and disabled persons in 1975 (Stone, 1980). Although these population groups were covered by public health insurance, the administration of their respective entitlements was as fragmented in 1997 as it was when the program expansions were made. However, mandatory membership in certain sickness funds based on social and occupational groupings was ended on January 1, 1997.

The 1883 law granted decentralized sickness funds full authority to determine which doctors could participate and to set the terms and conditions of their participation. The funds then dealt with physicians through offering individual contracts. The doctors grew increasingly dissatisfied with individual contracts, which limited access to the practice of medicine under the sickness funds. They mobilized and founded a professional association, the *Hartmannbund*, in 1900 and went on strike several times. Finally, in 1913, doctors and sickness funds agreed on a system of collective bargaining by which the distribution of licenses was to be based on the number of insured persons per district and doctors' remuneration became subject to collective bargaining between the sickness funds and doctors' associations. This 1913 agreement between doctors and sickness funds was integrated into the National Insurance Code (Alber, 1988, pp. 6-7). This approach to collective bargaining, though modified many times since 1913, continues to be practiced today.

The rise of Hitler in 1933 marked the beginning of another phase in the development of German health policy. In 1934, the Nazi regime dismantled the labor- and management-controlled self-governance structure of sickness funds and other insurance programs, appointing a director for each program who reported to the central authorities. A number of improvements in social and health insurance benefits and coverage and in need-based programs were made, as these served the political and ideological goals of the Nazi regime. Thus, in 1941, public health insurance coverage was extended to pensioners. In 1942, all wage earners, regardless of occupation, were covered by accident insurance, and the period of sick care was no longer limited. A 12-week fully paid and job-protected maternity allowance was provided (Alber, 1988, pp. 10-11). After the collapse of Germany in 1945, two separate German states evolved that pursued entirely different ideological goals and established different political regimes. In East Germany, the Communist Party gained a monopoly of power and control over all social and political institutions. The state became even stronger than it had been under the Hitler regime, extending its control over the whole economy and reducing the role of the private sector and private institutions to a minimum. West Germany moved away from Hitler's legacy of central control and administration, returning to the decentralized system of pre-Nazi days. Confronting a huge number of people in need of economic and social protection after the war, the Allies in the three occupation zones unwillingly allowed West German political leaders to restore statutory health insurance with the governance model of labor and management control (Hockerts, 1981). The influence of the medical profession had increased relative to employers and trade unions under the Hitler regime, and it continued to be strong because of the growing political influence of the medical profession after 1945 in the West.

Table 4.1 summarizes the major milestones in post-1945 federal health legislation (in West Germany) up to the present day. Note the emphasis on regulation of costs and the high frequency of federally mandated changes in the health care system.

Ideas and Values: Structure and Strategy

Three powerful ideas or principles underlie the development of German health insurance and medical care policy. They have shaped developments from 1883 to the present (Alber, 1988; Ashford, 1986; Baldwin, 1991; Mommsen & Mock, 1981). These principles have been institutionalized in law and in practice and have set limits on acceptable policy options.

The first of these principles is *solidarity,* which in health care elicits the willingness of the healthy to pay for the sick, the single for those with children, and the young for the old. This principle has been overriding and has been embedded in literally hundreds of decisions on financing, organizing, managing, regulating, and delivering medical care. Every federal, state, and local body—governmental and nongovernmental—is bound by the idea of solidarity, even though recently it is being redefined. German society has expressed its commitment to solidarity by offering universal coverage and comprehensive benefits to its population. These benefits are secured by the German constitution and court rulings. Thus far, they also have been safeguarded against the uncertainty and unpredictability of German electoral politics (Aichberger, 1994; Bundesministerium für Arbeit und Sozialordnung, 1993, 1995; Wasem, 1994). This has been achieved despite a fragmented federal system with multiple players, no one of which is in a position to dictate the terms of service delivery.

Although equal burden sharing between employer and employee—the core of solidarity—has weathered far worse political and economic crises in the past, this principle may currently be threatened. In July 1995, the Advisory Council for Concerted Action proposed to freeze the employer tax while making the employee tax contingent on the future stability of

TABLE 4.1. Milestones in Postwar Federal Social and Health Legislation in Germany

1951	Restoration of self-governing bodies for public health insurance
1953	Reestablishment of social courts
1954	Federal regulation of user charges
1955	Creation of regional and national sickness funds associations
1955	Federal regulation of relationship between doctors and insurance funds
1957	Reform of sickness insurance with partial wages during periods of disability
1969	Full disability wages for workers; constitutional reform strengthening the role of the federal government in the health sector
1970	Indexation of income ceiling for compulsory coverage; introduction of coverage for preventive medical checkups
1972	Compulsory sickness insurance for independent farmers; legislation and regulations assign the federal government and the *Länder* joint responsibility for capital financing of hospitals
1974	Federal regulation of hospital user charges (BPflV)
1975	Voluntary cost containment measures by doctors; a fee schedule is introduced
1977	Federal Cost Containment Act (KVKG)
1981	Hospital Cost Containment Act with decentralized rate setting (KHKG)
1982	Supplementary Cost Containment Act introducing copayments for the first time (except for 1931-1932)
1983	Amended budget act expanding copayments
1984	Amended budget act again expanding copayments
1985	The *Länder* become responsible for hospital capital financing
1986	Federal regulation on hospital rate setting introduces prospective budgets
1986	Act to improve sickness fund physician need planning
1988	Health Care Reform Act (GRG) extends preventive checkups and home care, institutes reference prices for pharmaceuticals, etc.
1993	Structural Health Care Reform Act (GSG) caps expenditures for office services, hospital budgets, and prescription drugs; mandates a new hospital rate-setting system (BPflV) to become effective January 1, 1996; restructures statutory health insurance and relations among sickness funds
1994	Amended regulations on hospital rate setting
1995	Statutory nursing care insurance introduced; amended regulations on hospital rate setting
1996	Further amendments to hospital rate-setting regulations
1996	Hospital Expenditure Stabilizing Law (limited to 1996); Health Insurance Contributions Reduction Act (KVBEG) lowers contribution rates starting in January 1997
1996	First Statutory Health Insurance Restructuring Act legislates increases in copayments when sickness funds need to increase contribution rates
1997	Second Statutory Health Insurance Restructuring Act abolishes budgets in ambulatory care and pharmaceuticals; new physician-specific "targets" will be negotiated between the two corporate actor groups of sickness funds and physicians

SOURCE: Alber (1988, p. 12) and Altenstetter (1987); updated by author.

health expenditures. Although this proposal has not been acted on, it could reduce the burden sharing in health care financing. Yet extensions of cost sharing since 1982 are not synonymous with abolishing solidarity, which remains high by international standards.

Reinforcing the principle of solidarity is a second principle known as *subsidiarity*. The application of this principle predates the unification of Germany in 1871 and lies at the heart of the political culture of German-speaking countries. It stands for power sharing, leaving the implementation of national policy to the smallest feasible political and administrative units and/or other voluntary forces in society. It thus provides a distinctive public-private partnership.[2] Subsidiarity means building social organizations and society from the bottom up rather than from the top down. Thus, the implementation of a national health care policy originates from the sickness funds, which evolved from decentralized, voluntary mutual aid societies that predated the Bismarck era (Bauer, 1990; Seibel, 1993; Tampke, 1981; Ullmann, 1981).

In Germany, the concept of subsidiarity is associated with regional identities and political forces that have survived more than a century of a tumultuous history and political instability, resisting the centralizing pressures of nation building and surviving totalitarian regimes. They are expressed in federal and regional power-sharing arrangements. Regional forces are strong and alive in post-1990 Germany and are expressed, among other ways, in the powers of the *Länder*.[3]

Paralleling the federal, state (*Land*), and local political authorities is an array of federally and regionally organized associations of doctors, dentists, pharmacists, sickness funds, and hospitals. Although their specific roles and responsibilities have changed over time, these nonstate, mostly decentralized intermediate bodies are the most important decision makers on vital issues of health policy. They are responsible for quality health care, they are accountable to the public and elected officials, and they have regulatory functions over their members.

The principles of solidarity and subsidiarity have been endorsed by the left, the center, and the right parties on the political spectrum (despite intermittent or temporary opposition by one or the other party) and are embedded in the constitution, the Basic Law of 1949. Earnings-related and insurance-based rights, including the redistributive elements and universal access to health care when needed, are contained in the bill of rights in the preface to the Basic Law and have again been sanctioned by the Social Security Code of 1988.[4]

German health policy has also been fundamentally influenced by a third principle, that of *corporatist organization*. German corporatism involves a dual form of political organization.[5] This entails representation based on occupational and professional groups and also representation based on elections. It is seen in the functional representation of employees and employers on the governing boards of sickness funds. It also serves as a device to organize regional and federal associations of the six types of nonprofit sickness funds and other nonprofit funds. These organizations are paralleled by the federal and regional associations of doctors and of other providers, which, together with the sickness fund associations, negotiate the terms of medical care.

This dual system of representation enhances effective participation in policy formulation and implementation by elected officials and by non-elected representatives of professional and occupational groups alike. It also contributes to the political feasibility and social acceptability of health care reforms, thereby strengthening the capacity of the federal system to formulate and implement health policy. The strong role of employers and employees in decision-making bodies counterbalances the roles of other organized and powerful groups, such as doctors, dentists, pharmacists, the pharmaceutical industry, and for-profit health insurance companies (Webber, 1991).

In consequence, a system of ground rules has evolved that cannot be altered or flouted without dismantling the whole health care structure: the healthy paying for the sick and the inclusion of employers and employees, provider groups, and nonprofit payer groups (i.e., the sickness funds) in the key decision-making bodies of the federal and regional governments and, to a lesser extent, in local decision-making bodies. No group can singlehandedly change rules, impose or raise fees, or raise contribution rates without the agreement of the other parties. All health care organizations and professional groups are bound by the same principles and rules (Altenstetter, 1985, 1987).

Within this framework of primary ground rules, a body of supplementary rules defines the specific responsibilities of providers, payers, employers, employees, and federal, state, and local governments and agencies. These supplementary rules enjoy as much political legitimacy as the constitution-backed primary ground rules. They reinforce each other and are sanctioned by federal and state legislation. They are also backed up by many court rulings, including those of the federal constitutional court. Examples of supplementary rules are the public health insurance law and the law pertaining to the practice of medicine and dentistry (Aichberger, 1994).

Reinforcing these values and principles, and securing their transfer into democratic Germany after 1918, are a body of law and a unique institution, the contribution of which to the development of the German welfare state has received scant attention. Parallel to the development of the four social insurance programs (including health), a body of social law, insurance law, and special legal and administrative procedures evolved from the 1880s onward and culminated in 1953 in the creation of a unique three-tiered social court system: local social courts of first instance, regional social courts of appeal, and a federal social court endowed with ultimate constitutional rule-making powers (Wannagat, 1965; *Sozialgerichtsgesetz* [SGG of 3 September 1953, as amended]). The social courts adjudicate and rule on social and health insurance matters, including social compensation, social and medical aid, and claims by providers against sickness funds. They are independent of the regular civil and criminal court system as well as the administrative courts that operate in some continental European countries where Roman law prevails.[6] The German system of codified social laws overseen by the social courts has fostered the durability of statutory health insurance in Germany. These judicial vehicles go a long way in explaining sources of resistance to the implementation of many provisions of the Health Care Structural Reform Act of 1993. Constitutional law, social law, and social (health) insurance law deserve attention by comparativists that they have not received in the past.

These social practices may appear outdated or undemocratic to those who have experienced another political tradition. But they do enjoy democratic and societal legitimacy. In the past, they offered flexible responses to rising health care costs and have adapted to medical progress while retaining health protection against unpredictable risks of life (White, 1995). Likewise, both the primary ground rules and the supplementary rules combine to provide a fairly stable legal and service framework for all players in the system, independent of the fluctuations, pressures, and dynamics of electoral politics. Critics emphasize the rigidities and constraints arising from this framework. But all Germans have a stake in the health care system as consumers, potential patients, voters, taxpayers, and premium payers. The overall salience of this fivefold role has made health policy prominent on the political agenda and has subjected all providers to continuing public scrutiny. Given the political sensitivity of health policy, one cannot predict how the "third phase" of health care reform will play itself out in the future.

Coverage for Hospitalization and Medical and Nursing Care

Operating by a system of consensus and cooperation rather than competition, the Germans have been able to accomplish three things.

First, while preserving the freedom of its population to choose their own doctors, the German system has delivered high-quality care to citizens on an almost universal basis: 88.5% of the population (or 72 million people) are included under the all-payer public health insurance program, with the remainder being either affluent citizens who are not required to join the public program and must be covered by private insurance (9.1%) or citizens covered by special schemes, such as those for the military or for higher civil servants (about 2.3%) (Bundesministerium für Gesundheit, 1995, p. 279). Only 0.1% of Germans carry no insurance. Of those covered by statutory health insurance, about 75% are compulsory members. Second, during the 1980s, Germany has kept health care expenditures under better control (decreasing from 8.4% to 8.1% of the gross domestic product spent on health care from 1980 to 1990) than most other OECD member states (OECD, 1990, 1992; Schieber, Poullier, & Greenwald, 1992; Schneider, 1995, p. 63). Third, doctors, though limited by fee schedules, have until recently retained clinical and professional autonomy (Altenstetter, 1989; Döhler, 1989, 1990).

Statutory health insurance continues to be the centerpiece of the German health care system. Financed in large part by mandatory insurance contributions and implemented through a mix of public and private providers, the multipayer public insurance system is decentralized and operated by six types of nonprofit statutory funds, the so-called "sickness funds."[7] These are supplemented by a few additional "substitute" nonprofit funds and extended by private health insurance.

All German workers earning less than a "ceiling" income are required to join a sickness fund.[8] Workers have been assigned to membership in fund- ... lity of residence, occupation, or employer. A varie ... ʻts maintain sickness funds; historically, these funds ... .ndec ... medieval guilds. In addition to these *In-* *nungs* ... *ʻen.* ... ʻ occupational funds for miners, sailors, and agricu ... worker not follow an occupation covered by on ... ʻe may be assigned to a "company fund" (*Betrie* ... .s were originated by industrial employers in the ... ʻred by an occupational fund or by a compai ... ʒned to a local fund (*Ortskrankenkasse*). Finally, ...ınd later blue-collar workers as well—were allowed ... ʻ covered by one of the "substitute" or *Ersatz* funds; these ori ... .ıs private insurance firms but have been made a part of the statutory health insurance system. Coverage for members of workers' families follows that of the breadwinner—and retired or unemployed workers retain membership in their sickness fund. As of January 1997, assignment to specific funds is no longer mandatory, and the funds can now compete for enrollment among all the working population.

Even though the official policy has stressed solidarity, social and occupational groups have not been treated equally by national policy. Social and occupational status determined whether workers were mandatorily insured in a specific sickness fund or, as in the case of white-collar workers and those with higher incomes, had the right to choose their insurance carrier or opt out of statutory health insurance.

In 1993, a total of 1,221 sickness funds existed in Germany. Forty-one percent of those enrolled in statutory health insurance belonged to the 269 local sickness funds (*Ortskrankenkassen*), 29% belonged to one of the 15 *Ersatz* funds, and 11% belonged to the 673 company-based funds. The remainder were enrolled in one of the occupational funds.

There has been a trend toward consolidation of the many small funds; thus, in West Germany, their numbers declined from 1,815 in 1970 to 960 in 1995 (Bundesministerium für Gesundheit, 1995, p. 280). Since that time, consolidation has progressed even faster.

Statutory health insurance continues to cover all medical and hospital bills. For inpatient care, patients paid a modest copayment of DM 10 per day for the first 14 days of hospitalization until January 1, 1993, when payment increased to DM 11 and then, in January 1997, to DM 12 per day in West Germany.[9] Copayments are also required for dental bills, eyeglasses, prescription drugs, and a variety of other services. Copayments for prescription drugs were introduced for the first time in 1982 (except for a short period in 1931-1932) and were increased in 1983, 1984, 1989, 1993, and 1997.[10] By international standards, these copayments are modest and until recently have not been a major tool for cost containment. Because balance billing and extra billing are not allowed, most patients do not pay for doctors' bills. Despite rising copayments, medical services remain almost free at the point of service delivery (Alber, 1992a; Knox, 1993; Schneider, 1991, 1995; Statistisches Bundesamt, 1992; see also Chapter 5 of this volume). This cannot be said about dental services.

Portability of coverage and eligibility for benefits is secured throughout the country and across all types of delivery sites. This has been independent of any regional or local reinterpretations by state or city politicians or by providers, insurance companies, or employers.

Registration at doctors' offices, hospitals, and specialized facilities takes only a few minutes, and individuals are then able to receive medical attention without delay. In 1993, a "smart card" replaced a voucher system that had served as identification and membership card for 100 years. It is a genuine passport to care practically everywhere, and no one can refuse a person in need of care without risking violating the law or the code of medical ethics. Universal coverage for comprehensive benefits is honored by any receiving doctor's or dentist's office or hospital.[11]

Human relations problems have occasionally led to gaps between entitlement and actual practice. A physician may have refused to treat a patient because of a personality clash or because a patient did not have the required "smart card" (or authorized form issued by the municipal offices for those on social aid). In such cases, a physician would not be reimbursed by the physicians' association. By the same token, patients may complain because they dislike a physician or because he or she refuses to prescribe medical treatment, sick leave, or prescription drugs that are considered medically unnecessary but that the patient views as an entitlement. These problem situations are increasing and are likely to affect doctor-patient relations adversely.

For some time, a system has been in place for the pooling of risks between the various sickness funds. An equalization mechanism for contribution rates across the general sickness funds assists those funds with a disproportionate number of high-risk groups, particularly elderly and chronically sick individuals. Therefore, Germany has not needed to pass additional need-oriented policy measures for such social groups as the unemployed, the poor or disabled, single mothers, children, or the elderly. It has thus avoided the inevitable expense and bureaucracy of administering separate programs to meet the needs of such needy groups. Supplemental tax funds are made available for the costs of maternity leave and allowances to the disabled. Even these funds have been pooled with public insurance funds. At the fund level, 95% of revenues comes from employer-employee contributions. When a fund cannot break even, it is faced with a choice: either restrict benefits or raise premiums. In theory, general sickness funds have been strong advocates of cost containment. In practice, however, the employer-employee-controlled boards have been willing to set higher premiums to compete with the substitute funds and private health insurers for higher-income groups by offering more comprehensive services than those mandated by federal law.[12] Because premiums are computed as a percentage of wages and salaries, funds that are successful in recruiting higher-income Germans and foreign residents are able to increase their revenues substantially.

By 1992, because of local decision making on contribution rates below a nationally set income ceiling, sickness fund premiums varied widely— from a low of about 6.5% to a high of about 14.5%. The Structural Reform Act corrected this inequity, mandating that contribution rates be equalized across all sickness funds, with adjustment for risk factors such as age, gender, and health risks.

For more than a century, the Germans have overemphasized statutory health insurance and curative medicine while underemphasizing health promotion and prevention.[13] Though proud of their health care delivery and insurance system, they have neglected social services, nursing, care for the chronically ill, and home care.[14] Deficits in long-term care and nursing services are hardly attributable to corporatist arrangements. Rather, they result from limited consumer power and from the low value placed on nursing care. Unequal power relationships in highly decentralized decision-making situations and difficulties in relationships between levels of government and between state-based and church-related institutions may also have contributed to this situation (Alber, 1995, pp. 136-141). This interpretation leaves out one important ingredient, however. Caregivers in Germany are for the most part women. Despite the recent political success of the advocates of statutory nursing insurance (enacted in 1995), nursing care remains gendered and often is discriminated against.

Medical Sectors

In Germany, the delivery of health services depends on a mix of providers ranging from single (medical and dental) entrepreneurs paid on a fee-for-service basis to large hospitals with salaried medical staffs. The supply of physicians in Germany is high: In 1988, West Germany had 2.9 physicians per 1,000 population (above the OECD average of 2.3). There were considerable regional variations; the most overdoctored regions are Hesse and Bavaria. With 11.5 physician contacts per year, Germans (and also Italians) visited their physicians more frequently than did other Europeans and about twice as frequently as did Americans. Nonetheless, physician expenditures per capita amounted to less than half ($193) of those in the United States ($414) (Schieber et al., 1991, p. 31).[15]

The ownership of hospitals in the former West Germany is the outcome of historical development and regional traditions rather than of conscious policy. There are three types of hospitals: public, nonprofit, and for-profit. In 1989, there were 1,046 public sector hospitals owned by the *Länder* or by local governments. They provided about 50% of all acute hospital beds. Nonprofit or community hospitals are typically run by religious orders affiliated with the Catholic or Protestant churches; these hospitals provided about 35% and for-profit hospitals about 15% of all acute beds. Whereas there were a total of 3,119 public and nonprofit hospitals in

1989, this number declined to about 2,354 in 1993; over the same period, the number of private for-profit hospitals has risen (Bundesministerium für Gesundheit, 1993, pp. 254-255, and 1995, p. 224). The pattern of ownership of special and long-term facilities varies from that of the acute care hospital sector, with for-profit institutions playing an increasingly more significant role.

By international standards, the ratio of hospital beds to population is high: 10.9 inpatient beds per 1,000 persons in former West Germany in 1988. The number of inpatient days per person per year was 3.5 in Germany compared to the OECD average of 2.8. The number of admissions as a percentage of the total German population was 21.5, significantly above the OECD average of 16.1. The average length of stay was 16.6 days—below the OECD average but more than double the American level. By international standards, the inpatient occupancy rate of 86.5% is fairly high (Beratungsstelle für Angewandte Systemforschung [BASYS], 1992a, 1992b; Schieber et al., 1992, p. 27). Since 1993, the length of stay has declined further, and ambulatory surgery is growing in importance, even though many legal and fiscal obstacles exist. For example, in 1996 in Bavaria, physicians performing outpatient surgery were refused appropriate reimbursement: A fee of DM 15 for an appendectomy is clearly inadequate!

Statutory health insurance provides the basic framework for ambulatory and hospital care. In former West Germany, these two sectors were never placed under one organizational umbrella controlled by the state. This separation of office and hospital medicine produced inefficiencies, duplications of tests and procedures, waste, and extra costs. The Health Care Reform Act of 1989 gave a clear political mandate to the respective *Land* associations of sickness funds, physicians, and hospitals to negotiate new public contracts that would better integrate office and hospital care. Because interfacing the two care sectors required coordinating investment, progress entailed negotiations with the *Länder*, which control capital expenditures for hospitals. The Health Care Structural Reform Act of 1993 therefore required the regional bargaining and negotiating associations of doctors, hospitals, and sickness funds and the responsible *Land* agencies to do what they had failed to do voluntarily. Progress in interfacing the office sector and the hospital sector depends on many factors. There is some evidence to suggest the existence of considerable variations in coordination efforts and actual cooperation across the care sectors and between them and *Land* agencies. Though legal hurdles have been eliminated, 4 years after the passage of the Structural Reform Act, the rules for implementing all its objectives in the 16 *Länder* are not yet even established. Likewise, important mandates of the 1989 Health Care Reform Act are not yet in place.

The East German Health Care System Before and After Unification

Health care delivery in the East was very different from that prevailing in the West (Freudenstein & Borgwardt, 1992; Light & Schuller, 1986; see also Chapter 6 of this volume). Delivery was hierarchically organized and centrally planned, with community-based or worksite-based health centers and dispensaries forming the basis of the delivery system. Health centers served between 20,000 and 50,000 people, depending on whether their location was urban or rural. Organizationally, health centers could be autonomous, affiliated with a hospital (when they were called *polyclinics*), or part of an enterprise. Health center staff included a team of general practitioners and a limited number of specialists. Dispensaries were smaller organizational units that operated primarily in rural areas; they typically had two physicians and a dentist on the staff. Like health centers, they could work independently, in close cooperation with a hospital, or in connection with a worksite. Doctors' and dentists' offices had been nationalized in 1956. In 1989, only 314 private doctors' and 447 dentists' offices existed along with socialized doctors' offices; these private offices provided 12.5% of all ambulatory care.[16]

The East German delivery system relied on district nurses, each of whom served about 1,000 to 1,500 people in rural areas and up to 8,000 individuals in urban areas. They were affiliated with the health centers or dispensaries. In 1989, over 5,585 nurse stations existed, including 124 church-related nursing care centers and 180 cancer treatment centers. Occupational health services were more important in the East than in the West. The former East Germany ran 1,967 worksite medical centers and 1,295 worksite nursing centers. Patients could choose their doctors by consulting them either at the worksite or at health centers.

Unlike the West, the East invested considerable resources in child-centered programs. This was related to the fact that 73% of women in the East were employed full time. Knox (1993, p. 245) described an elaborate system of financial incentives for childbearing. These included liberal paid maternity leaves, infant day care programs at the worksite, maternal and child health initiatives with financial inducements to encourage participation, school health programs, and child care accommodations for working mothers and their children. In 1976, these child care services reached more than 50% of children under 3 and 87% of children aged 3 to 6.

Although the two delivery systems differed considerably, they tended to allocate similar proportions of their resources to various categories of care. For example, West Germany allocated 17% and East Germany 12% to physician services. Hospital care consumed 34% in the West and 37% in the East. Hospitals in West Germany had higher staffing ratios, more staff, and more equipment. They also invested more in dental care (12%) than East Germany (6%) and more in medical aids (7% compared to 3% in the East). These data mirror differences in basic health care structures, price levels, and demands for health services, all of which were higher in the West than in the East (BASYS, 1992a). The departure from East Germany of about 1,800 physicians and dentists and about 5,000 nurses and other health workers after unification affected the hospital sector more than the office sector.

Hospital services in the former German Democratic Republic were the outcome of deliberate policy and ideological decisions. The framework hospital regulation of November 14, 1979, which served as the legal framework, linked hospital care organizationally with the ambulatory health centers and dispensaries. Planning for hospitals was entirely centralized, with the districts having no planning functions. The Communist Party decided on hospital policy and on the allocation of resources, whereas the Ministry for Health outlined the details of their mandates and the hospital doctors had to carry them out.

Before unification, 462 of the 539 hospitals were state run, 75 hospitals were operated by denominational groups, and 2 were private. State-run hospitals provided 93% of all beds. As the State Treaty of May 18, 1990, indicated, hospital care in unified Germany was to follow the Western model and adopt a similar mix of hospital sponsors (Bundesministerium für Gesundheit, 1993, p. 254; Stern & Schmidt-Bleibtreu, 1990). Since 1990, although the number of public hospitals in the East has been reduced to 341, they still provide about 93% of all inpatient care, and the 75 community hospitals and the 2 private hospitals provide the remaining inpatient care.

Barely 6 months after the events of November 1989, the political leaders of the two Germanies agreed that the West German approach to social union, employment, and the economy would be applied to newly unified Germany. This meant the emulation of the West German model of statutory health insurance as well as the fairly complex and heterogeneous organizational and financial arrangements that existed there

(Basic Law, Articles 17 through 25). The acceptance of this social model followed logically from the desire to make a transition to a free and social market economy. However, theoretically delivery of health and social services in East Germany did not necessitate that the old and the new *Länder* adopt identical structures and methods. Yet with extraordinary speed, and with practically no public debate, the two teams of civil servants from the relevant ministries prepared the State Treaty on Currency, Economic and Social Union and the common protocol that provided the policy and institutional framework to be adopted in the East (Stern & Schmidt-Bleibtreu, 1990). Many sector-specific provisions were phased in over the following years. Thus, a plethora of interim, transitional, and special provisions provided the basis for the administration of social and health care services in East Germany (Manow-Borgwardt, 1994; Stern & Schmidt-Bleibtreu, 1990).

Paradoxically, while they were being imposed on the East, fee-for-service medicine and the rigid separation of inpatient and outpatient care—distinctive features of the West German system—were coming under attack there. It was claimed that the West German system was too expensive, wasteful, inefficient, and duplicative of diagnostic and therapeutic services and that it was patient-unfriendly because of lack of continuity of care (Advisory Council, 1994; Akademie, 1987; Arnold, 1991; Arnold & Schirmer, 1990; Federal Ministry for Health, 1994; Sachverständigenrat, 1991, 1992, 1994, 1995; Stone, 1991; Thiele, 1990).

History tends to repeat itself, in particular when the balance of power tends to favor the stakeholders in the status quo. The situation between 1989 and 1991 is reminiscent of the period of 1945 and 1947 in the former West Germany, when the Allies allowed the health insurance program to be restored despite their own preferences (see Hockerts, 1981; Kirchberger, 1986; Leibfried & Tennstedt, 1986; Rosenberg, 1986). Whereas reconstruction was a primary goal in 1947, a wholesale transfer of institutions, rules, and procedures from West to East Germany was the goal in 1990. There was neither the time nor the political will to assess which norms, structures and practices should be retained and which should be abandoned. Though proposals for retaining elements of the East German system were presented by East German politicians and even accepted by the federal Ministry of Labor and Social Affairs (Robischon, Strucke, Wasem, & Wolf, 1994, pp. 23-29), West German stakeholders torpedoed their political acceptance in the East. The West German medical lobby, as well as the sickness funds and substitute funds, turned out to be powerful forces. Thus, the conflicts characteristic of the rivalry between the various sickness funds in West Germany reproduced themselves during the period of transition. (For details, see Manow-Borgwardt, 1993, 1994; Robischon et al., 1994; Wasem, 1992, 1993, 1997.) From a legal, regulatory, and administrative perspective, the integration of two health care systems under the umbrella of statutory health insurance was more or less complete by late 1992.

The State Treaty required a complete overhaul of a community-based and worksite-based health care system, described by Niehoff, Schneider, and Wetzstein (1992) as having been chronically "underfinanced, over-centralised and over-controlled" (p. 209). In addition, the complex contractual methods for negotiating prices and fees in the office sector were also introduced in the eastern part of Germany. In assessing the attempt to combine the two systems, Niehoff et al. commented:

> We have lost advantages and disadvantages. We got new advantages and new disadvantages. At least for the next few years we will find tendencies of having unified the disadvantages of the former GDR with the disadvantages of the FRG—certainly not for all the people in east Germany but possibly for at least a third of the population. (p. 213)

On January 1, 1991, statutory health insurance began to operate in the Eastern states.[17] Expenditures for the health care of East Germans were covered by different funding sources. To cushion the transition, the Structural Reform Act of 1993 made full allowance for the existence of differences in living costs and prices between the old and the new *Länder*. Whereas in the West commercial insurance was always limited to no more than 10% of the market, in the East it was elected by only about 0.5% of the population (BASYS, 1992a).

West German state hospital laws and federal regulations became effective in the East in several steps on January 1, 1991; after a transition period until January 1, 1994, the new *Länder* had to develop regional hospital plans to qualify for tax funding for hospital investment. Hospitals were to be brought up to the standard of those in the West.

To everyone's surprise, East German physicians made the transition to fee-for-service medicine more rapidly than expected and abandoned their employed positions in polyclinics and other health facilities, even though the conversion factor in the fee schedule for East German physicians was 45% less than it was in West Germany (Schneider, 1995, p. 80; Wasem, 1992, 1993). After July 1, 1991, employed East German physicians received only 60% or even less than the salaries of West German physicians. By 1991, 80% of all polyclinic-based physicians had become office-based physicians, and by 1993, only 5% were still employed by polyclinics.

Federal Health Policy Making and Implementation

The Basic Law of 1949 assigned the federal government exclusive authority for public health insurance matters and for setting broad policy in relation to benefits, eligibility, compulsory membership, covered risks, income maintenance during temporary illness, and employer-employee contributions to statutory insurance. Because the federal government has no authority over the hospital sector but is responsible for all matters pertaining to health insurance, the federal government and the *Länder* share authority. They jointly must set policy, including regulations on hospital rate setting and reimbursement to hospitals for inpatient care (Altenstetter, 1986b).[18] Federal regulations on internal hospital accounting were also strengthened and became law on January 1, 1993. Do such regulations represent an improvement over the previous accounting and management arrangements? The future will tell.

The federal government has the power to set policy but has none to implement policy. These powers are delegated by law to the sickness fund associations; to national associations of physicians, dentists, pharmacists, and nurses; and to the *Land*-based hospital associations. Together, federal provisions and rules (which cannot be passed without the consent of the *Länder,* as expressed in the *Bundesrat,* the upper house of parliament) provide a fairly prescriptive and all-inclusive set of mandates applicable to all stakeholders in the delivery system (Aichberger, 1994; Wasem, 1994).

Thus, an important characteristic of health policy making and implementation in Germany is the set of corporatist, intermediate arrangements that exist at national and regional levels (Gäfgen, 1988). The Federal Association of Sickness Funds and the Federal Association of Sickness Fund Physicians negotiate umbrella agreements based on federal guidelines for the delivery of medical care. These include fee schedules and relative value scales for close to 2,000 different medical procedures in a fee-for-service system. These schedules were overhauled in July 1996 and will be reviewed again in 1997.[19] Details have always been worked out by a little-known federal committee representing sickness fund physicians and the sickness funds. This committee has always made crucial decisions on health care behind closed doors.[20] In the final analysis, it agrees or disagrees with the political mandates for health care reform and cost containment coming from the Ministry of Health (and, before 1991, from the Ministry of Labor and Social Affairs).

The committee continues to set spending limits through a global budget that is now linked to the revenue base of the sickness funds. It decides on volume of services, quality criteria, and prices of office-based services. It determines the inclusion of new reimbursable medical procedures and preventive services (e.g., cancer screening and early screening of children) under statutory health insurance. It also develops guidelines for the diffusion and joint use of sophisticated medical technology and equipment in both office and hospital care sectors as well as for ambulance services, prenatal and postnatal care, hearing aids, and rehabilitation services. Some guidelines have the force of law, whereas others have not. Whether mandatory or voluntary, these guidelines are classic tools of procedural and substantive self-regulation within the context of broad federal legislation (Döhler, 1993; Döhler & Manow-Borgwardt, 1991, 1992; for a summary, see Aichberger, 1994; Bundesministerium für Arbeit und Sozialordnung, 1995).

Other important federal bipartite committees of sickness fund and provider representatives are the admission committee on access to medical practice within the framework of statutory health insurance and the evaluation committee, composed of seven representatives of sickness fund physicians and the funds. These all-payer negotiating and bargaining structures are allowed under German law (as in other continental European countries) but would be prohibited by current American antitrust laws.

The Advisory Council for Concerted Action in Health Care is another extra-parliamentary body playing an important role in health policy development since 1977. Chaired by the federal Ministry of Health after 1990, its 60 members have represented the most important parties with a stake in health care (Gäfgen, 1988; Henke, 1988).[21] Table 4.2 identifies the major stakeholders who traditionally were participants in debates about health care reform. However, in recent debates about the "third phase" of structural health care reform, this 60-member body has played a largely symbolic role while the Minister of Health has increasingly charged an eight-member expert committee with specific fact-finding missions and used the council's proposals as a testing ground for future legislation (Busse & Schwartz, in press).

At the state level, *Land* associations of sickness funds and of sickness fund physicians negotiate specific contracts, including those for reimbursement of all physicians in a region, and they enforce reference

TABLE 4.2. Core Members of Concerted Action in Health Care

Insurance Funds
1. Federal Association of the Local Sickness Funds
2. Federal Association of the Company-Based Sickness Funds
3. Federal Association of the Crafts' Sickness Funds
4. Federal Association of the Agricultural Sickness Funds
5. Miners' Sickness Fund
6. Sailors' Sickness Fund
7. Association of White-Collar Sickness Funds
8. Association of Blue-Collar Sickness Funds
9. Association of Private Insurance Companies

Doctors and Dentists
10. Federal Association of Physicians
11. Federal Association of Dentists
12. Federal Medical Chamber
13. Federal Dental Chamber

Hospitals
14. German Hospital Association

Pharmaceutical Sector
15. Federal Association of German Pharmacists
16. Federal Association of the German Pharmaceutical Industry

Trade Unions and Employer Organizations
17. German Trade Union Association
18. German White-Collar Trade Union
19. German Civil Servant Association
20. Federal Association of German Employers

Government
21. Federal Association of Municipalities
22. Land Ministries for Labor and Social Affairs
23. Federal Ministry for Economic Affairs
24. Federal Ministry of Health

SOURCE: Hoffmeyer (1994, p. 470).
NOTE: The council also includes nurses' representation. However, care representatives have typically been perceived as not having a financial stake in the most important agenda items ever since the council was set up.

standards for prescription drugs as well as procedures for economic monitoring of physicians.[22] In the past, the terms of regionally negotiated contracts were binding on all office-based physicians, dentists, and sickness funds on the same basis (Aichberger, 1994). However, over the last 20 years, ever stricter government-sponsored price controls have been imposed on all office-based providers and on a small number of employed hospital doctors who, unlike the majority, have been licensed to treat and bill outpatients.

These intermediate corporatist structures have been strengthened and their powers extended. Starting with the Health Insurance Cost Containment Act of 1977 and subsequent federal legislation, their roles and operational responsibilities have also been streamlined and standardized. Even arbitration continues to be handled by the respective groups rather than by the state.

Outside the framework of statutory health insurance are two other professional organizations: the Federal Chamber of Physicians and the Federal Chamber of Dentists. These chambers are responsible for deciding on access to medical and dental practice in general, licensing doctors and dentists, and setting quality standards for medical practice, specialization, and subspecialization. They interpret the code of professional ethics, and they have increasingly come under pressure to address quality assurance and health care technology more vigorously than they have in the past (Behaghel, 1994).

Professional self-policing has played an important role in stabilizing the growth of health expenditures in Germany. Over the last two decades, doctors and dentists have increasingly come under close scrutiny by the bipartite regional committees of doctors or dentists and sickness funds. Excess billing and prescribing practices are easily detected by means of statistical profiles of diagnostic and therapeutic practices; these serve to identify departures of individual practitioners from the group average.

Physicians who opt out of public health insurance and treat only patients with private insurance (a fairly limited number) are remunerated on the basis of another, more generous, federal fee schedule. Unlike the relative value scales under statutory health insurance, specific fees are assigned to about 7,000 items to cover current and future medical procedures. With proper justification for the need of procedures and tests, these physicians can charge up to 3.5 times the amount stipulated in the fee schedule. However, for laboratory services they can only charge 1.8 times the scheduled amount.[23]

Most hospital physicians are employed on a salaried basis and are not allowed to bill patients. A very limited number of senior hospital doctors may bill inpatients covered by private health insurance and those who buy private health insurance in addition to statutory insurance in order to retain their freedom of choice of doctors when hospitalized and to enjoy extra amenities (such as a private room and TV).[24] These doctors are reimbursed according to the more generous private fee schedule described above.

Land hospital associations and *Land* associations of sickness funds negotiate the general standards and conditions for hospital care and agree on criteria and procedures by which to monitor the appropriate and efficient delivery of quality inpatient care. Each hospital negotiates with the local sickness funds a contract for hospital care and the prices for inpatient services. In the early 1970s, hospitals became subject to some external budget controls and to certificate-of-need planning processes. Although the federal government and the *Länder* jointly financed investments and modernization of hospitals between 1972 and 1986, the *Länder* continue to be responsible for hospital capacity planning. After 1986, hospital investment financing again became the sole domain of the *Land* governments.

Hospital expenditures kept rising and in 1993 constituted 34.3% of total statutory health insurance expenditures compared to 17.5% in 1960 (Altenstetter, 1987, p. 512; Pfaff & Wassener, 1995, pp. 52, 55). In the early 1990s, responsible decision makers finally recognized that they could hardly stabilize the growth of health expenditures in the long run unless all care sectors were brought under the umbrella of the annual recommendations of the old-style Advisory Council for Concerted Action in Health Care. However, intentions do not always get translated into practice.

The Role of the *Länder*

Health policy formulation and implementation are conditioned not only by the existence of statutory insurance and its peculiar form of self-government but also by a unique version of federalism. "Vertical" or "cooperative" federalism assigns most policy-making responsibilities of national importance to the federal government and leaves the implementation of national policy to 11 (after 1990, 16) *Land* governments (Gunlicks, 1989, 1994; von Beyme & Schmidt, 1985).

To secure the political and administrative support of the *Länder* for national policy, the constitution assigns them an important role unknown in other federally organized systems. They effectively participate in the national legislative process through representation in the *Bundesrat,* the second chamber of Germany's parliament, and thus have strong veto powers over national policy. Although the *Länder* have no authority over health insurance matters, their veto powers are nevertheless very strong. Thus, between 1949 and 1992 no federal health legislation or regulation that touched on the vital interests of the *Länder* passed without undergoing substantial redrafting in the *Bundesrat.* The federal-*Land* coalition supporting the Health Care Structural Reform Act broke this established pattern of interest group domination for a brief time, but this fragile coalition between the federal government and the 16 *Länder* has already fallen apart. This enormous power of *Land* governments has been described by Scharpf and colleagues as a "cartel of the *Länder*" (Scharpf, Reissert, & Schnabel, 1976, p. 241). A "decision trap" inherent in German federalism (Scharpf, 1985) necessitates multilevel negotiations and makes for decisions reached at the lowest common denominator. These constitutional barriers to reform continue to be significant (Rosewitz & Webber, 1990).

Hospital laws of the *Länder* rather than federal law govern the hospital sector. The *Länder* own and partially finance medical school hospitals and teaching hospitals. They enforce accreditation and licensing of health facilities, as well as the qualification of health professions and of staff working in social services. Most important, they are responsible for the allocation and distribution of medical resources and capacities through hospital need planning. Finally, the *Länder* are responsible for policy development and implementation for social and nursing services. *Land* control over hospitals implies considerable regional variations in policy outcomes in response to federal guidelines.

For hospitals, the Health Care Structural Reform Act of 1993 introduced aggregate spending targets and spending caps in line with the revenue base of statutory insurance for the period of 1993 through 1995. They were to be lifted by January 1, 1996, when the new system of hospital rates came into effect. Trial aggregate spending targets were set for each hospital by the representatives of hospitals and sickness funds.[25] Moreover, more stringent capital spending controls were imposed on hospital construction and purchase of medical equipment. The 1993 act abolished the entitlement of hospitals to full payment of costs while retaining the principle of "dual financing," by which investments are tax financed by the *Länder* and inpatient care is financed by statutory and private insurance.[26]

This new regulation introduced a more complex method of reimbursing hospitals. Since 1994, instead of three broad categories of hospital retrospective per diem rates, reimbursement has been based on a mix of these old, retrospective per diem rates and prospective cost-per-case payments negotiated locally for each hospital. This reimbursement formula includes (a) diagnosis-related groups (DRGs) that cover the full treatment of a case (with the possibility of an extra payment if a patient is hospitalized for an unusual length of time for medical reasons)—to date, there are 40 DRGs; (b) special payments for surgery and treatments before and after surgery—to date there are 104 different special or cost-by-case payments; (c) departmental per diem allowances that reimburse the hospital for all nursing and medical procedures; and (d) a basic per diem allowance for all nonmedical procedures and accommodations. According to close observers of hospital policy,

> It is too early to tell how new arrangements in the hospital sector, both already introduced (e.g, prospective payments which are set by the federal Ministry of Health) and planned (e.g., state-wide budgets for hospitals) will influence not only the quantity and quality of the services but also the clinical freedom of the physicians. (Busse & Schwartz, in press)[27]

The reform of hospital rate setting aimed to contain rising hospital costs. This increase was thought to be related to four root causes: (a) limited information about the flows of services and costs; (b) few incentives for economic management of hospitals; (c) negative incentives because costs were covered retroactively on the basis of length of stay and number of patient cases, rather than efficiency; and (d) lack of continuing care between office and hospital medicine (Pfaff & Wassener, 1995, pp. 11, 36-37).

The Health Care Structural Reform Act has five additional provisions affecting the hospital sector: (a) Hospitals are allowed to receive funds from private sources; (b) chief hospital physicians who have signed contracts for treating private patients after 1993 must, on average, return a third of revenues from this source to the hospital; (c) hospitals are to create new jobs, in particular in nursing care, while adjusting to the new rate structure; (d) patients are to pay increased copayments when hospitalized; and (e) hospital investment programs in the new *Länder* were to be financed through a flat fee of DM 8 per day of hospitalization, to be paid for by statutory or private insurance.

As has happened when previous health insurance reforms were legislated, enabling regulations and ordinances to implement these changes have been delayed for months and even years. Though newly amended rate schedules and related ordinances are available, other regulatory measures necessary for the implementation of hospital reform are still missing. Meanwhile, as a result of administering a diversity of hospital rates, total administrative costs in hospitals have risen (Pfaff & Wassener, 1995).

Further Effects of the Structural Health Care Reform Act

The provisions of the act and those of its "third phase" have not been made in a policy or institutional vaccuum; they build on existing decision-making and implementation structures, a federally organized polity, and a corporatist tradition. The Structural Reform Act has not scrapped statutory health insurance, nor has it eliminated the multipayer approach to financing health care or the portability of entitlements. The basic framework for policy making and organization of the delivery system remains in place. So do all the ground rules and primary and secondary rules in that no single actor or group can change them single-handedly without the support of a legitimate majority. Even Health Minister Seehofer needs political allies to add new rules to an already complex set of regulations and to translate new policy language into results.

Unlike previous reforms, however, the Health Care Structural Reform Act has not only reproduced the organizational and regulatory status quo but also launched substantial restructuring. This has been the result of implementing regional budgets for hospitals and ambulatory care in 23 regions, the reorganization of sickness funds, and the reform of the hospital sector within the context of established regulatory regimes.

According to Schulenburg (1996), Germany is moving either toward a

> tax-financed national health service under total control of the government, or to a competitive health insurance scheme with multiple choice for the insured, freedom of pricing for everyone and selective contracting between the sickness funds and suppliers of health services. Recent experience shows that it is impossible to provide high quality medical care efficiently at stable cost in a mixed system; that budgets, price regulations and governmental interventions are easier to impose than to remove; and that interventions induce the need for further interventions. This has proved even more the case during the difficult economic times since Germany's reunification in 1990. (n.p.)

Besides increased state intervention, what other key issues are raised by the Structural Reform Act of 1993 and were not addressed previously? Four developments deserve attention: (a) the organizational reform of sickness funds, (b) social or "soft" rationing, (c) regional budgets for paying physicians, and (d) new contractual relations between providers and sickness funds.

Organizational Reform of Sickness Funds

Reorganization of statutory health insurance produced immediate effects. The act stipulated free choice of sickness funds by consumers, mandated open enrollment for substitute funds, and made open enrollment optional for company funds. In anticipation of January 1, 1997, the date when the new provision on free choice of insurance carrier was to come into effect, preparations to facilitate increased competition were underway in statutory public and private health insurance circles. Freedom of choice of sickness funds indeed appears to end a 100-year tradition in which membership was stratified along age, social, and occupational lines. However, it is possible that a new stratification by income will result, which may create worse disparities among Germans than have the old patterns of stratification.

Sickness funds now compete with other insurance carriers for new members by offering highly variable service packages, some aspects of which are summarized in Table 4.3. Such competition has led the press to label funds as "regular funds," "superfunds," "sensational funds," and/or "five-star funds." ("Wer hat das bessere Angebot?" 1996).

The act was intended to strengthen the purchasing power of payers through organizational consolidation. The number of general sickness funds decreased from 269 in January 1993 to 94 in April 1994. Consolidation proceeded at such a speed that by April 1995 a single *Land*-wide fund existed in all regions except for Bavaria and Lower Saxony, which kept their systems of 39 and 35 individual sickness funds; Saxony, which retained 3; and Saxony-Anhalt, which retained 2 (National Economic Research Associates [NERA], 1995, pp. 123-124).

Concomitant with this reorganization of the sickness funds was the extension of a risk adjustment mechanism that had been operational in general sickness funds before 1993. Now risk adjustment mechanisms have been extended to cover all types of public insurance carriers. The objective is to equalize the widely differing contribution rates to the funds. These new mechanisms were put in place for all contributors to statutory insurance as of January 1994 and for pensioners as of January 1, 1995. Did they achieve their intended goal? According to NERA, the answer is yes and no. Differentials in contribution rates continue to exist, though at a somewhat reduced level. Why? Not all variables factored into the German risk adjustment mechanism are direct measures of risk. Others include age, gender, number of dependents (who are automatically insured), and income levels.

> Regional variations in health care costs are not adjusted. Income levels, or more precisely, *income levels for which members of the statutory health insurance funds have to pay insurance premiums,* add a degree of complexity to the system which is absent in other countries that operate a risk-adjustment mechanism and which do not adjust for income levels. The old German health care system not only encouraged selection by health risk, but also by income levels. (NERA, 1995, p. 127)

TABLE 4.3. Recent Competitive Strategies of Sickness Funds: New Benefits Offered

Optional Benefits	*Range of Discretionary Decisions*
Preventive care for mothers	Payment in full or partial subsidy
Vaccinations (except for trips abroad)	Payment in full, a fixed subsidy, or no subsidy at all
Home nursing care	Basic nursing care and household help (including preparation of meals) paid by the fund, which determines the duration of benefits
Household help	Payment in full; duration highly variable
Transportation	Payment in full, a fixed subsidy, or no subsidy at all
Kuren (spas) and rehabilitation	Payment in full, a fixed subsidy, or no subsidy at all
Medical services while abroad and not otherwise covered	Fund may pay for special needs (e.g., a child's heart surgery)
Indemnity reimbursement by fund rather than direct service benefit (*Sachleistungen*)	Bills must be paid in full by patients and are then reimbursed by the fund
Deductibles and reduced contribution rates	Patients who do not see a physician during a certain time period will receive refunds worth several months' contributions (variable)
Medical aid, massages	Full payment, a fixed fee, or no subsidy at all
Trial prices (e.g., for alternative medicine, holistic medicine)	Fund can decide to pay for unconventional procedures and therapies
Contribution rates	Trial-phase rules may apply, or contribution rates are returned if patient has sparingly used medical services

SOURCE: "Wer hat das bessere Angebot?" (1996, p. 319).

As a result of the new risk adjustment system, some Germans find their contribution rates rising while others find them decreasing.

NERA (1995) suggested that four issues remain on the agenda for future decisions concerning risk adjustment: the inclusion of additional risk factors, whether pensioners should receive different treatment under statutory insurance, the need for more transparency, and the effects of a fixed adjustment process on competition. Moreover, it cited some obstacles to further progress:

The German health care system is riddled with regulations which prohibit sickness funds from concluding individual rather than the collective contracts they are compelled to support. Similarly, regulations at present do not encourage the establishment of new, and possibly more cost-effective provider models, such as Health Maintenance Organisations. (p. 145)

This assessment says much about the effects of the coexistence of a strong regulatory state and corporatist, self-regulatory traditions.

Social or "Soft" Rationing

According to the Advisory Council for Concerted Action (1996), the third-phase reforms will lead to additional "soft rationing," which involves shedding or transferring of non-illness-related services out of statutory insurance; differentiation between a basic mandatory benefit package and optional benefits; choice of adding or dropping additional benefits; and use of clinical guidelines (health care technology assessment) as a basis for further restructuring the current fee-for-service reimbursement scheme.

Regional Budgets

By far the most far-reaching effects have been generated by the introduction of regional budgets linked to the revenue base of statutory health insurance for reimbursing hospitals and providers of ambulatory care. Between 1993 and 1997, regional budgets for office medicine were subdivided into separate budgets for medical services, prescription drugs, and medical aids and patient support devices; there have been also smaller budgets for early screening and treatment. Over a 15-year period, the worth of relative value points declined from 12.7 Pfennig to 6.45 Pfennig (in the first quarter of 1996). This decline led to waves of protests that erupted in the summer and fall of 1996 and may lead to a total revamping of the fee schedule. Meanwhile, the serious press in Germany reported that patients experience situations in which they are informed that the physician has reached the ceiling of total points assigned to each specialty group and will therefore not be reimbursed for any additional services. If patients are willing to pay out of pocket, they may receive services or prescription drugs that were always covered in the past.

In the hospital sector, administrative costs have risen, and hospital rate setting has become highly conflictual. Litigation and conflict resolution by arbitration have increased. Before 1993, arbitration was necessary in about 100 cases per year in the old Länder. By 1996, there were about 330 cases, affecting almost 10% of the total number of hospitals in Germany ("Schiedsstellenverfähren im Bundesgebiet," 1996).

The Second Statutory Health Insurance Act, which was adopted in March 1997, did away with regional budgets for physician care and pharmaceuticals. An era, lasting from 1977 to 1997, in which the burden for cost containment was placed on the providers of care while primarily shielding patients from excessive cost sharing, has come to an end. Copayments seem to have become politically acceptable instruments of cost containment (Busse & Howorth, in press).

Selective Contracting

Whereas other aspects of the third-phase reforms were quickly put in place, there has been a slow take-off of new individual and selective contracts complementing the existing collective federal and regional contractual arrangements. Thus, although these new contracts are theoretically important for restructuring the system, it is not yet possible to assess their effects.

Conclusion

In evaluating the impact of the Structural Reform Act, we need to distinguish between words and achievements. A need for cost controls arising from ever-rising health expenditures and the high costs of German unification prompted the adoption of the act. As well as controlling costs, it sought to develop a better interface between hospital and ambulatory care sectors and to use new contracts constructively in opening up old monopolies of power. Rhetoric about competition and management has been abundant in health policy discourse since 1993. It has been complemented by a neoliberal market orientation, which, with increasing global pressures, has found favor in many political circles in Germany. Though some analysts have jumped to the conclusion that Germany indeed has a health care system that operates on the basis of competition, other observers, including myself, feel that it is too early to assess the record of the Structural Reform Act. A primary reason is the short time span since its passage. Another reason is that analyses of the interaction between central instructions and local adaptations (in which regional and local actors bring their own rationale to the negotiating table) are a prerequisite for an assessment of the effects of the act. Yet empirical analyses of local delivery conditions and of health policy processes are missing.

Four key questions arise for the future. Will Germans be as satisfied with their health care system as they have been in the past? Will they be better served by market-based competition than by the historic policy based on a national consensus about solidarity and cooperation? Will market making replace the "public-political" (Streeck, 1995, p. 27) and corporatist institutional arrangements that are the subject of this chapter? Finally, will the health care system remain as cost-effective by international standards as it has been in the past? The jury is still out.

Unlike the political regime, which has collapsed several times in this century, the three core values of solidarity, subsidiarity, and functional representation continue to undergird the German health care system, even though new policy values—competition, individual freedom, and rights to contract freely—are now competing with them. By international standards, the German system is equitable. Germans are not unduly suffering from cost containment, despite increasing cost sharing. The retention of generous benefits in the basic service package may possibly work against the rise of a new three-class system consisting of (a) those who can afford only the basic package of benefits; (b) poor retirees, unemployed, recipients of social aid, and voluntary members of general sickness funds who are exempt from rising copayments; and (c) higher-income and educated groups who can afford extra coverage.

Corporatist power-sharing arrangements among the major stakeholders of payers and providers, with the balance of power shifting according to circumstances, have been characteristic of the German system. Corporate groups also shared responsibility and accountability for collective federal and regional contracts. Though theoretically the new forms of contracting are meant to unfreeze the monopoly of power of current stakeholders, in practice, if implemented on a large scale they will tend to diffuse responsibility and thus reduce accountability.

To balance centralizing and centrifugal forces and to meet the diverse needs of the state, of a differentiated and complex society, and of the rights of individuals, corporatist negotiations have been considered essential. During most of this 100-year history, the medical profession was given the responsibility for defining the state of the medical art that should be covered by statutory insurance. Yet the politics of the stakeholders has dynamically changed, and bitter conflicts have threatened the historic pattern of corporatist cooperation. The strength of the German approach in what Schulenburg (1994) called the "miracle of German cost containment policy" (p. 1476) over the last two decades derived from its sector-specific intermediate institutions. Between 1975 and 1993, they did reasonably well in sustaining cost containment efforts and stabilizing, controlling, and monitoring health spending. Intrusive micromanagement interventions in the practice of medicine and doctor-patient relationships were largely absent in the past.

Cost controls were easier to implement in Germany than in any other of the leading industrial countries between 1970 and 1990, when the two Germanies united. They were effective for at least three reasons. First, all office-based providers were paid by the same fee schedule according to relative value points.[28] Second, most hospital doctors continue to be salaried following a public service schedule (which is cheaper than fee for service). The only exception was a small number of chiefs of departments who charged extra. And third, in the past all holders of public health insurance have enjoyed the same or very similar benefits everywhere in Germany. Most important, cost containment and universal coverage have not been seen as mutually exclusive. With risks pooled under universal health insurance rather than separated into several independent programs for specific population groups, German health policy makers have not needed to agonize over how to integrate separate programs with other elements of the health care system.

Where is the system going? A few observations are fairly clear. Despite the same policy language, symbols, and metaphors and the propagation of globalizing "myths" (Marmor, 1997, pp. 351-354; Stone, 1997, pp. 137-162), the words *competition* and *managed care* do not mean the same thing in Germany as in other countries, such as the United States or Great Britain, "that have historically relied less on public-political and more on private contractual economic governance" (Streeck, 1995, p. 27).

In contrast to the United States, in which there has been a tremendous transfer of power to market-based commercial health care organizations and an information-rich marketplace, no such transfer of power has occurred in Germany. Universal access to services has been maintained, and the responsibility of the *Länder* to secure hospital care has not been repealed, nor have the responsibilities of other corporatist, intermediary bodies. There really is no rapidly evolving marketplace, and full disclosure of information has not been attained, even though it is increasing. Accounting remains nontransparent for most health care organizations, notably in the hospital sector. Whatever competitionlike or managed care-like activities are practiced, they are embedded in Germany's distinct regulatory context, with its unique collective bargaining tradition based on cooperation and strong corporatist representation.

Statutory health insurance, although enriched with competitive elements, remains anchored in a self-regulatory, corporatist middle ground between market and state (White, 1995). The direction of change has been toward more state intervention while emphasizing competition both in rhetoric and action. Until the fiscal constraints of German unification are no longer as strong as they currently are, it will be difficult to tell whether this should be seen as a transitional stage. Meanwhile, cost shifting from public budgets to statutory insurance and in turn to the private purse is indeed a distinct feature of the 1990s.

Finally, old antagonisms between providers and public and private insurance carriers, between family physicians and specialists, and between wholesale and retail pharmacists, although rooted in a conflictual history over 100 years, have escalated to a new level because of the Health Care Structural Reform Act and subsequent legislation and regulations. New divisions are emerging between family doctors and specialists, between hospital- and office-based physicians, between young and old doctors, between the medical profession and pharmacists, and between the pharmaceutical industry and providers of care. A major divide has developed between the leadership and the membership of the regional physicians' associations; this has led to demonstrations and to one-day strikes by some specialty groups. Some physicians are even considering returning their license to practice medicine. Health Minister Seehofer's power, which reached a zenith in 1993, is declining. He is losing political credibility for having sacrificed too much to the rationale of coalition politics and to the pressures of the Free Democratic Party for more competition. Even Chancellor Kohl's initial strong support for his Minister of Health is fading away.

The Health Care Structural Reform Act and decisions of the "third phase" have created many losers and few winners while leaving a myriad of unresolved policy issues. The new government after the federal elections in 1998 will have to resolve them, while possibly facing worse fiscal constraints than does the current government. Because support for universalism in medical care entitlements remains high among the public, it will be necessary to reconcile the high expectations of a "culture of solidarity" with the maintenance of comprehensive medical protection in a competitive health care system. Otherwise, the voters may punish the government in power. On the other hand, seeking to reform statutory health insurance and the practice of medicine while handling the fiscal constraints of unification and coping with fiscal requirements for European economic and monetary union will be a major challenge. Germany may indeed have reached its limits in resources and wealth. However uncertain the future, given demographic and expenditure trends and the move toward European union, the new challenges to the regulatory regimes will necessitate new adaptations within the existing political and institutional order.

Notes

1. A national law on miners in 1923 centralized the administration of social and health insurance programs for all miners. Instead of 110 separate associations, one central agency assumed responsibility for the administration of programs against the risks of disability, old age, and disease.

2. The Oxford English Dictionary, noting that the term has been much used in Catholic social thought, defines *subsidiarity* as "the quality of being subsidiary; specifically the principle that a central authority should have a subsidiary function, performing only those tasks which cannot be performed effectively at a more immediate or local level." It should not be confused with a British notion of the term, which denotes the principle of parliamentary sovereignty.

3. The importance of regional forces has historical roots. The German nation-state, created in 1871—late by comparison with other European nation-states—evolved out of numerous autonomous political units: four kingdoms, five grand duchies, 12 duchies, 12 principalities, and three free cities, each with rich and distinct political, religious, and social traditions. Although they came to be overshadowed by centralizing forces through national party and interest group formation from 1871 onward, many of these pre-1871 regional distinctions survive in the present-day *Länder*.

4. This code (SGB V) is the most important piece of federal legislation since 1911, when the social insurance programs and health insurance (enacted between 1883 and 1889) were integrated into a unified national social insurance code (RVO).

5. Corporatism characterizes the political culture of continental European countries and after the collapse of communism is resurfacing in some central European countries. This form of representation is little practiced in Anglo-Saxon countries but must not be confused with the typical form of lobbying.

6. A distinguishing feature of Roman law is codification, ranging in Germany from the civil code to the social insurance code and many others. In 1949, the Basic Law institutionalized, among other fundamental goals, the goals of a social market economy and a "sozialer Rechtsstaat" (a social state of the rule of law) and reinforced these entitlements and rights (article 20 Abs. 1, article 28 Abs. 1, Satz 1 GG; Zacher, 1985).

7. For a concise description of this system before 1993, see Glaser (1991, pp. 501-506).

8. The ceiling has been increased numerous times. In 1992, it was set at DM 61,200 per year (or DM 43,200 in former East Germany), and in 1995 it was increased to DM 70,200 (or DM 57,600 in the East) (Bundesministerium für Gesundheit, 1995, p. 311; Hoffmeyer, 1994, pp. 438, 495).

9. The copayment was reduced from DM 10 to DM 8 in East Germany.

10. For more details and data on cost-sharing regulations between 1977 and 1997, see Busse and Howorth (1997, pp. 16-18).

11. The same standards, medical and financial alike, apply to rehabilitation, workers' compensation insurance, unemployment, disability, and public assistance at the point of entry

to the delivery system. In contrast, the way in which patients' entitlements are administered is variable.

12. Being outside the statutory health insurance framework, substitute funds and private health insurance have been able to remunerate physicians at a higher rate than have the statutory sickness funds.

13. For recent changes in perceptions of priorities, see Busse and Schwartz (in press).

14. On German satisfaction with health care delivery, see Iglehart (1991). On social and nursing services for the chronically ill and aged, see Alber (1992b), Hollingsworth (1992), and Hollingsworth and Hollingsworth (1992).

15. When East and West German data are compared, East Germany had an even higher physician-per-population ratio (Beratungsstelle für Angewandte Systemforschung [BASYS], 1992a, pp. 23-26, 41).

16. About 70% of all dental services were provided in health centers. The rest were provided in dispensaries and worksite health centers (BASYS, 1992a, pp. 18-23).

17. The general sickness funds set up one locality-based fund with some 200 offices serving the 12 districts. The West German substitute funds opened 501 offices in East Germany, and by March 1991 about 3.76 million East Germans had joined the substitute funds. By mid-1991, about 50 company-based funds had been set up. From January 1, 1991, they were exempt from the fixed 12.5% contribution rate that applied to the sickness funds in the former GDR and could set rates depending on the situation of the company. About 1.3 million East Germans joined them.

18. Such regulations were issued in 1986 and have been issued annually since January 1, 1994.

19. For details and empirical data on the most recent changes, see Busse and Schwartz (in press).

20. Since January 1, 1997, its leadership has been assumed by three retirees who previously held important positions in the Ministry of Labor and Social Affairs, the federal association of sickness funds and the legal division of this bipartite federal committee.

21. Before 1990, the Advisory Council for Concerted Action was chaired by the federal Ministry of Labor and Social Affairs.

22. Public contracts on dental services are negotiated between the federal committees of dentists and sickness funds and at the state level by the *Land* associations of dentists and sickness funds.

23. A similar fee schedule is in place for dentists in private insurance practice.

24. About 8.5% of those covered by statutory insurance also purchase private health insurance.

25. Their role in direct local negotiations over price, volume, and quality of inpatient care was strengthened by the Structural Reform Act.

26. This dual mode of financing was adopted in 1972 and was supported by the same hospital policy community that for the last few years has recommended a shift to "one-pipe" financing (*monistische Finanzierung*) of individual hospitals in order to give payers more influence over financing inpatient care. However, these plans, which were originally addressed in the so-called "Lahnstein compromise" in the summer of 1992, proved highly contentious, and "one-pipe" financing was dropped from the Structural Reform Act.

27. For updates on policy developments and future plans for the hospital sector, see Busse and Schwartz (1997) and Busse and Howorth (in press); for a study of the implementation of the Hospital Financing Law of 1972 in two German regions, see Altenstetter (1985).

28. The importance of the organization of the medical profession in Germany and France in recent health care reforms is discussed by Hassenteufel (1996).

References

Advisory Council for Concerted Action in Health Care. (1994). *Health care and health insurance: Expert opinion report 1994* (abbreviated version). Bonn: Author.

Advisory Council for Concerted Action in Health Care. (1995). *Health care and health insurance 2000: A closer orientation towards results, higher quality services and greater economic efficiency. Summary of the special expert report.* Bonn: Author.

Advisory Council for Concerted Action in Health Care. (1996). *The health care system in Germany: Cost factor and branch of the future: Vol. 1. Demographics, morbidity, efficiency reserves and employment. Special report 1996. Summary.* Bonn: Author.

Aichberger, F. (1994). *Sozialgesetzbuch: Reichsversicherungsordnung mit Nebengesetzen, Ausführungs- und Verfassungsvorschriften.* Munich: C. H. Beck.

Akademie für Ärztliche Fortbildung der DDR. (1987). *Sozialökonomische Grundlagen für den Schutz der Gesundheit für alle Bürger in der Deutschen Demokratischen Republik.* Berlin: Ärztebuchverlag Berlin und Medizinischer Fachverlag Leipzig.

Alber, J. (1988). Germany: Growth to limits. In P. Flora (Ed.), *The western European welfare states since World War II* (Vol. 2, pp. 1-154). New York: Walter de Gruyter.

Alber, J. (1992a). *Das Gesundheitswesen der Bundesrepublik Deutschland: Entwicklung, Struktur und Funktionsweise.* Frankfurt: Campus.

Alber, J. (1992b). Residential care for the elderly. *Journal of Health Politics, Policy and Law, 17,* 929-957.

Alber, J. (1995). A framework for the comparative study of social services. *Journal of European Social Policy, 3,* 131-149.

Altenstetter, C. (1985). *Krankenhausbedarfsplanung: Was brachte sie wirklich?* Munich: Oldenbourg.

Altenstetter, C. (1986a). German social security programs: An interpretation of their development. In D. E. Ashford & E. W. Kelley (Eds.), *Nationalizing social security in Europe and America* (pp. 73-97). Greenwich, CT: JAI.

Altenstetter, C. (1986b). Reimbursement policy of hospitals in the Federal Republic of Germany. *International Journal of Health Planning and Management, 1,* 189-211.

Altenstetter, C. (1987). An end to a consensus on health care in the Federal Republic of Germany? *Journal of Health Politics, Policy and Law, 12,* 505-536.

Altenstetter, C. (1989). Hospital planners and medical professionals in the Federal Republic of Germany. In G. Freddi & J. W. Björkman (Eds.), *Controlling medical professionals: The comparative politics of health governance* (pp. 157-177). Newbury Park, CA: Sage.

Arnold, M. (1991). *Health care in the Federal Republic of Germany.* Cologne: Deutscher Ärzte-Verlag.

Arnold, M., & Schirmer, B. (1990). *Gesundheit für ein Deutschland Ausgangslage: Probleme und Möglichkeiten der Angleichung der medizinischen Versorgungssysteme der Bundesrepublik Deutschland und der DDR zur Bildung eines einheitlichen Gesundheitswesens.* Cologne: Deutscher Ärzte-Verlag.

Ashford, D. (1986). *The emergence of the welfare states.* Oxford, UK: Basil Blackwell.

Baldwin, P. (1991). *The politics of social solidarity and the class bases of the European welfare state, 1875-1975.* Cambridge, UK: Cambridge University Press.

Bauer, R. (1990). Voluntary welfare association in Germany and the United States of America: Historical development. *Voluntas, 1,* 97-111.

Behaghel, K. (1994). *Kostendämpfung und ärztliche Interessenvertretung: Ein Verbandssystem unter Streß.* Frankfurt: Campus.

Beratungsstelle für Angewandte Systemforschung. (1992a). *Die alten und neuen Bundesländer.* Augsburg: Selbstverlag.

Beratungsstelle für Angewandte Systemforschung. (1992b). *Internationaler Vergleich von Gesundheitssystemen* (3rd ed.). Augsburg: Selbstverlag.

Bundesministerium für Arbeit und Sozialordnung. (1993). *Übersicht über die Soziale Sicherheit: Textergänzung.* Bonn: Author.

Bundesministerium für Arbeit und Sozialordnung. (1995). *Sozialgesetzbuch: Referat Öffentlichkeitsarbeit.* Bonn: Author.

Bundesministerium für Gesundheit. (1993). *Daten des Gesundheitswesens: Ausgabe 1993* (Schriftenreihe des Bundesministeriums für Gesundheit, No. 25). Baden-Baden: Nomos.

Bundesministerium für Gesundheit. (1995). *Daten des Gesundheitswesens: Ausgabe 1995* (Schriftenreihe des Bundesministeriums für Gesundheit, No. 51). Baden-Baden: Nomos.

Busse, R., & Howorth, C. (in press). Cost-containment in Germany 1977-1997. In E. Mossialos & J. LeGrand (Eds.), *Health expenditure in the European Union: Cost and control.* Aldershot, UK: Ashgate.

Busse, R., & Schwartz, F. (1997). Financing reforms in the German hospital sector: From the full cost cover principle to prospective case fees. *Medical Care, 35*(10), OS40-OS49.

Busse, R., & Schwartz, F. (in press). Decision-making and priority-setting in public health and health care in Germany. In W. W. Holland, E. Mossialos, P. Belcher, & B. Merkel (Eds.), *Public health decisions: Methods for priority setting in the EU member states.* Luxembourg: Office for Official Publications of the European Communities.

Döhler, M. (1989). Physicians' professional autonomy in the welfare state: Endangered or preserved? In G. Freddi & J. W. Björkman (Eds.), *Controlling medical professionals: The comparative politics of health governance* (pp. 178-197). Newbury Park, CA: Sage.

Döhler, M. (1990). *Gesundheitspolitik nach der Wende: Policy Netzwerke und ordnungspolitischer Strategiewechsel in Großbritannien, den USA und der BRD.* Berlin: Sigma Bohn.

Döhler, M. (1993). Ordnungspolitische Ideen und sozialpolitische Institutionen. In R. Czada & M. Schmidt (Eds.), *Verhandlungsdemokratie, Interessenvermittlung, Regierbarkeit* (pp. 123-141). Opladen: Westdeutscher Verlag.

Döhler, M., & Manow-Borgwardt, P. (1991). *Korporatisierung als gesundheitspolitische Strategie* (MPIFG Discussion Paper 91/9). Cologne: Max-Planck-Institut für Gesellschaftsforschung.

Döhler, M., & Manow-Borgwardt, P. (1992). Gesundheitspolitische Steuerung zwischen Hierarchie und Verhandlung. *Politische Vierteljahresschrift, 33,* 571-596.

Döhler, M., & Manow-Borgwardt, P. (1995). *Formierung und Wandel eines Politikfeldes: Gesundheitspolitik von Blank zu Seehofer* (MPIFG Discussion Paper 95/6). Cologne: Max-Planck-Institut für Gesellschaftsforschung.

Federal Ministry for Health. (1994). *The health care system of the Federal Republic of Germany.* Bonn: Osang.

Franco, C. (1992). *The German health care system* (Congressional Research Service, 92-543 EPW). Washington, DC: Library of Congress.

Freudenstein, U., & Borgwardt, G. (1992). Primary medical care in former East Germany: The frosty winds of change. *British Medical Journal, 304,* 827-829.

Gäfgen, G. (1988). *Neokorporatismus und Gesundheitswesen.* Baden-Baden: Nomos.

Gesetz zur Sicherung und Strukturverbesserung der gesetzlichen Krankenversicherung (Gesundheitsstruktur-gesetz of 21 December 1992. (1992). *Bundesgesetzblatt, 1,* 2266-2334.

Giaimo, S., & Manow, P. (1997). Institutions and ideas into politics: Health reform in Britain and Germany. In C. Altenstetter & J. W. Björkman (Eds.), *Health policy reform: National variations and globalization* (pp. 175-202). New York: Macmillan.

Glaser, W. (1991). *Health insurance in practice.* San Francisco: Jossey-Bass.

Gunlicks, A. (1989). Federalism and intergovernmental relations in West Germany: A fortieth year appraisal. *Publius: The Journal of Federalism, 19*(4), 1-15.

Gunlicks, A. (1994). German federalism after unification: The legal/constitutional response. *Publius: The Journal of Federalism, 24*(2), 81-98.

Hassenteufel, P. (1996). The medical profession and health insurance policies: A Franco-German comparison. *Journal of European Public Policy, 3,* 461-480.

Henke, K. (1988). Funktionsweise und Steuerungswirksamkeit der Konzertierten Aktion im Gesundheitswesen (KAiG). In G. Gäfgen (Ed.), *Neokorporatismus und Gesundheitswesen* (pp. 113-157). Baden-Baden: Nomos.

Hinrichs, K. (1995). The impact of German health insurance reforms on redistribution and the culture of solidarity. *Journal of Health Politics, Policy and Law, 20,* 653-687.

Hockerts, H. (1981). German post-war social policies against the background of the Beveridge Plan: Some observations preparatory to a comparative analysis. In W. J. Mommsen & W. Mock (Eds.), *The emergence of the welfare state in Britain and Germany 1850-1950* (pp. 315-339). London: Croom Helm.

Hoffmann, W. (1996, September 27). Sägen am System: Bonns geplante Gesundheitsreform stellt das Prinzip der Solidarität in Frage. *Die Zeit,* p. 27.

Hoffmeyer, U. (1994). The health care system in Germany. In U. K. Hoffmeyer & T. R. McCarthy (Eds), *Financing health care* (Vol. 1, pp. 419-512). Dordrecht, the Netherlands: Kluwer Academic Publishers.

Hollingsworth, E. (1992). Falling through the cracks: Care of the chronically mentally ill in the United States, Germany, and the United Kingdom. *Journal of Health Politics, Policy and Law, 17,* 899-928.

Hollingsworth, R., & Hollingsworth, E. (1992). Challenges in the provision of care for the chronically ill. *Journal of Health Politics, Policy and Law, 17,* 869-898.

Iglehart, J. (1991). Health policy report: Germany's health care system. *New England Journal of Medicine, 324,* 503-508, 1750-1756.

Jérôme-Fourget, M., White, J., & Wiener, J. (1995). *Health care reform through internal markets.* Washington, DC: Brookings Institution.

Kirchberger, S. (1986). Public-health policy in Germany, 1945-1949: Continuity and a new beginning. In D. Light & A. Schuller (Eds.), *Political values and health care: The German experience* (pp. 185-238). Cambridge, MA: MIT Press.

Knox, R. (1993). *Germany's health system: One nation, united with health care for all.* Washington, DC: Faulkner & Gray.

Leibfried, S., & Tennstedt, F. (1986). Health insurance policy and Berufsverbote in the Nazi takeover. In D. Light & A. Schuller (Eds.), *Political values and health care: The German experience* (pp. 127-184). Cambridge, MA: MIT Press.

Light, D., & Schuller, A. (Eds.). (1986). *Political values and health care: The German experience.* Cambridge, MA: MIT Press.

Manow-Borgwardt, P. (1993). *Gesundheitspolitische Entscheidungen im Prozeß der Deutschen Einigung.* Unpublished doctoral dissertation, Freien Universität, Berlin.

Manow-Borgwardt, P. (1994). Die Sozialversicherung in der DDR und der BRD, 1945-1990: Über die Fortschrittlichkeit rückschrittlicher Institutionen. *Politische Vierteljahresschrift, 35*(1), 40-61.

Marmor, T. (1997). Global health policy reform: Misleading mythology or learning opportunity. In C. Altenstetter & J. W. Björkman (Eds.), *Health policy reform: National variations and globalization* (pp. 348-364). New York: St. Martin's.

Mommsen, W., & Mock, W. (1981). *The emergence of the welfare state in Britain and Germany 1850-1950.* London: Croom Helm.

National Economic Research Associates and Pharmaceutical Partners for Better Healthcare. (1995). *Risk-adjustment and its implications for efficiency and equity in health care systems.* London: Author.

Niehoff, J., Schneider, F., & Wetzstein, K. (1992). Reflections on the health policy of the former German Democratic Republic. *International Journal of Health Sciences, 3,* 205-213.

Organization for Economic Cooperation and Development. (1990). *Health care systems in transition.* Paris: Author.

Organization for Economic Cooperation and Development. (1992). *The reform of health care: A comparative analysis of seven OECD countries.* Paris: Author.

Organization for Economic Cooperation and Development. (1994). *The reform of health care systems: A review of seventeen countries.* Paris: Author.

Organization for Economic Cooperation and Development. (1995). *Internal markets in the making: Health systems in Canada, Iceland and the United Kingdom.* Paris: Author.

Pfaff, M., & Wassener, D. (1995). *Das Krankenhaus im Gefolge des Gesundheits-Struktur-Gesetzes 1993.* Baden-Baden: Nomos.

Robischon, T., Stucke, A., Wasem, J., & Wolf, H. G. (1994). *Die Politische Logik der deutschen Vereinigung und der Institutionentransfer: Eine Untersuchung am Beispiel von Gesundheitswesen, Forschungssystem und Telekommunikation* (MPIFG Discussion Paper 94/3). Cologne: Max-Planck-Institut für Gesellschaftsforschung.

Rosenberg, P. (1986). The origin and the development of compulsory health insurance in Germany. In D. Light & A. Schuller (Eds.), *Political values and health care: The German experience* (pp. 105-126). Cambridge, MA: MIT Press.

Rosewitz, B., & Webber, D. (1990). *Reformversuche und Reformblockaden im deutschen Gesundheitswesen.* Frankfurt: Campus.

Sachverständigenrat der Konzertierten Aktion. (1991). *Das Gesundheitswesen im vereinten Deutschland.* Baden-Baden: Nomos.

Sachverständigenrat der Konzertierten Aktion. (1992). *Ausbau in Deutschland und Aufbruch nach Europa: Vorschläge für die Konzertierte Aktion im Gesundheitswesen.* Baden-Baden: Nomos.

Sachverständigenrat der Konzertierten Aktion. (1994). *Gesundheitsversorgung und Krankenversicherung 2000: Eigenverantwortung, Subsidiarität und Solidarität bei sich ändernden Rahmenbedingungen.* Baden-Baden: Nomos.

Sachverständigenrat der Konzertierten Aktion. (1995). *Gesundheitsversorgung und Krankenversicherung 2000: Mehr Ergebnisorientierung, mehr Qualität und mehr Wirtschaftlichkeit.* Baden-Baden: Nomos.

Scharpf, F. (1985). *The joint decision trap: Lessons from German federalism and European integration* (Discussion Paper IIM/LMP #85-1). Berlin: Wissenschaftszentrum.

Scharpf, F., Reissert, B., & Schnabel, F. (1976). *Politikverflechtung: Theorie und Empirie des kooperativen Föderalismus in der Bundesrepublik.* Kronberg: Scriptor.

Schieber, G., Poullier, J.-P., & Greenwald, L. (1991). Health care systems in twenty-four countries. *Health Affairs, 10*(3), 22-38.

Schieber, G., Poullier, J.-P., & Greenwald, L. (1992). U.S. health expenditure performance: An international comparison and data update. *Health Care Financing Review, 13*(4), 1-89.

Schiedsstellen verfähren im Bundesgebiet. (1996, February 1). *PKV Publik,* No. 1, pp. 10-11.

Schneider, M. (1991). Health care cost containment in the Federal Republic of Germany. *Health Care Financing Review, 12,* 87-101.

Schneider, M. (1995). Evaluation of cost-containment acts in Germany. In Organization for Economic Cooperation and Development (Ed.), *Health: Quality and choice* (pp. 63-81). Paris: Editor.

Schulenburg, J. M. G. von der. (1994). Forming and reforming the market for third party purchasing of health care: A German perspective. *Social Science and Medicine, 39,* 1473-1481.

Schulenburg, J. M. G. von der. (1996, April). German health policy at the crossroads [Pfizer Forum Europe, 1-page insert]. *Economist,* n.p.

Seibel, W. (1993). Government/third sector relationship in a comparative perspective: The cases of France and West Germany. *International Journal of Voluntary and Non-Profit Organisations: Voluntas, 1,* 41-60.

Statistisches Bundesamt. (1992). *Datenreport 1992: Zahlen und Fakten über die Bundesrepublik Deutschland* (No. 309). Bonn: Bundeszentrale für politische Bildung.

Stern, K., & Schmidt-Bleibtreu, B. (1990). *Staatsvertrag zur Währungs-, Wirtschafts- und Sozialunion mit Vertragstext, Begründung und Materialien.* Munich: C. H. Beck.

Stone, D. A. (1980). *The limits of professional power.* Chicago: University of Chicago Press.

Stone, D. A. (1991). German unification: East Meets West in the doctor's office. *Journal of Health Politics, Policy and Law, 16,* 401-412.

Stone, D. A. (1997). *Policy paradox: The art of political decision making* (2nd ed.). New York: Norton.

Streeck, W. (1995). *German capitalism: Does it exist? Can it survive?* (MPIFG Discussion Paper 95/5). Cologne: Max-Planck-Institut für Gesellschaftsforschung.

Tampke, J. (1981). Bismarck's social legislation: A genuine breakthrough? In W. J. Mommsen & W. Mock (Eds.), *The emergence of the welfare state in Britain and Germany 1850-1950* (pp. 71-83). London: Croom Helm.

Thiele, W. (1990). *Das Gesundheitswesen der DDR: Aufbruch oder Einbruch? Denkanstöße für eine Neuordnung des Gesundheitswesens in einem deutschen Staat.* Sankt Augustin: Asgard-Verlag.

Ullmann, H.-P. (1981). German industry and Bismarck's social security system. In W. J. Mommsen & W. Mock (Eds.), *The emergence of the welfare state in Britain and Germany 1850-1950* (pp. 133-149). London: Croom Helm.

U.S. General Accounting Office. (1993). *German health reforms: New cost control initiatives* (GAO/HRD-93-103). Washington, DC: Author.

von Beyme, K., & Schmidt, M. (1985). *Policy and politics in the Federal Republic of Germany.* New York: St. Martin's.

Wannagat, G. (1965). *Lehrbuch des Sozialversicherungsrechts.* Tubingen: J. C. B. Mohr.

Wasem, J. (1992). *Poliklinik in die Kassenarztpraxis: Versuch einer Rekonstruktion der Entscheidungssituation ambulant tätiger Ärzte in Ostdeutschland* (MPIFG Discussion Paper 92/5). Cologne: Max-Planck-Institut für Gesellschaftsforschung.

Wasem, J. (1993). Strategische Planung oder ungesteuerte Kettenreaktion? Zur Erosion der poliklinischen Einrichtungen in Ostdeutschland nach der Vereinigung in *Gesundheitsmärkte. Jahrbuch für Kritische Medizin, 19,* 39-52.

Wasem, J. (1994). Sozialpolitische Grundlagen der gesetzlichen Krankenversicherung. In B. Schulin (Ed.), *Handbuch des Sozialversicherungsrechts: Vol. 1. Krankenversicherungsrecht* (pp. 80-112). Munich: C. H. Beck.

Wasem, J. (1997). Health care reform in the Federal Republic of Germany: The new and the old Länder. In C. Altenstetter & J. W. Björkman (Eds.), *Health policy reform: National variations and globalization* (pp. 161-174). New York: St. Martin's.

Webber, D. (1991). Health insurance reform in the Federal Republic of Germany. In C. Altenstetter & S. A. Haywood (Eds.), *Comparative health policy and the New Right* (pp. 49-90). New York: St. Martin's.

Wer hat das bessere Angebot? (1996). *Focus, 42,* 318-319.

White, J. (1995). *Competing solutions: American health care proposals and international experience.* Washington, DC: Brookings Institution.

Zacher, H. (1985). *Einführung in das Sozialrecht der Bundesrepublik Deutschland* (3rd, rev. ed.). Heidelberg: R. V. Decker & C. F. Müller.

CHAPTER 5

Health Care Cost Containment in Germany

BRADFORD KIRKMAN-LIFF

The health care system of Germany is based on private practice physicians, on community, church, and municipality-affiliated hospitals, and on a large number of nonprofit and for-profit insurers and autonomous sickness funds. Before reunification, some 92% of the West German public obtained health services through the approximately 1,240 sickness funds. These individuals and their families are obligated to become members because they fall below certain income levels (approximately $41,000 in 1993) or are in certain occupational classifications. The cost of the sickness fund is paid by an income-adjusted premium, half paid by the employee and half paid by the employer. Approximately 7% of the population purchase private health insurance. Less than 0.5% of the German public is uninsured. It is a pluralistic, private system, yet it ensures universal coverage and contains costs. One contributing factor to this achievement is that policymakers in Germany have consistently focused on health care cost containment over the last two decades.

The remainder of this chapter will be in six sections. Germany's approach to controlling the costs of health care will first be reviewed, including the activities of Concerted Action in Health Care. The next two sections will examine the specific cost control mechanisms for ambulatory care physicians and hospitals, respectively. The fourth section will discuss the 1993 Health Care Reform Act and show how its actions build on the past control activities. The fifth section will present an analytical summary of German experiences with cost containment, and the last section will attempt to derive lessons for cost containment in the United States.

The English-language literature on Germany has grown in the last few years. Though much of the material in this chapter is drawn from my own interviews and research in Germany, a number of other sources were used; these should be consulted for more details.[1]

Global Budgeting in the German System

One of the underlying principles of the German health system is self-government by corporate parties. This system involves two steps. First, private sector bodies are created that represent the collective interests of groups of private organizations or individuals and are governed by their members. These bodies are similar to trade associations such as the American Medical Association in the United States. The second step is the devolution of governmental power and responsibility to these bodies. They are charged with performing legal, regulatory functions over their members. These bodies also have official standing in the complex negotiations over the financing of the health care system and are an important tool in cost containment. Because all parties (insurers, physicians, hospitals, employers, unions) are organized into these bodies, they form a structure of countervailing power against one another. This approach has been described as corporatism.

Nonetheless, the need for more effective cost containment efforts led in 1977 to the creation of an advisory group called Concerted Action in Health Care. This is a forum for all parties, composed of 68 members from a number of provider, insurer, employer, union, and governmental organizations. The forum meets twice a year and has a standing staff of six university professors who serve 3-year terms. This advisory committee to Concerted Action in Health Care is seen as one of the most prestigious in the German health care policy community: it is equivalent to being on the President's Council of Economic Advisors in the United States. Concerted Action in Health Care has a very specific duty: to maintain stability in the contribution rates for the sickness funds. To achieve this goal, expenditure controls must be placed on the funds, and that in turn requires changes in provider payment methods.

At the meetings of Concerted Action, there are formal reviews of macroeconomic trends in health care that lead to discussions that build consensus on policy changes. The advisory committee usually prepares draft policy documents. When consensus is reached, advice and guidelines, which are technically nonbinding, are given to participating organizations. These include aggregate growth rates for prices, expenditures, and premiums. More important, Concerted Action in Health Care endorses reports, prepared by its staff, on payment reforms. These reports are circulated before the meetings, are revised, and represent consensus documents. They are often forwarded to the government, which uses them as the basis for legislation. This was the process used to change physician reimbursement from fixed fee-for-service payments to variable payments from capitated pools.

The recommendations of the Concerted Action in Health Care were translated into legislation by Parliamentary committees and passed as Cost Containment Acts. Such acts were passed in 1977, 1981, 1982, 1983, 1984, 1985, 1986, 1989, 1992, and 1993. Many of these acts contain only minor adjustments to the basic services covered by sickness funds and to the magnitude of copayments for sickness fund members. Some of these laws allowed changes in the form of the contracts between providers and insurers. Most of this legislation is viewed as having originated with Concerted Action in Health Care and thus is thought to reflect the consensus of the major stakeholders in the health care system.

Cost Controls for Ambulatory Care Physicians

Cost control over ambulatory care physicians is achieved by means of a number of corporatist mechanisms. All German physicians who practice outside hospitals must belong to two different bodies. First, to be licensed, they must join the physicians' chamber for the state in which they practice. The physicians' chamber is somewhat like a state medical licensure board in the United States, but whereas in the United States the board is a government agency with physician representatives, in Germany the physicians' chamber is a private body, organized and controlled by physicians, which has been given governmental authority. The physicians' chamber in each state develops a "Professional Medical Code" that has the legal standing of an enforceable set of laws. The chambers are responsible for professional licensure, discipline of physicians for unethical practices, and monitoring of residency programs.

The second corporatist body to which ambulatory care physicians must belong is the regional sickness fund physicians' association. Created in 1933, these associations are somewhat analogous to American independent practice associations (IPAs) that contract with health maintenance organizations. Unlike American IPAs, however, there is only one sickness fund physicians' association in each region, and all the sickness funds in the region must contract with it for ambulatory care for their members. Between 1933 and 1965 and since 1986, the associations negotiate with the sickness funds over the capitation rate to be paid to the associations by the funds for each covered member. (The 21-year period between 1965 and 1986 saw a number of different payment mechanisms, none of which failed to control costs as well as capitation.) Since 1986, there has been a higher capitation rate for retirees than for those who are working or their dependents. This capitation is used to fund the payments made by the associations to their members for care provided to sickness fund members. The associations manage the capitation fund, monitor physician practice patterns, and discipline physicians who exhibit high-cost practice patterns. Each of these activities will be described in detail below.

The way in which the sickness fund physicians' association pays physicians from the capitated pool is an important element in cost control. Ambulatory care physicians send their bills to their associations, using a standardized fee schedule expressed in "points," not actual currency amounts. Most of the associations split the capitation into several pools—usually three—for basic services, laboratory services, and other services. All of the points of all of the physicians in the region are aggregated in these separate pools, and the total number of points is divided into the total amount placed into each pool to obtain a conversion factor. These conversion factors differ between the pools and also differ across regions. The conversion factors are then applied to each physician's individual billing to determine the amount to be paid to that physician.

Under this system, once the capitation rates are negotiated, the sickness funds know exactly what their costs for ambulatory care will be. The physicians, on the other hand, do not exactly know what the conversion factor will be and thus do not know exactly what their income will be for their volume of services.

An important aspect of the system is that the associations, and not the sickness funds, pay the physicians and monitor their practice patterns. Due to the nature of the capitated pool, when a physician exploits the system by ordering extra laboratory tests or treatment for his or her patients, the other physicians in the region, and not the sickness fund, lose income to that physician. As a physician-controlled organization, the sickness fund physicians' association is also seen as the appropriate body for practice pattern review. Using elaborate information systems, the associations develop practice profiles for each physician, comparing him or her to peers in the region, as defined by specialty and practice size. Some 10 or more components of the practice are examined. Those physicians who exceed the average production levels by 40% are notified that their fees will be reduced in the components where the high production occurred unless they can convince a panel of physicians and sickness fund representatives that the higher production was justified. About 7% of German physicians receive such notices in a year, and about 2% (about one third of those receiving notification) have their fees reduced.

The 1989 Cost Containment Act created medical service organizations to undertake broader utilization review activities. These activities include concurrent review of hospital stays and appropriateness of "spa cures," as well as assistance with other peer review efforts. There has thus far been no assessment of the effectiveness of these new organizations.

Cost Controls for Hospitals

German hospitals are predominantly owned by local and regional government (51%), but there are large numbers of community and church nonprofit hospitals (35%) and private for-profit hospitals (14%). The current structure of the hospital payment system was created in 1972. It separated the financing of capital costs from operating costs, placing the former in the hands of governments and the latter in the hands of the sickness funds and private insurers. The capital financing was and is allocated according to regional hospital need plans, established by the state governments, with relatively little input from the hospitals themselves.

Operating costs were fully paid until 1985, when a major reform of that method occurred. A global budget system was created. The hospitals negotiate an operating cost budget with the dominant sickness funds and private insurers in their region. This budget also includes a projected daily "fixed-cost break-even volume."[2] The operating cost budget is divided by the fixed-cost break-even volume to obtain a per diem reimbursement rate. If a hospital's actual volume is greater than its break-even volume, then it receives only 25% of the per diem rate for those patient-days in excess of the break-even volume. On the other hand, if the actual volume is less than the break-even volume, then the hospital receives 75% of the per diem rate for those days between its actual volume and the break-even volume.

This structure requires the hospitals and the payers to negotiate both the fixed-cost break-even volume and the appropriate operating cost budget for that volume. There are no standards, and the parties are free to negotiate whatever they agree is an appropriate settlement. The sickness funds have a major constraint in the pressure to have no increases in their contribution rates, and the hospitals have salaried medical staffs that want to expand their services. Compulsory arbitration exists in cases when agreement is not possible, but both sides to the negotiations view compulsory arbitration as an admission of failure and fear that an arbitration settlement could be worse for them than a negotiated settlement.

The 1993 German Reforms

The recession of the early 1990s, coupled with the far higher than expected costs of reunification, caused the sickness funds to increase their contribution rates by an average of an additional 1% of their members' income. Given other inflationary pressures and an increase in unemployment, the government felt that significant cost containment was necessary. Moreover, for the first time since it was founded in 1977, Concerted Action in Health Care was unable to come to a consensus on a comprehensive package of reforms. After a closed meeting of the political parties, the government responded with a set of emergency global budget controls. The controls involve eight short-range and two long-range components.

First, the contribution rates of the sickness funds were to be frozen for 3 years. The only growth in income for the funds would be due to increases in the employed population and in the incomes of the employed. This severe limitation on the capacity of the sickness funds to pay providers would normally be difficult to sustain, but other elements made such cost containment feasible.

Second, and related to the reduced financial capacity of the sickness funds, non-negotiable global budgets were to be established for different health sectors: ambulatory care physicians, hospitals, prescription drugs, and dentists. The sickness funds would thus be able to operate within their restricted resources because the provider sectors would know that they could not negotiate for additional resources. These global budgets are set by the government, but the process by which they are developed reflects the traditional consensual process, although in a less public and formal manner. A number of the corporatist parties make their views known privately to the government during the budget determination process, and all provide vocal comments after the figures are released.

Third, the imposition of strict budgets on the ambulatory care physicians has been accompanied by stricter financial sanctions on high-volume physicians. Doctors' practice patterns will be reviewed more frequently, and those physicians who exceed the average production levels by 25% or more will be notified that their fees will be reduced in the components in which the high production occurred. The penalties for excessive unjustified volumes will be harsher, and physicians can have all reimbursement for high-technology services suspended if they do not have proper authorization for those technologies.

Fourth, strict regulations for planning physician numbers were established. Defined physician/population ratios for each specialty are compared to the current distribution in defined geographical areas. For those specialties in which the current physician/population ratios of a geographical area exceed the standards, that geographical area will be closed to the establishment of new practices by physicians of those specialties.

Fifth, the method of hospital reimbursement was changed. Hospitals have moved from a per diem payment system to a prospective payment that sets fixed prices by service or admission diagnosis for a large portion of their activities. During the transition, hospitals were to be given strict global budgets, with no additional payments even if their volume of activities should increase.

Sixth, hospital-based physicians were allowed to provide some ambulatory care services. In Germany, it has long been contended that the division between ambulatory care and hospital physicians reduces quality and increases costs because of extensive duplication of laboratory tests and radiology examinations. The inability of hospital physicians to see their patients in an ambulatory context after discharge has resulted in longer than necessary lengths of stay. By allowing hospital physicians to see recently discharged patients, it is hoped that length of hospital stay can be reduced.

The seventh change was a major political victory over the very strong German pharmaceutical industry. Mandated price reductions for both prescription and over-the-counter drugs were imposed, and physicians and the pharmaceutical industry were placed at risk for the total expenditures on pharmaceuticals. If the volume increases to such an extent that the total costs for drugs increase (despite mandated price reductions), the higher costs will be balanced by first a reduction in physician fees and then payments to be made by the pharmaceutical industry. Patient cost sharing for prescription drugs has also been increased.

The eighth and last short-term change is a reduction in dental fees and the imposition of some practice-monitoring systems as used with ambulatory care physicians.

These eight policies are being implemented by the Ministry of Health, which has assumed some of the regulatory oversight functions that the Ministry of Labor Affairs formerly exercised over the sickness funds. The traditional corporatist bodies are also involved in the implementation of the policies. Thus, the associations of sickness funds, the sickness fund physicians' associations, and the physicians' chambers retain an important role in achieving the cost containment goals.

Two long-term changes are intended to change the overall structure of the system so as to encourage more effectiveness and efficiency. The first involves equalization of the contribution rates that are paid by employers and employees to the various sick benefit funds. To make this possible, funds will either receive transfers from other funds or give transfers to other funds based on the age and sex distribution of the sickness fund's members, the number of insured dependents, and the fund's payroll tax base. The equalization will not result in completely equal rates, and in fact some variation in rates is desired so that the more efficient funds will be able to offer lower rates and so attract new members. This relates to the second long-term change. The insured will be able to choose among funds once a year, rather than staying in one fund for the entire period of employment with an employer. Some minor forms of competition will be allowed, such as expanded provision of health promotion and wellness services. It is hoped that extra services and lower contribution rates offered by the more efficient funds will enhance competitive adjustments and thus result in long-term gains in cost containment.

It is difficult to assess the true magnitude of the effects of these reforms at the present time. It is reported that physicians reacted to being placed at risk for the total expenditures on pharmaceuticals with two strategies. Many significantly reduced their prescription volumes, especially for drugs for which there were over-the-counter near-equivalents. It is also reported that physicians started to admit patients to hospitals for pharmaceutical treatments that previously would have been taken at home. Both strategies apparently led to a reduction in total outpatient prescription drug costs, for outpatient drug costs were substantially below the budget. Increased patient cost sharing for prescription drugs may also have had a role in this cost reduction.

It is too early to say if the 1993 reforms have destroyed the concept of consensus building among stakeholders through the Concerted Action in Health Care mechanism. German corporatism in health care is very resilient: It has survived defeat in World War I, depression, Nazism, defeat in World War II, and national division. It should be able to survive reunification.

Summary of the German Experiences

There are a number of explanations for Germany's relatively great success in health care cost containment. First, cost containment is achieved through a two-sided approach. On one side, extensive macroeconomic analysis of health care costs is performed by the staff of Concerted Action in Health Care, resulting in guidelines communicated to the various parties for use in their negotiations. The goal of Concerted Action is to link insurance premium rate increases to the growth rate of average wages in order to achieve stability in rates. Because insurance premium rate increases determine the ability of insurers to pay physicians and hospitals, provider payment increases become linked to the growth rate of average wages. On the other side, the government, often acting on the recommendations of Concerted Action, has repeatedly been willing to pass cost containment acts that annually adjust the structure of the system. These yearly system revisions have affected covered benefits, patient cost sharing, and provider payment mechanisms. The combination of global negotiations and regulatory enforcement acts as a "one-two punch" to restrain cost increases.

Second, implementation of national/regional price agreements that limit income growth among insurers, physicians, and hospitals is achieved by appropriate volume-monitoring systems and capacity-planning systems. Simply setting prices fails to lower costs because volume may increase. Volume, price, and capacity must all be addressed.

Third, the containment of expenditures was least effective when insurers did not cooperate on uniform provider payment methods. For example, when the substitute funds chose to pay ambulatory physicians higher fees than did the other funds, cost containment in that sector was weak.

Fourth, government can distance itself from negotiations but still exert influence on outcomes through the mechanism of quasi-governmental advisory bodies. These bodies are simultaneously representative bodies, composed of members from the interested parties, and directive agencies, translating goverment policy into guidelines for the negotiations. The 1993 reforms build on the past successes of these structures but do entail an unusual degree of government involvement. The combined effect of economic recession and high unification costs led to this deviation from the usual role.

Lessons for Cost Containment in the United States

The German (and other European) experience reveals that explicit public discussion about underlying values is essential if a consensus is to be reached on strategies to achieve universal coverage and cost containment. The German system is based on a set of mutual obligations and responsibilities, as well as a shared belief in solidarity. With consensus on these matters, cost containment strategies can be crafted that have support because they are congruent with the value system. The political debate in 1993-1994 over American health care reform indicates that we are far from reaching consensus on values and strategies; until we reach it, cost containment may be very difficult to achieve on a systemwide basis.

The German experience indicates that mechanistic global budgeting is not necessary to achieve cost containment. It is also politically unacceptable in both the United States and Germany. Rather, the German strategy is global negotiations to build consensus on broad macroeconomic policy on health care. This may also be the right strategy for the United States, where such a strategy would involve linking rates of increases in both insurance premiums and provider payments to general economic growth, and could involve an expanded role for the Prospective Payment Assessment Commission and the Physician Payment Review Commission. Proposals to combine their functions in one commission mirror the broad responsibility of Concerted Action in Health Care in Germany. What is required is open and honest debate among national trade associations and other interest groups about macro-level health cost trends to set goals for local institutions.

The German experience shows that regional negotiations among insurers, providers, and purchasers are essential in developing fee schedules and budgets that adequately compensate all providers while ensuring that both medical care and administrative costs are controlled. Such negotiations must occur in a context in which all parties are aware of—and bound by—national targets for growth in premiums and prices. This is especially applicable to determination of local capitation rates. The growth of multiple-employer insurance-purchasing coalitions in the United States may evolve into an American version of German-style private sector negotiation.

Global negotiations require that insurers and providers understand that one party's revenue is another party's cost. Cost containment means revenue curtailment. This issue must be faced head-on. The entire health sector must learn to act responsibly by exercising self-restraint on the rate of cost increases and not becoming an excessive burden on the rest of society. All parties must remember that the only feasible alternatives to global negotiations are either invasive central government regulation or continued cost inflation.[3]

Notes

1. For the English literature, see Altenstetter, 1987; Henke, 1986; Knox, 1993; Light and Schuller, 1993; Schneider, 1991; Stone, 1979; Stone, 1980; U.S. General Accounting Office, 1993; Webber, 1991.

2. This is an estimate of the number of patients per day at which the hospital could expect to break even on fixed costs.

3. Recent American experience has shown, however, that a rigorous campaign by payers to control costs through the mechanism of managed care may also be able to reduce medical cost inflation.

Bibliography

Altenstetter, C. (1987). An end to consensus on health care in the Federal Republic of Germany? *Journal of Health Politics, Policy and Law, 12,* 505-536.

Henke, K. (1986). A "concerted" approach to health care financing in the Federal Republic of Germany. *Health Policy, 6,* 341-351.

Knox, R. (1993). *Germany's health system.* Washington, DC: Faulkner & Gray.

Light, D., & Schuller, A. (1993). *Political values and health care: The German experience.* Cambridge, MA: MIT Press.

Schneider, M. (1991). Health care cost containment in the Federal Republic of Germany. *Health Care Financing Review, 12,* 87-101.

Stone, D. (1979). Health care cost containment in West Germany. *Journal of Health Politics, Policy and Law, 4,* 176-199.

Stone, D. (1980). *The limits of professional power.* Chicago: University of Chicago Press.

U.S. General Accounting Office. (1993). *1993 German health reforms: New cost control initiatives* (GAO/HRD-93-103). Washington, DC: Author.

Webber, D. (1991). Health insurance reform in the Federal Republic of Germany. In C. Altenstetter & S. A. Haywood (Eds.), *Comparative health policy and the new right* (pp. 49-90). New York: St. Martin's.

CHAPTER 6

German Unity and Health Care Reform

BRADLEY SCHARF

The creation and consolidation of the communist German Democratic Republic (GDR) had been ridden with tensions, setbacks, rebellions, and repression. But by the mid-1970s the country enjoyed a period of relative prosperity, tranquillity, and pragmatic partnership between the narrow Politburo oligarchy and the emerging postwar generation of institutional leaders. Entering the 1980s, however, the communist regime undertook a misbegotten strategy of economic and social modernization that depended too much on external capital and too little on internal political and economic innovation. In the face of economic stagnation, the regime tried vainly to sustain its ambitious program of social benefits, which was correctly perceived to be the basis of the state's fragile legitimacy. By the middle of the decade, the corrosion of economic management and social services had become virtually universal and was easily recognized by the majority of citizens in everyday life. Health care was among the most visible areas of decline.

In the course of German unification, health care for the people of the eastern *Länder* (states) would change dramatically. This chapter focuses on (a) East German assessments of their previous health care system, (b) the failure of proposals to "merge" the two German health care systems, and (c) subsequent East German assessments of their "new" health care system. The failure to retain elements of GDR health care illustrates the difficulty of reform in the presence of entrenched interest groups. The unique experience of East Germans as consumers under two very different systems sheds some light on the relative merits of alternate forms of health care delivery.

Assessment of East German Health Care

From the earliest days, comprehensive health care was a central element in the East German package of promised social benefits. Basic principles included (a) universal medical coverage through a regionally based public health service;[1] (b) a coordinated and interactive network of leading hospitals, secondary hospitals, polyclinics, and miniclinics (*Ambulatoria*); and (c) a strong emphasis on preventive care and early diagnosis, facilitated by service delivery in schools, at the workplace, and in residential complexes. The few systematic attempts to measure public opinion in this authoritarian state found relatively high regard for health care achievements well through the 1970s and early 1980s. Even as late as early 1988, when general public skepticism toward the state had sharply increased, the majority of people surveyed (64%) expressed satisfaction with medical services. By 1989, however, the continuing trend toward public discontent enveloped all areas of regime performance. With increasingly visible shortcomings, satisfaction with health care fell to 41.9%, still a modest decline compared to the broad, spiraling popular turn against the government (Gensicke, 1992).[2]

Chief among citizen complaints were the physical deterioration of hospitals (Dankel, Böhm, & Müller, 1990, pp. 84-90; Sachverständigenrat, 1991, pp. 127-128), the recurrent shortage of specialty (i.e., imported) medications and simple outpatient supplies,[3] and longer waiting times for elective surgery. The elderly and others with chronic or compound medical problems objected to the multiple sources of care: sometimes two or more general practitioners—due to rotating clinic service and high rates of work absences—and perhaps two or more specialty care teams if, for example, the patient had both cardiovascular and gastrointestinal conditions (Harych, 1990; Knoch, 1990; von Appen, 1990).

In April 1990, after the path toward unity had been chosen but few concrete steps had been taken, a survey of Dresden residents nevertheless evoked positive assessments of East German health care from 43.3% of respondents, a surprisingly affirmative result in view of deteriorating conditions and the fact that, even compared to other GDR regions, investment in Dresden area hospitals had long been below average. At the same time, Dresden respondents were evenly divided in their expectations about the coming adoption of the West German health care system. And, in a remarkable departure from past experience, 61.4% expressed a willingness to make out-of-pocket contributions as a way to restore the fiscal viability of the health service (Belau, Böhm, & Müller, 1990.

A large, representative survey in May 1990 yielded an even more affirmative result: Two thirds of the respondents said they were "very satisfied" or "satisfied" with the medical care that they received through their worksite *Ambulatoria* (Hofemann, 1993, p. 27). But soon the momentum of unification altered the prevailing mood, and on the eve of Economic and Social Union, July 1, 1990, an Emnid-Institut survey revealed a poignant dimension of East German public opinion: Though not explicitly rejecting their own system, by a ratio of 65% to 18% East Germans now expressed the belief that health care in the Federal Republic would be superior to the GDR system (*Der Spiegel,* 3 July 1995, p. 43).

Proposals for a Health Care "Merger"

Although the occasion of German unity evoked press comment about a new *Stunde Null*—a "zero-hour," or new beginning, a term generally used to describe the immediate postwar period—there is little to justify such a view of the actual unification process. The GDR had indeed come to an end, but the Federal Republic scarcely hesitated in its grappling with the political agenda of the day. In absorbing the former GDR and accepting six new federal states,[4] the Bonn government eventually had to come to grips with more limited resources and increased demands. Yet the pattern of political contest in the enlarged Germany was characterized by far more continuity than change. A new beginning never took place.

Health care reform had long been on the agenda in the Federal Republic. As early as 1977, the Social Democratic-Liberal coalition government initiated the first of several measures to control rising costs in outpatient care, followed by a reform of hospital payments in 1981. Beginning in 1984, the new Christian Democratic-Liberal coalition government carried the reforms forward, culminating in the Health Care Reform Law of 1988. However, because many participants in the policy process regarded the reforms as incomplete, the *Bundestag* (Federal Assembly) created a special commission to recommend structural changes in the delivery and financing of health (Alber, 1990, pp. 46-49; Frerich & Frey, 1993, pp. 264-277). This report was completed in February 1990, shortly before the March elections in East Germany, which confirmed a rapid course toward German unification. Thus, the "annexation" of *East* Germany became the paramount issue just as the prolonged debate over *West* German health care was approaching a new round of confrontation. Not surprisingly, forces advocating divergent goals in West German health reform sought respective allies in the "new states."

The central issues in the West German health care reform controversy were (a) alleged inequities in the system of differentiated consumer payments to a multitude of sickness funds; (b) continued reliance on fee-for-service principles of remuneration, with a consequent disproportionate growth in medical specialties with higher income potential and a corresponding neglect of preventive care; (c) fragmentation of the entire system of health care delivery, with barriers between outpatient care, hospital care, and rehabilitative-convalescent care. Additional criticism focused on the high frequency and high costs of drug prescriptions and on physicians' indifference to principles of holistic medicine—that is, the general neglect of the emotional and social factors affecting health (Manow-Borgwardt, 1993a, pp. 47-74; Stange, 1994, pp. 291-297).

Unified Regional Sickness Funds

Social policy specialists in the opposition Social Democratic Party (SPD), closely allied with General Local Sickness Funds (AOK), aimed to reduce the cost discrepancies among the many different kinds of funds by promoting cost equalization and larger risk pools. Building on the East German practice of a single, unified sickness fund—in contrast to the West German funds differentiated by class and occupational status—the SPD and AOK proposed transforming the East German sickness fund into six unified funds organized by *Land,* initially as a transitional measure. This proposal quickly evoked the vigorous opposition of the more numerous specialized sickness funds, who saw it as effectively precluding their expansion into the new *Länder* (Stange, 1994, pp. 308-310). Lacking strong support from the (essentially West) German Labor Federation (DGB), which was itself divided by occupation and economic sectors, and from the states and cities of the East, which were in a frenzied state of transition and lacked qualified health-related personnel, the unified-funds proposal was soon discarded (Manow-Borgwardt, 1993a, pp. 5-62).[5]

The swift victory of the major sickness funds is an almost prototypical example of the power of semipublic institutions in the network of German corporatism and their ability to avert policy change that might undermine the prior corporatist balance (Döhler & Manow-Borgwardt, 1992). The subsequent advance of the sickness funds into the new territories enabled them to play a pivotal role in resisting efforts to retain other features of the East German health care system.

Retaining the Polyclinics

A more protracted battle took place over the future role of East Germany's ubiquitous polyclinics in any future system of outpatient care. Before unification, there were 626 polyclinics[6] and another 154 company-polyclinics.[7] In addition, there were more than 1,020 miniclinics (*Ambulatoria*) and 364 company-miniclinics (Sachverständigenrat, 1991, pp. 1-14). In principle, a polyclinic employed at least 50 physicians divided among at least six medical specialties. By sharing equipment and administrative overhead, significant efficiencies could be achieved. Because the bulk of income for polyclinic physicians was a monthly salary, the polyclinics resembled U.S.-style institutional health maintenance organizations[8] in their reliance on salary or capitation compensation rather than fee for service and in their relative emphasis on primary care and preventive medicine. During the 1980s, East German reforms aimed to better develop the polyclinics' potential for more integrated care between primary care physicians and specialists, as well as among specialists themselves.

Despite the chronic financing shortfalls, incomplete reforms, spreading environmental hazards, and mounting personnel shortages, East Germany's polyclinic system delivered a quality of care that compared favorably with West German results on some health indicators (Korbanka, 1990, pp. 120-140; Sachsverständigenrat, 1991, pp. 104-114). Because most shortcomings were identified as financial rather than structural, a post-unity increase in capital outlays to West German levels promised significantly improved results. Consequently, East German health officials and some West German Social Democrats urged that the polyclinics be retained as part of a "pluralistic" approach to health care delivery in the new *Länder.* Among the sickness funds, too, there was some initial interest in preserving the polyclinics as a form of competition with the traditional German medical practice. Although the Unity Treaty stipulated independent medical practice as the preferred delivery mode for primary health care in the long run, subsequent implementing regulations allowed for polyclinics to continue at least through an expected 5-year transition period (Stange, 1994, pp. 305-307).

But once again, corporatist power coalesced to conquer the polyclinic challenge in nearly every arena. The most vigorous opposition to polyclinics came from the Association of Sickness Funds Physicians, which regarded them as a potential threat both to their treasured autonomy in making medical decisions and to their reliance on fee for service to support substantial incomes (Hofemann, 1993). Both the 1988 Health Care Reform and numerous new reform proposals represented an erosion of professional autonomy and a slowdown in the growth of physicians' income; thus, the Physicians' Association was especially wary of any institutional innovation that might disrupt their professional unity.

The frontal assault on the polyclinics took the form of publicly ridiculing their lack of modern equipment and their "outmoded" forms of treatment. The more extreme view condemned the polyclinics as an alien, Soviet invention—although polyclinics had been a growing German phenomenon in the pre-Hitler era and now exist in many places throughout western Europe and North America.

A more devastating, and possibly unintended, blow to the polyclinics resulted from their ambiguous financial situation. The polyclinics faced a tremendous need for short-term capital improvements, as well as a predictable income to cover their operating costs. Given the mammoth infrastructure needs and uncertain revenues of local governments, public investment plans to modernize health care were not forthcoming; in any case, hospitals, not outpatient care, took priority. Of course, private financing was available in principle, but uncertainty over the meaning of the 5-year transition in health care made banks reluctant to grant long-term credit to the polyclinics. On the other hand, for a physician willing to set up an independent practice and affiliate with a sickness fund, the fund itself could assure the bank of an applicant's creditworthiness (Hofemann, 1993, pp. 31-33; Stange, 1994, pp. 312-316).

In addition, there emerged a major discrepancy in projected physicians' incomes between the fee-for-service schedule of the sickness funds and the capitation method of compensating polyclinic physicians. The semipublic sickness funds quickly negotiated a fee-for-service schedule for the new Länder that assured physicians a predictable income, which was only somewhat less than West German levels. But compensation formulas for polyclinic physicians, requiring formal government action, were delayed more than once; when the formulas were finally adopted, they could be expected to yield far lower incomes than the fee-for-service mode (Stange, 1994, pp. 312-313; Wasem, 1993).

Coinciding with the polyclinics' financial uncertainties was the growing perception that the only secure future for physicians lay in joining the Association of Sickness Funds Physicians and entering into a collective contract with the sickness funds. In turn, the sickness funds did nothing to discourage the belief that their need for new physicians was limited and that those who waited too long to join might be left out. Wherever a handful of East German physicians abandoned a polyclinic to found a private practice, others were increasingly likely to follow. As a result, even the better equipped polyclinics found themselves below the threshold of personnel needed to deliver basic health care services. Scarcely 22 months after the Social Union and 19 months after formal unification (October 3, 1990), the fraction of East German physicians in independent practice had soared from 2% to 89% (Hofemann, 1993, pp. 37-38). Of the 11% remaining in polyclinics and miniclinics, many were entering their last years of medical practice and felt no need to abruptly alter their professional habits or acquire new management skills. This chain reaction (Wasem, 1993) has been described by some Western sources as a voluntary choice, with East German physicians simply voting their preference for a "market" approach to health care. If so, it was a choice exercised with no practical alternative.

East Germans and Their New Health Care System

The living circumstances and attitudes of people in the new Federal states have been closely monitored by the Sozialwissenschaftliche Forschungszentrum (SFZ), staffed chiefly by former researchers of the Institute for Social Policy in the East German Academy of Sciences. Assessments of health care were hesitant in the first year of the transformation; then they grew generally more positive. In the transition year of 1991, the SFZ *"Sozialbarometer"* reported that 33% of East Germans were satisfied with their health care, whereas 22% were dissatisfied; thus, health care satisfaction ranked sixth among the 12 items surveyed.[9] One year later, the reported level of satisfaction had jumped to 58%, compared to only 9% dissatisfied; this raised health care to third place among the 12 items. By

1994, further change was nearly imperceptible: 57% and 11% (*Sozialreport,* 1994:3, pp. 3-9).

This positive view is altered somewhat when one considers the responses by East Germans over the age of 60. A parallel SFZ survey of this age group reported health care satisfaction at 49% in 1990 and 1991, increasing to 58% in 1992 but dropping markedly to 35% in 1995. Although declines were registered also for other survey items, the 23% shift in health care satisfaction was unmatched. This downward trend was amplified when a somewhat larger group, those over the age of 50, were asked about their *expectations* of change: With regard to health care, scarcely more respondents expected improvement (36%) than those (33%) who expected deterioration (*Sozialreport,* 1994: 4, pp. 6-9). These findings for seniors were echoed by a later study of all adult ages: Expectations of improved health care fell from a high of 61% in 1991 to only 34% by 1995 (*Sozialreport,* 1995:2, pp. 3-8).

However, none of these emergent downward trends presaged the startling result of the 1995 *Emnid* survey that dramatically reversed the East Germans' earlier comparative assessment of East and West German health care arrangements. Whereas the 1990 survey revealed a 65-to-18 preference for the West German system of health care, the 1995 survey showed a 67-to-23 preference for the previous East German system (*Der Spiegel,* 3 July 1995, p. 43). Although the survey also revealed other areas of public life in which East German attitudes had shifted toward more positive judgments on the past and more negative judgments on the present, the negative shift in the realm of health care was by far the largest.

The causes of this abrupt decline in the evaluations of health care in the new federal states are not self-evident. *Der Spiegel* cited West German scholars in attributing East German attitudes to a generalized "nostalgia" for a GDR past that never was or to a kind of "selective memory" that exaggerates the good and minimizes the bad in past experience. In this view, East Germans are compensating for the loss of identity that came with assimilation into the much larger Federal Republic or, perhaps, for a growing sense of frustration over the failure to assert control over their personal futures.[10] The SFZ *Sozialbarometer* reveals a creeping alienation among the Easterners, who express declining satisfaction with the quality of German public administration and the character of German democracy (*Sozialreport,* 1994:3, pp. 8-9; 1994:4, pp. 6-7). To a significant degree, then, the present negative views of their new health care system probably reflect a broader East German sense of disenchantment and disappointed expectations.

On the other hand, this generalized interpretation does not explain why East German attitudes toward health care are particularly volatile and why there has been a particularly emphatic shift in assessments of health care performance. Clearly, one must take into account the role of practical experience. Apart from housing and daily shopping, health care represents a realm of sometimes frequent and always immediate experience, and it is an especially important part of life.[11] Therefore, one should expect that judgments about health care will typically be concrete.

Unfortunately, none of the surveys currently available attempts to investigate more closely the components of declining health care satisfaction. I can offer only some impressions gathered from a dozen acquaintances during a visit to the new federal states in late 1994.[12] All of those questioned were present or former academics or administrators concerned with some dimension of social policy; compared to the "average" citizen, my acquaintances presumably held higher expectations of health care delivery and were probably more assertive consumers.[13]

Five of the 12 continued to receive health care from the same physicians they had visited before the transformation, and they reported high levels of satisfaction. In each case, the physician had created an independent practice in or near the old polyclinic building. Each claimed that doctor-patient relations remained as collegial as before, although there were sometimes longer waits for appointments. Most also enthusiastically reported a notable improvement in the physical appearance and equipment in the doctor's office.

All of the others had to find new physicians. Except for one young administrator who chose a remaining Berlin polyclinic out of conviction, all others had located physicians in private practice. Although none of my acquaintances or their family members had experienced especially serious medical problems, four reported episodes of dissatisfaction. The common complaint was that office personnel were inflexible in scheduling appointments and did not seem especially "customer oriented." In general, too, the time allotted for office visits was very brief, and physicians seemed reluctant to provide full explanations for medical procedures. In one case, the doctor insisted on repeated visits and tests for a minor problem, which my respondent inferred had more to do with the physician's compensation formula than with standards of care. In a case involving an adolescent family member, an acquaintance expressed dismay at the poor communication between the primary care physician and a specialist, and he objected to the need to transport his ailing child to another part of the city before receiving appropriate treatment.

This unsystematic and highly biased sample does little more than suggest possible avenues for research. At first glance, however, there is some reason to believe that East Germans are experiencing some of the negatives in the conventional German health care system that reformers have long highlighted. Although not addressed by my informal survey, general East German attitudes toward health care may also be affected by negative assessments of health and social provisions for the very young. The implementation of the Health Care Structural Reform Act of 1993 may also change East German perceptions, particularly with respect to the incentives to guide physicians toward less interventionist and less medication-dependent care.

Notes

1. The state-run public health service was supplemented by health activities sponsored by some of the larger employers, who set up clinics at the workplace. Because these employers were also owned by the state, it is accurate for most purposes to regard the entire network as a single integrated system.

2. For example, satisfaction with the environment dropped from 66% in 1987 to 12% in 1989. Only housing and children's services ranked higher than health care in both surveys.

3. Physicians sometimes urged patients to use personal contacts in the West to secure medication. With the growing shortages of surgical dressings, crutches, and other small necessities, outpatients were increasingly left to their own devices (Günther, 1990, p. 51).

4. This involved the transformation of East Germany's 14 counties into five reconstituted *Länder*, plus the newly unified city-state of Berlin. From 1949 to 1990, West Berlin existed under Allied control and thus was not a fully constituent part of the Federal Republic.

5. The local sickness funds, however, did adhere to their regionalization concept in East Germany. Rather than developing many local funds, they organized only six—one for each of the new *Länder*.

6. Polyclinics were not evenly distributed throughout the GDR; there were 41 polyclinics in East Berlin alone.

7. Large, multibranch state companies sometimes helped to fund and organize polyclinics for their employees, especially when companies were established in areas that initially lacked an infrastructure of urban services.

8. An institutional (or staff-model) HMO delivers prepaid care in its own centralized facility, unlike network HMOs, which are merely prepayment insurance arrangements that contract with physicians in independent practice.

9. For all *Sozialbarometer* results, the positive answers are *very satisfied* and *satisfied;* negative answers are *very dissatisfied* and *dissatisfied.* Neutral answers and no responses are not reported.

10. The Emnid Institut survey provides further clues: Large majorities of East Germans defiantly assert pride in their former lives as GDR citizens and judge that the Bonn government has done far too little to promote the equalization of living conditions between East and West (*Der Spiegel,*, 3 July 1995, pp. 49-52).

11. The *SFZ Sozialbarometer* routinely confirms that "a healthy life" ranks near the top of personal values and that the maintenance of future health lies among the leading areas of worry (*Sozialreport,* 1994:4, pp. 5-6).

12. At the time, health care was not a principal focus of my research but only a secondary interest. Consequently, I made no attempt to administer a systematic set of questions.

13. All had university degrees; most were PhDs. Ten were former members of the ruling SED party, one was a former member of the East German Liberal Democrats, and one was a new member of the post-SED Party of Democratic Socialism. During my previous (pre-1989) visits to the GDR, all of these ·acquaintances had expressed political views consistent with those of progressive German or Swedish Social Democrats.

References

Alber, J. (1990). *Das Gesundheitswesen der Bundesrepublik Deutschland.* Frankfurt: Campus.

Belau, D., Böhm, B., & Müller, P. (1990). In W. Theile (Ed.), *Das Gesundheitswesen der DDR: Aufbruch oder Einbruch?* (pp. 42-44). Skt. Augustin: Asgard.

Dankel, G., Böhm, B., & Müller, P. (1990). Bau und Instandhaltung von Einrichtungen des Gesundheits- und Sozialwesens: Zu einigen Aspekten der Kapazitätsermittlung und Bauplanung. In W. Theile (Ed.), *Das Gesundheitswesen der DDR: Aufbruch oder Einbruch?* (pp. 84-91). Skt. Augustin: Asgard.

Döhler, M. (1993). Ordnungspolitische Ideen und sozialpolitische Institutionen. In R. Czada & M. Schmidt (Eds.), *Verhandlungsdemokratie, Interessevermittlung, Regierbarkeit* (pp. 123-141). Opladen: Westdeutscher Verlag.

Döhler, M., & Manow-Borgwardt, P. (1992). Korporatisierung als gesundheitspolitische Strategie. *Staatswissenschaften und Staatspraxis, 3*(1), 64-106.

Frerich, J., & Frey, M. (1993). *Handbuch der Geschichte der Sozialpolitik in Deutschland: Vol. 3. Sozialpolitik in der Bundesrepublik Deutschland bis zur Herstellung der Deutschen Einheit.* Munich: R. Oldenburg.

Gensicke, T. (1992). Mentalitätswandel und Revolution: Wie sich die DDR-Bürger von ihrem System abwandten. *Deutschland Archiv, 25,* 1266-1282.

Günther, E. (1990). Sozialversicherung und ärztliche Tätigkeit. In W. Theile (Ed.), *Das Gesundheitswesen der DDR: Aufbruch oder Einbruch?* (pp. 45-52). Skt. Augustin: Asgard.

Harych, H. (1990). Zur Zukunft der Polykliniken und der ambulanten Versorgung in der DDR. In W. Theile (Ed.), *Das Gesundheitswesen der DDR: Aufbruch oder Einbruch?* (pp. 99-104). Skt. Augustin: Asgard.

Henke, K., & Leber, W. (1994). Territoriale Erweiterung und wettbewerbliche Neuordnung der gesetzlichen Krankenversicherung (GKV). In K.-H. Hansmeyer (Ed.), *Finanzierungsprobleme der deutschen Einheit II* (pp. 12-61). Berlin: Duncker & Humblot.

Hofemann, K. (1993). Die Privatisierung der ambulanten Versorgung: Vom Niedergang der poliklinischen Versorgung in den neuen Ländern. *Jahrbuch für Kritische Medizin: Gesundheitsmärkte, 19,* 24-38.

Jacobs, K., & Schräder, W. (1993). Gesundheitszentren im Land Brandenburg: Zur Modernisierung ambulanter Angebotsstrukturen zwei Jahren nach der deutschen Vereinigung. *Jahrbuch für Kritische Medizin: Gesundheitsmärkte, 19,* 53-65.

Knoch, H. (1990). Das ambulante Operieren. In W. Theile (Ed.), *Das Gesundheitswesen der DDR: Aufbruch oder Einbruch?* (pp. 109-114). Skt. Augustin: Asgard.

Korbanka, C. (1990). *Des Gesundheitswesen der DDR. Darstellung und Effizienzanalyse.* Cologne: Müller Botermann.

Kurz-Scharf, I. (1994). Sozialbarometer. *Sozialreport [SFZ], 3,* 3-7.

Manow, P., & Giaimo, S. (1995, August-September). *Welfare state regimes, globalization, and health care reform.* Paper presented at the annual meeting of the American Political Science Association, Chicago.

Manow-Borgwardt, P. (1993a). *Gesundheitspolitische Entscheidungen im Prozess der deutschen Einigung.* Unpublished doctoral dissertation, Freie Universität, Berlin.

Manow-Borgwardt, P. (1993b). Gesundheitspolitische Entscheidungen im Vereinigungsprozess. *Jahrbuch für Kritische Medizin: Gesundheitsmärkte, 19,* 8-23.

Perschke-Hartmann, C. (1994). *Die doppelte Reform: Gesundheitspolitik von Blüm zu Seehofer.* Opladen: Leske & Budrich.

Sachverständigenrat für Konzertierte Aktion im Gesundheitswesen. (1991). *Das Gesundheitswesen im vereinten Deutschland.* Baden-Baden: Nomos.

Scheuch, K. (1990). Bewahrenswertes im Betriebsgesundheitswesen und der Arbeitsmedizin der DDR. In W. Theile (Ed.), *Das Gesundheitswesen der DDR: Aufbruch oder Einbruch?* (pp. 127-133). Skt. Augustin: Asgard.

Schmidt, P., Hess, C., Laetz, T., & Perez, J. (1994). *German health reforms: Changes result in lower health costs in 1993.* Washington, DC: U.S. General Accounting Office.

Schwarz, F., & Busse, R. (1994). Die Zukunft des deutschen Gesundheitssystem: Vorschläge, Mythen und Aussichten. In B. Blanke (Ed.), *Krankheit und Gemeinwohl* (pp. 403-421). Opladen: Leske & Budrich.

Sozialreport 1994. (4th quarter). Sozialbarometer: Uber fünfzigjährige—ihre Zufriedenheiten, Hoffnungen und Ängste, pp. 4-9.

Stange, K. (1994). Verpasste Reform der ambulanten Versorgung? Die Transformation des Gesundheitssystems in den neuen Bundesländern. In B. Blanke (Ed.), *Krankheit und Gemeinwohl* (pp. 291-325). Opladen: Leske & Budrich.

Statistisches Bundesamt. (1994). *Datenreport 1994.* Bonn: Bundeszentrale für politische Bildung.

Von Appen, D. (1990). Anspruch und Wirklichkeit: Gesundsschutz und ambulante Betreuung. In W. Theile (Ed.), *Das Gesundheitswesen der DDR: Aufbruch oder Einbruch?* (pp. 105-108). Skt. Augustin: Asgard.

Wasem, J. (1993). Strategische Planung oder ungesteuerte Kettenreaktion? Zur Erosion der poliklinischen Einrichtungen in Ostdeutschland nach der Vereinigung. *Jahrbuch für Kritische Medizin: Gesundheitsmärkte, 19,* 39-52.

White, J. (1995). *Competing solutions: American health care proposals and international experience.* Washington, DC: Brookings Institution.

Winkler, G. (1993). Sozialbarometer. *Sozialreport [SFZ], 3,* 4-7.

Winkler, G. (1995). Sozialbarometer. *Sozialreport [SFZ], 2,* 3-7.

PART III

The Canadian Experience

CHAPTER 7

Canadian National Health Insurance

Evolution and Unresolved Policy Issues

CATHERINE A. CHARLES
ROBIN F. BADGLEY

The quest to make access to good health care more equitable was the basis for the gradual development of legislation establishing a Canadian national health insurance program. Its cornerstones were the federal Hospital Insurance and Diagnostic Services Act (1957) and the Medical Care Act (1966). The intent of these measures was reaffirmed by Allan J. MacEachen, Minister of National Health and Welfare, when he introduced the Medical Care Act of 1966 in the House of Commons. He then stated that the government recognized "the fundamental principle that health is not a privilege but rather a basic right which should be open to all" (Canada, House of Commons, 1966a, p. 7545). The provisions of the new act would "insure access to medical care to all of our people regardless of means, of pre-existing conditions, of age or other circumstances which may have barred such access in the past" (p. 7549). The act's terms were fully adopted across Canada by 1971.

Between 1960 and 1970 the share of health expenditures relative to the gross domestic product (GDP) for Canada rose from 5.5% to 7.3%, then leveled out during the mid-1970s and subsequently climbed to 10.1% in the early 1990s before dropping back to 9.5% in 1995 (National Forum on Health, 1997, p. 12; Organisation for Economic Co-operation and Development [OECD], 1988, p. 42). Opinion polls show that Canadians, for the most part, are highly satisfied with their health insurance program (Blendon, 1989; Blendon & Taylor, 1989; Coutts, 1995; Little, 1991), a public program that a succession of federal Ministers of Health and external sources, such as the U.S. General Accounting Office, have rated as being "one of the best in the world" (Bégin, 1988; Canada, House of Commons, 1989, p. 30; Canada, House of Commons, 1995d, p. 15526; Lalonde, 1988).

In recent years, the United Nations Development Programme has consistently ranked Canada near the top internationally on its composite measure of social progress—national income level, adult literacy, and average life expectancy (United Nations Development Programme, 1991, p. 15). Comparatively, Canada has had—and still has—a "generous" health system. Compared to 22 Western industrial nations assessed by the OECD, Canada ranked second at the beginning of the 1960s in its spending on health care as a share of its GDP (OECD, 1988, p. 42). During the next decade, its position dropped to between sixth (1975) and seventh (1980) place, rebounded to between second and third place during the late 1980s and the early 1990s, and ranked fifth in 1995.

With all of the provinces having joined the national program by the early 1970s, the latter part of the decade was a time of expansion and consolidation. The use of health services, the supply of health personnel, and the size of health expenditures as a share of government budgets grew substantially. There was also a deepening concern about growing health care expenditures and the erosion of the philosophical principles on which national health insurance had been founded. Subsequently, the federal government responded by enacting four major legislative changes. First, the Federal-Provincial Established Programs Financing Act of 1977 modified the structure of federal- provincial co-financing arrangements and set limits on the share of the federal contribution. Second, the Canada Health Act of 1984 clarified and strengthened the conditions on which federal payments to the provinces were contingent by imposing financial penalties to ensure reasonable access to health care without economic impediment. Third, the 1990 Federal-Provincial Fiscal Arrangements Act, which was reconfirmed in the 1991 federal budget, limited the per capita cash and tax transfer increases to the provinces until 1994-95 to a level well below the annual rate of growth in provincial spending on health care and advanced education (Canada, House of Commons, 1991a, 1991b, 1991c). Fourth, this precedent was extended under the deficit-reducing targets of the 1995 federal budget, which resulted both in cutbacks and a major restructuring of transfer payments to the provinces. As of April 1996, the Canada Health and Social Transfer consolidated federal contributions for the Canada Assistance Plan with federal contributions for health and postsecondary education. Preserving the objectives and standards of the Canada Health Act while affording more provincial flexibility for initiating social security reforms, funding under this new arrangement represented a phased-in reduction of about 3% in aggregate provincial revenues (Canada, House of Commons, 1995a, pp. 11257-11260; Canada, House of Commons, 1995c, pp. 13103-13106).

During the first 15 years of national health insurance, there was little official review of a number of salient social policy issues relating to federal-provincial cost sharing for health care. For instance, the 1985 Macdonald Commission (Royal Commission on the Economic Union and Development Prospects for Canada, 1985, Vol. 2, Chapter 1), the most comprehensive review of federal- provincial fiscal relations in half a century (since the 1940 Royal Commission on Dominion-Provincial Relations [Rowell-Sirois Commission]) sketched only recent trends in the evolution of government financing of health care. The Report of the 1985 Neilson Task Force (Task Force on Program Review, 1985) noted that up to that time "no formal evaluation of EPF has been done" (p. 69).

During the 1990s, there was widespread and growing support for a reduction in the size of governments and for the elimination of deficit spending from the public purse. Within the context of this evolving change in philosophy about the financing of public programs, it became broadly accepted that major structural changes were required if an affordable Canadian public health insurance program with its current objectives was to be preserved. This perspective was epitomized by former Health Minister Diane Marleau's assessment in 1995 that "it is not more money that is needed in the system; it is a different way of spending" (Canada, House of Commons, 1995d, p. 15524).

Faced with increasing financial pressures, provincial governments shifted their focus from custodians of expansion to managers of a largely supply-side retrenchment of health resources. The changes that evolved included the widespread reduction and, in some cases, reallocation of funding from hospitals to community and social services; the devolution of authority from provincial governments to regional levels; the broader acceptance of a needs-based planning and funding approach for health services, coupled with the development of better health information systems for planning and performance evaluation; an erosion of the autonomy of the medical profession; and a withdrawal by government from the direct delivery of certain services in favor of a role as strategic manager of the core business of health care. Relative to these emerging trends, this review traces the development of national health insurance legislation in Canada and describes the continuing social policy debate over the funding and restructuring of health services.

Evolution of the National Health Insurance Program

The historical record shows that the interplay of social, economic, and political forces has greatly affected the timing and nature of government involvement in funding health care in Canada. The main contours of the health care system have been molded by a long-standing debate over the division of constitutional responsibilities between the federal and provincial governments, the balancing of public and private sector input, and the state of the economy at different points in the country's history.

The precedent of colonial or provincial assemblies providing financial support for charities and hospitals was well established before Confederation in 1867. With the exception of the Maritime colonies, which had enacted legislation in the tradition of the Elizabethan Poor Laws, the regimes in Lower and Upper Canada were then providing a substantial share of the funding for the maintenance of hospitals and the care of the indigent sick (Province of Canada, 1894, pp. 113-175). Under the terms of the British North America Act of 1867, which established the constitutional division of authority, health care was designated primarily as a provincial responsibility, with residual powers accruing to the federal government. The conventional interpretation for this assignment of powers, as reflected in the accounts of several subsequent royal commissions (Royal Commission on Dominion-Provincial Relations, 1940; Royal Commission on Health Services, 1964; Royal Commission on the Economic Union and Development Prospects for Canada, 1985), is that minimal provincial funding was given to health care in the 1800s and that the health needs of the population were largely met by families and charities. In fact, however, Ontario and Quebec were already active in the funding of health care at this time. With the assumption of provincial debts by the federal government under the terms of Confederation

(1867), these provinces had sufficient tax revenues to increase their contributions for health services.

In Ontario, eight of nine hospitals received legislative grants-in-aid in 1866, which, in the case of the Kingston General Hospital, accounted for about 90% of its operating budget (Gibson, 1935). Five years later, the revenues of the 10 hospitals in Ontario were heavily dependent on government support: 64.2%, provincial legislature; 12.9%, municipalities; 10.3%, paying patients; and the remainder from endowments and public subscriptions (Ontario Legislative Assembly, 1873, pp. 66-67). Sir John A. Macdonald, who represented Kingston in the Legislative Assembly and subsequently in Parliament as the new dominion's first prime minister, was well informed about his local hospital's reliance on public funding, which he deemed "unwise" and serving to cool "the enthusiasm of charitably minded citizens" (Kennedy, 1955, p. 44).

As the country's population grew and its economic base expanded, the level of financial support for hospitals provided by the Quebec and Ontario governments declined, but a similar sequence of events evolved during the early development of western Canada. Replacing the tradition of more substantial government support that had developed in the colonial period and had continued following Confederation, what gradually evolved was a residual concept of social welfare—namely, that the needs of individuals were properly met by their families or marketplace forces. Under this philosophy, social welfare programs, including health care, were to be initiated only as a residual obligation of government at times when the viability of the family and the economy was in jeopardy (Wilensky & Lebeaux, 1965, p. 139).

The British North America Act assigned major taxing powers to the federal government, an arrangement that, in light of the recently concluded American Civil War (1861-1865), was intended to create a strong and unified nation. As social priorities and economic circumstances changed through time, this meant that the provinces had jurisdictional authority for health care but lacked the taxing power to finance large-scale health insurance programs. In turn, the federal government, with its broad taxation powers, lacked the constitutional authority to operate such programs directly. Much of the history of government health insurance programs in Canada, particularly since the 1930s, has revolved around attempts to resolve this constitutional dilemma.

By World War I, the costs of health care were largely borne by individuals and municipalities, with some provincial support. The first federal proposals for a national health insurance program were made in 1919 by the Liberal Party (King, 1973). However, no action was taken.

The devastating impact of the Great Depression of the 1930s on the health of the poor was documented in several studies. In the classic report, *Health and Unemployment: Some Studies of Their Relationships,* Marsh, Grant, and Blackler (1938) concluded that "if medical care is a contingency left to each individual to secure as best he can, it becomes a function of the distribution of wealth" (p. 216). During this period, the federal government's attempt to introduce relief measures was rejected by the Judicial Committee of the British Privy Council on the grounds of infringing on provincial jurisdictional rights. In response, the Royal Commission on Dominion-Provincial Relations (Rowell- Sirois) was appointed to review how deadlocks in constitutional negotiations might be resolved. Several public medical relief programs were also started in the 1930s, and health insurance legislation was enacted but not implemented in Alberta. A similar measure was thwarted by the opposition of the medical profession in British Columbia.

The commission tabled its report in 1940 at the beginning of World War II. It concluded that the introduction of a national health insurance program was feasible, being contingent on federal contributions, with the provinces retaining responsibility for the administration of services (Grauer, 1939; Royal Commission on Dominion-Provincial Relations, 1940). Looking ahead to the end of the war, Ian MacKenzie, the federal Minister of Pensions and National Health, initiated discussions at the Dominion Council of Health in May 1941 on national measures to strengthen public health and medical care (MacKenzie, 1944). An Advisory Committee on Health Insurance was struck in February 1942. It presented a comprehensive draft health insurance bill in March 1943, whose terms were endorsed by 15 national health organizations, including the Canadian Medical Association (Special Committee on Social Security, 1943).

The legislative social security proposals presented to a series of federal-provincial conferences between August 1945 and May 1946 were influenced in part by the signing of the Atlantic Charter, a utopian vision of the postwar world, and a growing recognition of the extent of illness and its effects (reflected in statistics presented by Marsh and his colleagues on the rejection rate of armed forces recruits during World War II). Under the terms of this comprehensive legislative package, the provinces would cede personal income and corporate taxes in exchange for the federal administration of a national social security program, including health insurance. These proposals were accepted by all of the provinces except Quebec and Ontario. Their rejection stemmed from their refusal to relinquish taxation powers under their jurisdiction and to separate taxing from spending authority between levels of government. This setback was seen by Prime Minister Mackenzie King as a temporary roadblock. He confided in his diary at the time that "I had never dreamt a national programme . . . to be a matter of a year or two but that it would take years to establish a national minimum" (Pickersgill & Forster, 1970, p. 216).

Though no further attempts were made to enact comprehensive national health insurance, what evolved over the next two decades was the phased introduction of a national program. During the late 1940s, it was estimated that there was a national shortage of about 60,000 hospital beds, and a Gallup poll in 1947 found that two thirds of Canadians wanted more hospitals and free clinics (Taylor, 1973). In 1948, the federal government introduced one component of its earlier proposals, which provided health grants for hospital construction, health personnel training, and the mounting of health surveys to identify needs for planning services. As Willard (1959) noted, "From the inception of the program to September 30, 1959, assistance had been approved for 48,599 active treatment beds, 8,058 chronic and convalescent beds, and 10,575 bassinets" (p. 608).

During the 1940s and 1950s, voluntary health insurance plans (sponsored primarily by local medical and hospital associations) spread rapidly. Provincially sponsored and funded health insurance programs for low-income and high-risk groups were also developed. Saskatchewan under the Co-operative Commonwealth Federation (CCF) government, led by Tommy Douglas, implemented the first universal, publicly funded hospital insurance plan in 1947. Comparable programs were started by British Columbia in 1949 and Alberta in 1950.

In 1953, the federal government expanded its program of health grants to include maternal and child health, rehabilitation, and diagnostic and radiological services. Though views in the federal cabinet were sharply divided on the issue, during the election of that year, the Liberal government promised to introduce national hospital insurance when a majority of the provinces were prepared to join such a scheme. No action was taken due to Prime Minister St. Laurent's philosophy that "the federal government should not undertake responsibilities in any field better handled by the provinces" (Martin, 1985, p. 23). His assumption that the major provincial players would not willingly cede powers was challenged when the Conservative government of Ontario endorsed a national program. Hospital operating expenditures in Ontario had risen by 175% (nominal dollars) between 1947 and 1954. An initial annual surplus of 3.3% had fallen to a 3.7% deficit during the same 8-year period (Canada, House of Commons, 1957a, pp. 2646-2647).

The financial formula of the Hospital Insurance and Diagnostic Services Bill tabled in Parliament in the spring of 1957 was designed to redress the regional imbalance in the distribution of hospital services, particularly in the Maritimes (Canada, House of Commons, 1957a, pp. 2642-2681; 1957b, pp. 3096-3124; 1957c, pp. 3237-3252; 1957d, pp. 1235-1270; 1957e, pp. 1283-1301). The debate focused on two key issues: the exclusion from coverage of services already provided for by the provinces (tuberculosis sanatoria and mental health facilities) and whether adoption of the act should be contingent on its acceptance by a majority of the provinces (six), or those representing a majority of the population. No attention was paid to the implications of introducing national hospital insurance before full medical care coverage or the potential displacement impact of the excluded services being rechanneled to fall within the orbit of insured hospital benefits.

The legislation was unanimously enacted by Parliament on April 10, 1957 (Canada, 1957). The election, two months later, of a minority Conservative government delayed its implementation until July 1958. An immediate by-product was the decision in 1959 of the CCF socialist government of Saskatchewan to act on its long-standing pledge to develop a medical care insurance program, a step facilitated by the infusion of new federal funding for hospital insurance. This triggered an acrimonious confrontation with the Saskatchewan medical profession and led to the federal government appointment in 1961 of the Royal Commission on Health Services (Royal Commission on Health Services, 1964) to inquire into the country's future need for health services. Following a bitter doctors' strike of 23 days, Saskatchewan's pioneering universal medical care plan started in 1962 (Badgley & Wolfe, 1967).

During the next 6 years, the country was led by a succession of three minority governments. In the first of its two terms in power, the Liberal government was divided between extending social security programs and maintaining the stability of government expenditures. Two events that tipped the balance in favor of the former were the prospect of a continuing electoral stalemate at the polls and the 1964 Hall Report, which called for a national medical care insurance program. According to Prime Minister Pearson, the government's commitment to introduce such legislation during the 1965 federal election was to ensure that the socialist "NDP doesn't make all the running with social welfare issues. . . . We have stolen some of their clothes while they were bathing in holy water" (quoted in Munro & Inglis, 1975, p. 200).

The intent of the social reform legislation tabled in Parliament during 1965-66 (Medical Care Bill, Canada Assistance Plan, increased Guaranteed Income Supplements for the Aged, and the Health Resources Fund Bill) was "the elimination of poverty among our people" (Canada, House of Commons, 1965, p. 2). To be eligible for federal funding for medical

care, provinces had to insure comprehensive coverage of medically necessary services, accessible to provincial residents on uniform terms and
conditions with portability of benefits and public administration. The new
measure was also intended to redress regional disparities in the distribution of services "irrespective of ability to pay" (Canada, House of Commons, 1966a, pp. 7544-7545).

To permit the development of provincial programs during the first 5
years of their operation, the co-financing agreement was to remain
open-ended. Thereafter, according to Mitchell Sharp, then Minister of
Finance, the terms of the funding arrangement would be revised to accord
with the equalization formula of payments made by the federal government to the provinces for established co-financed programs (Canada,
House of Commons, 1966b). The Medical Care Act was passed by a vote
of 177 to 2 on December 6, 1966, with its terms coming into force on
July 1, 1968. By 1971, all provincial governments had joined the national
program.

From Cost-Shared to Block Funding

The 1964 Hall Report (Royal Commission on Health Services, 1964)
had forecast that following the introduction of national health insurance,
there would be an initial increase in government expenditures for health
care, followed by a leveling off as unmet needs were provided for.
However, the cost-sharing formula established by the 1966 Medical Care
Act soon came under attack. Concerned about the open-ended nature of
the funding formula and rising expenditures, the federal government
began to lobby for a change that would limit federal expenditures for
health care to the annual growth rate of the GDP instead of increasing in
line with provincial health care expenditures (Carter, 1977). The provinces, in turn, argued that the 50-50 cost-sharing arrangement restricted
their flexibility to provide less costly services because federal funds were
tied to specific programs (e.g., insured benefits for hospital and medical
care).

After protracted negotiations, the federal government introduced the
Federal-Provincial Fiscal Arrangements and Established Programs Financing Act (EPF) in 1977, a measure encompassing both health and postsecondary education. Under the new financing formula, the provinces received a per capita block grant (cash) linked to changes in the growth of
the population and the GDP, plus a transfer of tax points from the federal
government. Equalization payments were made to the poorer provinces
to apportion the yield of the tax transfers relative to the national average.
Per capita grants (increased annually according to GDP increases) were

also provided for extended health care benefits, and provinces were offered a transitional allocation so that they would not suffer financially as a result of the new fiscal changes (Parliamentary Task Force on Federal-Provincial Fiscal Arrangements, 1981, p. 68). The new formula realized the federal intent of developing a funding mechanism on which Ottawa's contribution would be calculated independently of provincial health spending, and the change to block-grant funding gave the provinces greater flexibility to support a broader range of health care programs.

Though moving toward a policy of equalizing federal assistance across provinces, the EPF arrangements initially favored certain wealthier provinces, where the tax points transferred from the federal government yielded a "fiscal dividend" (MacEachen, 1981, p. 37). In 1982, the method of calculating the federal contribution was changed to eliminate this advantage. Under the new method, the federal per capita grant became the residual of the yield from the tax points and the equalization formula up to a maximum amount such that the total dollars per capita provided by the federal government would be equal across all provinces.

Three major issues emerged during the late 1970s and the early 1980s in response to the perceived impact of the new EPF fiscal arrangements: (a) allegations that the federal government's share of the funding for provincial health insurance programs was declining under EPF; (b) charges that the shift to block funding had diminished the federal presence in health care and that some provinces were allowing the program's conditions to erode; and (c) the contention that provincial governments were diverting federal funds intended for health care to other programs.

The debate over underfunding centered, in large part, on an alleged decline in federal funding to the provinces under EPF. Provincial governments and the Canadian Medical Association were major advocates of the underfunding claim (Baltzan, 1982, pp. 9-11). The Canadian Hospital Association argued that more information was needed before a claim of underfunding could be proved or disproved (Canada, House of Commons, 1984). A central issue often lost in the debate over underfunding was the nature of the policy outcomes to be achieved from federal-provincial cost-sharing arrangements. As well, there was sharp disagreement between federal and provincial governments over the validity of statistics relating to changes over time in the share of the federal contribution to the provinces under EPF as a proportion of total provincial health spending (Alberta Hospitals & Medical Care, 1983; National Health & Welfare Canada, 1983).

A second issue was the alleged increase in physician extra billing and user fees. The federal government feared that private funding of health care (e.g., through extra billing and user charges) was increasing, leading to divergent standards of accessibility and an erosion of the federal government's role in maintaining this national standard. To preserve the principles initially established for national health insurance, the federal government subsequently introduced the Canada Health Act in 1984 (see next section).

Allegations that the provinces were diverting federal funding intended for health care to other purposes became the third contentious issue during this period because under block funding, federal contributions were no longer tied to specific programs. To review this matter and other related issues, the federal government turned in 1979 to Mr. Justice Hall, who had chaired the 1964 Royal Commission on Health Services. Completed in 1980, Hall's report concluded that the allegations of provincial diversion of funds were unfounded. The report, however, provided scant evidence either to support or to refute this conclusion (Hall, 1980). Two other reviews published in the early 1980s significantly contributed to the debate over underfunding and accessibility. The report, *Health: A Need for Redirection,* prepared by a task force of the Canadian Medical Association, found that "nearly all Canadians are in favour of our universal publicly funded health care system" (Canadian Medical Association, 1984a, p. xii). On the question of underfunding, the task force concluded:

> Because the evidence is contradictory and inconclusive, the Task Force does not support the contention that there is underfunding generally in Canada. However, the regional disparities in the range of health care services available point to the need for additional assistance to be given to the poorer provinces. (Canadian Medical Association, 1984a, p. 116)

The task force noted that continued restraints on capital expenditures might adversely affect the quality of medical services and that because of projected increases in the elderly population, a policy of deinstitutionalization should be devised if health care costs were to remain a manageable share of the GNP. What constituted a "manageable" share of the GNP was not specified.

A second report, *Fiscal Federalism in Canada* (Parliamentary Task Force, 1981), was prepared in 1981 by an all-party parliamentary task force. This committee's mandate was to review the programs authorized by the EPF Act, "focusing, in particular, on fiscal equalization, the tax collection agreements, the Canada Assistance Plan and Established Programs Financing" (Parliamentary Task Force on Federal-Provincial Fiscal Arrangements, 1981, pp. xiii-xiv). The majority of members of the Parliamentary Task Force recommended that extra billing by physicians be banned, that provinces develop mechanisms to ensure reasonable compensation for physicians, and that, when negotiations failed, the issues in dispute be submitted to binding arbitration. The Task Force concluded that, in aggregate, Ottawa's funding for health care was adequate but that there should be no further reductions in federal support.

Despite this latter recommendation, the federal government announced plans during the 1980s to limit increases in transfer payments to the provinces. Under the federal Expenditure Control Plan, major cash and tax transfers to the provinces for social programs were projected to be limited to an annual growth of about 3.7%. In contrast, all other federal program spending was limited to a 3.4% annual increase up to 1995-96 (Canada, House of Commons, 1991a, pp. 17684-17697; Canada, House of Commons, 1991b, pp. 18653-18657). Because the growth rate of the federal transfers for health fell short of annual increases in provincial health care spending (which, in the case of Ontario had increased at an average yearly rate of 11.3% during the 1980s) (Ontario Ministry of Health, 1992, pp. 6-7), the federal decision was criticized by the provinces as representing the death knell of national health insurance. A continuing decline in the federal contribution as a proportion of total provincial health care expenditures was seen to lessen the federal government's leverage to persuade provinces to maintain national program standards.

The Canada Health Act, 1984

The Canada Health Act developed by the federal government was designed to make provincial governments recommit themselves to the principle of health insurance as a national program providing medically necessary health care accessible to all on uniform terms and conditions regardless of ability to pay. The act, passed in 1984, clarified and strengthened the existing principles of the national health insurance program and provided explicit financial sanctions for provinces failing to meet these. These provisions were clearly influenced by the reports of the 1980 Hall Commission and the 1981 Parliamentary Task Force.

Deputy Prime Minister Allan J. MacEachen wrote in 1981 that "there is every reason to believe that federal-provincial agreement [on the Canada Health Act] can be reached quickly" (MacEachen, 1981, p. 38). In fact, the debate over the substance and justification of the new bill was protracted and acrimonious. Major concerns raised by the provinces included allegations that the bill represented an infringement on provincial jurisdiction over health; that the bill did not address a major problem, underfunding; and that the federal government had not sufficiently consulted with the provinces in developing the proposed legislation and in responding to their proposals (Canada, House of Commons, 1984a).

The Canada Health Act of 1984 replaced the Hospital Insurance and Diagnostic Services Act and the Medical Care Act. To be eligible for the full federal cash contribution for insured health services, the provinces had to meet the program's clarified conditions of universality, comprehensiveness, accessibility, public administration, and portability. In some cases, these conditions were strengthened. The new universality criterion, for example, required provinces to insure all eligible residents instead of 95%. More important, if a province continued to allow extra billing and user fees, the act provided for a nondiscretionary reduction in the cash portion of the federal contribution by the amount charged through these practices.

Setting in motion a new era in federal-provincial legislative and fiscal relations, the act reasserted the national presence in health care, reaffirmed the conditions of the original health insurance legislation, and provided clear-cut and forceful federal fiscal sanctions against defaulting provinces (Canada, House of Commons, 1984b). The act also fueled the long-standing debate over federal-provincial constitutional jurisdiction in health affairs.

Staunchly opposed to the act, the Canadian Medical Association and the Ontario Medical Association challenged its legality, although both associations subsequently withdrew their challenges. From a different perspective, the act was also sharply criticized for its failure to expand the scope of insured services and to address directly ways of improving effectiveness and efficiency in the provision of health care.

Under the Canada Health Act, provinces "must provide for insured health services on uniform terms and conditions and on a basis that does not impede or preclude, either directly or indirectly whether by charges made to insured persons or otherwise, reasonable access to those services by insured persons" (Clause 12). The act had a substantial impact. Following its passage, several provinces (e.g., Nova Scotia, New Brunswick, Ontario, Manitoba, Saskatchewan, and Alberta) banned extra billing, although other provinces (e.g., Quebec and British Columbia) had already taken legislative steps in this area before passage of the act (Government of Saskatchewan, 1985a, 1985b; Health and Welfare Canada, 1985a, 1985b; Heiber & Deber, 1987). Provinces still allowing extra billing following enactment of the act faced considerable fiscal pressure to terminate this practice but in turn had to contend with formidable opposition (as in the case of Ontario in 1986) from the medical profession.

Although extra billing and user charges had not been completely eliminated across Canada, by the late 1990s the Canada Health Act had largely attained its intended purpose of minimizing the extent of these practices. In the mid-1990s, a highly visible and acrimonious controversy took place between the federal and Alberta governments over the issue of user fees. Approximately 35 clinics in Alberta providing a hybrid of services and procedures were charging patients a "facility fee" to offset overhead costs (Gray, 1996). Meanwhile, physicians practicing in these facilities were billing the provincial medical care program for their fees. In 1995, federal Minister of Health Diane Marleau warned the provinces that such charges collected in addition to public funding were contrary to the principles of the Canada Health Act (Canada, House of Commons, 1995a, pp. 11256-11257). In October 1995, Ottawa began withholding its share of federal transfer payments to the Alberta government in proportion to the "overhead" charges levied to patients by the clinics. Eventually, the Alberta government backed down but placated the clinics by agreeing to pay the facility fee out of provincial government funds. Although the federal government was able to stem provincial challenges to the Canada Health Act principles during this period, such challenges will undoubtedly persist.

The gradual chipping away of the public system of national health insurance has been further underscored by the recommendation in 1995 from all provincial health ministers that the concept of "medically necessary services" under the terms of the Canada Health Act be explicitly defined ("How Medicare Can Be Saved," 1995). This would enable the provincial governments to off-load to the private sector those services not defined as medically necessary. A definition of *medically necessary services* as the minimum federal floor of service entitlement has now become the provinces' preferred ceiling of service entitlement on the grounds that this is all that provincial governments can afford (Charles, Lomas, Giacomini, Bhatia, & Vincent, 1998). The meaning of *medical necessity* and the development of appropriate processes and structures to define it have become contentious health policy issues in the 1990s, engaging the attention of many national health care stakeholders such as the Canadian Medical Association (Canadian Healthcare Association, 1996; Canadian Medical Association, 1994a; Health Action Lobby, 1994; Wilson, Rowan, & Henderson, 1995).

Canada Health and Social Transfer, 1996

The events dominating the political landscape during the first half of the 1990s were the continuing specter of Quebec's potential separation from Canada; the recession, which dampened the rate of the economy's growth below that of public sector spending; and a strong neoconservative populist shift in outlook among the electorate, demanding less taxation and supporting a sharp reduction in government spending. Journalist Peter Newman (1995) described the decades after World War II as an era during which government promised entitlement to "universal access to government largesse from womb to tomb" (pp. 290-291). As this generous package of benefits became more deeply entrenched, it was also increasingly subsidized by deficit financing by the provincial and federal governments.

The annual rate of increase in total national public health care spending averaged 11.2% between 1975 and 1991, then dropped to about 3% between 1992 and 1994 (Health Canada, 1996a, pp. 24, 34). The comparable rates for provincial government health expenditures averaged between 7% and 18% during most of this period before leveling off to an average increase of 4.8% in 1992, 1.1% in 1993, and −1.0% in 1994. Despite a decline in these rates during the 1990s, they continued to outstrip the annual rate of growth in the Canadian economy. Faced with public debt levels that during the decade had doubled at the federal level and tripled in the instance of Ontario (Eves, 1995), Canadian jurisdictions responded in the mid-1990s by either tabling balanced budgets or implementing deficit reduction plans.

The 1995 federal budget projected a decrease in spending of 7.3% between 1995 and 1998, which, if maintained, would reduce Ottawa's annual borrowing requirements to about 1.7% of GDP (Canada, House of Commons, 1995a, pp. 11251-11260; Canada, House of Commons, 1995c, pp. 13103-13105). The federal deficit budget reduction plan also included decreases in federal transfer payments to the provinces for health, postsecondary education, and welfare by 8.5% for 1996-97 and 15.2% for 1997-98. These reductions were criticized by those seeking to preserve the country's social safety net as destroying national programs and standards. Opposition was rather more muted than might have been expected, however, for the cuts levied were lower than those imposed on other sectors and on the administration of the federal government itself (Hurley, Bhatia, & Markham, 1995).

The new consolidated block payment program, called the Canada Health and Social Transfer, was introduced in April 1996. It has continued the policy started a decade earlier of partially deindexing each federal transfer to the provinces as well as continuing to channel payments by means of ceded tax points and cash transfers. The overall objectives of the Canada Health Act are retained within the framework of the 1996 legislation, although the former act's nondiscretionary economic sanctions were replaced by penalties to be determined in each instance at the discretion of the federal Cabinet.

After a decade and a half of fairly consistent increases in the share of total national health expenditures to the GDP, Canada appears to be entering a period of stabilization at a lower level of health spending. The recent cutbacks in federal transfers are in tune with historical trends that have seen the federal government's share of provincial health expenditures decline from 38% in 1988 to 33% in 1994 (Canada, House of Commons, 1995b, pp. 11851-11853; 1995c, pp. 13092-13094). Should further cuts occur, the fiscal power of the federal government to monitor provincial adherence to the national health insurance standards will decrease. Concerns raised by a number of health-related organizations about this issue have led the federal government to establish a guaranteed cash floor below which cash transfers to the provinces will not be allowed to fall. The intent of this policy is to preserve the federal government's role as the guardian of national program standards.

Health Resources

Hospital Services

Hospitals across Canada are in the process of seeing their position as the centerpiece of the health care system diminishing. John Stoeckle (1995) observed in his perceptive essay "The Citadel Cannot Hold" that hospitals are gradually becoming "an adjoining, participating institution available for the acute and seriously disabled and sick" with the center shifting to "community practices and to their missions" (p. 13). The changes perceived as reducing the need for inpatient beds and enabling shorter hospital stays include location of substantially more diagnostic technology in nonhospital community sites, a substantial increase in the use of day surgery, more extensive use of quickly performed testing procedures, greater reliance on rehabilitative follow-up care, more efficient hospital administration, and changes in community care. The growing belief among provincial governments that the overall level of hospitalization of the population can be contained without serious jeopardy to health status has led governments to make substantial funding cuts in this sector while redirecting funds to other health priorities.

Changes over time in public expenditures on hospital care are reflected in trend statistics. Between 1974 and 1994, the number of hospital beds and patient days per 100,000 population declined respectively by 17.1% and 23.6%. While the average public sector health expenditure per patient-day in hospital rose from $223.89 in 1975 to $827.61 in 1994, total spending on hospitals as a share of total health expenditures declined from 45.0% to 37.3% (Health Canada, 1996a, pp. 18-19; Health Canada, 1996b, Tables 4c, 6b).

Before the introduction of public national health insurance, Canada and the United States spent approximately the same proportion of their national incomes on health care (Evans, Lomas, & Barer, 1989; Health Canada, 1996a, Figure 1). Subsequently, the United States has spent proportionately more, particularly since the end of the 1980s. One factor contributing to this difference is that Canadian provincial governments have been responsible for approving and funding almost all of each hospital's operating budget. Before the recent development of regional boards mandated to allocate funds across health services within their jurisdiction, annual budgets were negotiated between the ministry and each hospital. In addition, all new capital plans, renovations, and technology acquisitions were approved by provincial health ministries. This centralized control meant that hospitals, in general, lacked access to other major sources of funds for expanding operating programs, equipment, technology, and capital projects (Ball, 1991). In their day-to-day operations, hospitals were limited to operating within the overall global budget negotiated with each provincial health ministry and often dictated by government-wide Treasury Board guidelines.

The situation in Ontario exemplifies some of these more general hospital funding trends. In 1992, the provincial government announced that hospitals would receive only a 1% increase in funding over the next year, followed by a 2% increase over the following 2 years, despite increases to hospital costs deriving from a wage settlement with the Ontario Nurses Association and meeting pay equity obligations. Government attempts to control hospital costs subsequently led to several reactions from the hospital sector: (a) an accumulation of annual deficits with the (increasingly futile) hope that these would be picked up by provincial governments; (b) attempts to introduce more rational planning into the hospital system through mechanisms such as clinical budgeting, physician impact analysis, utilization reviews, quality assurance, an expanded role for physicians as resource managers, and a variety of joint planning ventures between hospitals (for articles reviewing these strategies, see Botz & Singh, 1985; Carlow & Rea, 1988; Charles & Roberts, 1994; Linton, Butts, & Atkinson, 1987; Linton & Peachey, 1989; MacLeod & Deane, 1984; McCutcheon, 1988; Murray, Jick, & Bradshaw, 1984; Ontario Hospital Association, 1991; Parfrey, Gillespie, McManamon, & Fisher, 1986); and (c) the downsizing of hospitals through bed closures and staff cutbacks.

In tabling its 1995 financial plan to achieve a balanced budget by the year 2000, the newly elected Conservative government in Ontario introduced a stiffer program of cutbacks in hospital funding than its New Democratic Party (socialist) predecessor. Overall, government expenditures were projected to be cut by 28% (Ontario Ministry of Finance, 1995). Though the government promised to retain the 1995 level of provincial government health spending, payments to hospitals specifically were scheduled to be scaled back by 18% between 1995 and 1998 (5% in 1996-97, 6% in 1997-98, and 7% in 1998-99). In line with the shift toward providing more day surgery and ambulatory services, the provincial government subsequently set a goal of reducing the number of acute care beds to 2.5 per 1,000 population for 1997 (Canadian College of Health Service Executives, 1997, p. 30). With about 20% of the province's hospital beds already withdrawn from use, this goal suggested the prospect of extensive hospital closures and mergers, personnel reductions in the provincial Ministry of Health, and lower staff-to-patient ratios. The government's Health Services Restructuring Commission, empowered to close hospitals, recommended in 1997 that Toronto's hospitals be cut from 44 to 32 (Health Services Restructuring Commission, 1997). Though the amount of the savings in expenditures remains to be seen and may not be of the magnitude envisioned (Markham & Lomas, 1995), the Ontario government has maintained that it will use the hospital savings realized to improve access to services for rural and northern communities, expand community home care services, and meet the growing demand for long-term care facilities (Ontario Ministry of Health, 1996b; Wilson, 1996).

In addition to facing budget cutbacks, hospital governance has been radically restructured by reforms involving the regionalization of health and social services. In 9 of the 10 provinces, much of the decision-making responsibility for allocating health care resources has been devolved to regional boards. Involving provincial governments from across the political spectrum, these steps included

- The closure of 52 of 132 hospitals by a social democratic government in Saskatchewan and the consolidation of over 300 health boards into 30 district boards ("Again, Common Sense," 1996)
- The dissolution of 51 hospital boards into eight regional hospital corporations by a middle-of-the-road government in New Brunswick (Reamy, 1995)
- The creation of 17 regional health authorities by a conservative government in Alberta (Alberta Health, 1995, p. 3)

In its 3-year Business Plan for 1995-98, Alberta's provincial government called for "sustaining essential treatment services under a value-for-money orientation to the health system" within a framework of an integrated service delivery organized on a regional basis (Alberta Health, 1995, pp. 3, 15). The regional health authorities established in 1995 are "responsible for allocating funds for a wide range of health services" with hospitals to be managed jointly in conjunction with home care and community mental health services (Alberta Health, 1995, p. 16).

Though it is clear that provincial government priorities have shifted to the community health sector, the extent to which such downsizing policies at the level of individual hospitals have been preceded by sufficient evaluation of health resources and displacement consequences is not fully known. Many of these decisions appear to be a somewhat quick and arbitrary response to fiscal constraints. As pressures to control expenditures continue, the hospital sector's domain is likely to become further eroded in terms of its share of total health spending and its autonomy of governance.

The new regional health boards developing across Canada are in different stages of implementation. For the most part, they receive global budget funding from their respective provincial governments, usually based on (but somewhat lower than) historical spending levels for the population being served. (Lomas, Woods, & Veenstra, 1997). Though some provinces have expressed interest in a needs-based per capita funding approach, the Saskatchewan government has moved the furthest in this direction.

Regional boards established by the provinces are typically delegated responsibility for planning, priority setting, allocating funds, and managing services within a provincially defined set of core program areas. The scope of services included within the mandate of each board varies by province, from hospital care only in New Brunswick to a range of health and social services in Prince Edward Island. As of the late 1990s, no province had included doctors or drugs in the devolution process. The relationship of doctors to the regional boards varies by province. Medical associations such as the Canadian Medical Association (CMA) have encouraged doctors to become well positioned to influence regional board activities (Canadian Medical Association, 1995).

Physicians' Services

During the 1970s and 1980s, per capita public expenditures for physicians' services in Canada increased steadily from $78.12 in 1975 to $229.87 in 1985 to $307.97 in 1989. This represented an annual percentage increase of 9% to 11% (1975-1979); 13% to 15% (1980-1983); and 5% to 10% (1984-1989). Nationally, public sector expenditures on physicians' services per capita reached a high of $364.64 in 1992 but subsequently declined to $349.50 in 1994. In 1993 and 1994, for the first time in the history of the national medical care program, the annual percentage change in per capita physician expenditures decreased rather than increased (Health Canada, 1996b, Tables 4c, 6b). Physician expenditures as a proportion of total Canadian health expenditures remained fairly stable between 1974 and 1994 at approximately 15%.

At the inception of the national medical care program, provincial governments, for the most part, adopted the schedule of physician service benefits used up until that time by the voluntary medical care insurance plans developed by physicians in most provinces. Each medical association negotiated with its respective provincial government the size of the overall fee increase for physicians' services. Allocations of the fee increase across medical fee items for each specialty were undertaken internally by each provincial medical association.

Early efforts by the provincial governments to contain the costs of medical care were directed at attempts to negotiate smaller increases in the overall price of medical services (i.e., in the overall fee increase). Over time, however, provincial governments learned that this would not, in and of itself, control total government medical care expenditures because increases due to expansion in the average quantity of services delivered per physician and in physician supply were not taken into account. Public expenditures for medical care remained unpredictable and open-ended, with frequent cost overruns absorbed by the respective provinces.

By the mid-1980s, provincial governments began intensifying their efforts at cost control by focusing during fee negotiations on the average incomes of physicians—the product of fee (price) and quantity (utilization) increases (Lomas, Charles, & Greb, 1992). The negotiation of an agreed-on allowable percentage increase in the utilization component (as well as in the price component) for medical care expenditures reflected the provincial governments' desire to bring more predictability to the funding of these services. The alleged causes of "overutilization"—that is, unanticipated cost increases over and above the agreed-on targets—became and remained a contentious issue. Provincial governments argued that cost overruns were due to physician overservicing for which physicians should be held responsible. For their part, the medical associations laid the blame on population increases, sicker populations, and patient demand, insisting that these were costs that the government and not the profession should bear. By 1992, six provinces (Prince Edward Island, New Brunswick,

Quebec, Ontario, Saskatchewan, and British Columbia) reported having some form of expenditure target (soft cap) for setting the overall provincial medical care budget, with various formulas put in place to deal with situations of cost overruns due to unexpected utilization increases. These formulas specified how much of the unanticipated costs over and above the target should be absorbed by the government and how much should be absorbed by the profession in the form of clawbacks or price discounts (holdbacks) for physicians (Lomas et al., 1992).

The attempts by provincial governments to contain costs were not entirely successful (Katz, Charles, Lomas, & Welch, 1997). Nor were individual thresholds for physician incomes imposed by several governments during the late 1980s and early 1990s. Such policies still did not address expenditure increases resulting from an expanding physician supply. To close the circle around physician expenditures, the provincial governments increasingly pushed for "hard" caps—that is, a predetermined maximum annual budget for medical care expenditures. Under this funding arrangement, physicians would have to pay back to the provincial governments all expenditures above the cap through clawbacks or further price discounts on physician fees. Because the cap represents a closed predictable funding system, it provides a much stronger mechanism for the provincial control of medical care expenditures.

As of 1995, all provincial governments had implemented some version of expenditure caps for physician services. In Ontario, for example, during fiscal year 1994-95, physicians exceeded the 3-year social contract hard cap reached with the then New Democratic Party government by more than $300 million. About $122 million was recovered by the provincial government when physicians faced an across-the-board 2% clawback effective June 1, 1994. A 6% holdback of fees was imposed in December of that year. An additional monthly 10% clawback was imposed to pay back the remaining $179 million.

The imposition of hard caps places total responsibility for any cost overruns in the medicare budget on the medical profession's shoulders and shifts the major focus of economic disputes from government-medical association negotiations to intraprofessional negotiations (Katz et al., 1997). Medical associations now face extremely difficult and often acrimonious decisions with respect to allocating fee decreases rather than fee increases. How to make such decisions equitably and harmoniously has proven to be elusive.

Faced with clawbacks and holdbacks, some physicians have been more willing than in the past to consider alternative payment systems to fee for service. In Ontario, for example, several academic health sciences centers have negotiated alternate funding arrangements with the provincial government. A discussion document released by the Ontario Medical Association (OMA) in 1996 recommended that patients register with a particular family physician (patient rostering) and that physicians be paid on a modified fee-for-service system based on the population of patients whom they serve (Graham, 1996). Other federal-provincial and medical association reports have also recommended patient registration with a primary care organization and the payment of such organizations on a capitation or blended-funding basis (College of Family Physicians, 1995; Forster et al., 1994; Kilshaw, 1995).

From the beginning of the national medical care program, individual physicians ceded economic autonomy to set their own fees to provincial medical associations that negotiated fee increases on their behalf. Through this process, the collective economic autonomy of the profession was enhanced at the expense of individual physician autonomy. To the extent that global medical care expenditure caps and individual caps are now being imposed on the medical profession unilaterally by provincial governments, the profession's collective economic autonomy has also been undermined.

Increasingly, medical associations have lost ground in their power struggles with provincial governments. In 1996, for example, the Ontario government passed Bill 26, which rescinded all existing economic agreements with the Ontario Medical Association and gave the Health Minister new and far-reaching powers to establish unilaterally the global medical care expenditure cap, set fees, and determine which physicians were eligible to receive payments on the basis of geographic and practice criteria. This legislation further restricted the professional association's power by eliminating binding arbitration for most disputes (Katz et al., 1997).

The OMA has also lost influence with its rank-and-file members, largely because of its inability to gain concessions in fee negotiations with either the New Democratic Party government or the subsequent Conservative government in power in Ontario through the 1990s. This failure at the bargaining table has splintered the profession into different factions, each pursuing its own economic interests. In addition, the OMA adopted a policy in the late 1980s to support voluntary clinical guidelines in order to prevent external government implementation of utilization controls (Rappolt, 1997). However, physicians did not adopt a united approach to this policy, despite OMA leaders' pleas for support.

By implementing hard caps on medical care budgets, provincial governments went a long way toward controlling medical care expenditures because physicians alone became responsible for paying back cost overruns. At the same time, as medical associations struggled to allocate fee decreases, an expanding physician supply under a capped system had painful implications for physicians' incomes (Katz et al., 1987). Under this new fiscal reality of the mid-1990s, physicians have gradually become less resistant to government proposals both to limit physician supply and to impose financial disincentives for physicians (especially for new physicians) to practice in overserviced areas.

Physician Resources

In 1964, the Royal Commission on Health Services (Vol. 1, Chapters 2, 7) had projected a shortage of physicians and recommended a substantial increase in medical school facilities, training grants for medical students, and additional programs for postgraduate study. Although these policies were actively followed during the 1960s and 1970s, hindsight reveals the inaccuracy of the assumptions on which the projections were based. The Hall Commission had estimated that by 1971 Canada would have a deficit of 2,228 doctors unless special measures were taken to maintain its prevailing physician-to-population ratio of 1:857. In fact, this ratio for the nation dropped steadily from 1:977 in 1951 to 1:857 in 1961, 1:661 in 1971, and 1:518 in 1990 (Department of National Health and Welfare, 1984; "How Many Doctors," 1991).

The Federal-Provincial Advisory Committee on Health Manpower concluded in 1984 that "from 1961-80 the physician supply increased 105 percent, . . . whereas . . . the population increased only 33 percent over the same period" (Executive Summary, p. i). The committee projected a 12% surplus of physicians by the year 2000, a trend that is also evolving in several other Western industrial nations. In a 1991 review commissioned by the Provincial-Territorial Conference of Ministers of Health, Barer and Stoddart (1991) reiterated that "physician supply in Canada is, and has been for some time, increasing far faster than the size of the population" and that there did not appear to be "any compelling reason for this to continue" (p. 4c-6). The authors argued that physician resources should be matched with needs and that policy initiatives in this area required "Nationally co-ordinated provincial/territorial policies built upon a commonly understood policy objective and framework" which up until then had been lacking (p. 3-2).

Following release of the Barer and Stoddart report, the Provincial/ Territorial Conference of Ministers of Health (1992) agreed in 1992 on a policy statement regarding strategic directions for Canadian physician resource planning, part of which called for a reduction by the fall of 1993 of Canadian medical school entry size by 10%, and a similar reduction in national postgraduate medical training positions.

Medical school enrollment was reduced in a number of provinces in keeping with the Health Ministers' policy statement. In Ontario, for example, with five medical schools, a decision was made that the University of Toronto Medical School would absorb the total 10% reduction in provincial medical school enrollment, resulting in 75 fewer entrants to that program. As part of this agreement, the medical school was allowed to keep its base budget even though the enrollment had dropped. These funds were used to strengthen the research and educational capacity of other programs in the Faculty of Medicine by adding staff positions in community health, health administration, and clinical epidemiology.

In general, provincial governments did not keep their commitment to move toward a national policy on physician supply but rather responded in an individual way to their most pressing physician resource concerns by working with their respective medical associations. These policies took four general forms: (a) differential fees for new entrants to medical practice, (b) billing number restrictions, (c) restrictions on graduates of foreign medical schools, and (d) adjustments such as those noted above to medical school enrollment (Barer, Sanmartin, & Lomas, 1995). Both the imposition of differential fees and the restriction of billing numbers tended to target new physicians entering practice. For example, in Prince Edward Island, new physicians without hospital privileges were to be paid 50% of negotiated fees. In British Columbia, starting in February 1994, physicians granted new billing numbers were to be paid at 50% of the prevailing fee schedule. New Brunswick refused access to public plan payment to new physicians who could not obtain hospital admitting privileges, and in Nova Scotia, new billing numbers were restricted to physicians who agreed to practice in areas of need (Barer et al., 1995). Global expenditure caps encouraged medical associations to become more supportive than in the past of these supply-side controls because they realized that an increase in physician supply translated into less space for each physician to graze in the "medical commons" (Grumbach & Bodenheimer, 1990).

The fact that many of the above policies were directed at recent medical graduates created tensions within the medical profession because new physicians felt that their earning power was being sacrificed so that currently practicing physicians could maintain their incomes. The combination of global expenditure caps and an increasing physician supply also led to greater interest among medical associations (and governments) in removing or delisting certain services from public health insurance coverage. Making such services available though the private sector is appealing to physicians because it provides them with an additional source of income outside the constraints (e.g., income caps) of the public system.

Accessibility and Health Status

One of the principal objectives of the 1966 Medical Care Act that was reaffirmed by the 1984 Canada Health Act was to reduce regional disparities in accessibility to health care. Since the inception of this program, gains have been made in achieving this objective in terms of the leveling out of regional differences in the supply of health personnel across the country. This composite trend, however, masks what is in fact a patchwork quilt of benefits whose provision is affected by the relative availability of specialized measures and clinical practice styles, different provincial policies on the coverage of selected services, and the comparative wealth of the region where a person lives. Following the national program's phasing in, there was a substantial leveling out in terms of per capita health expenditures. Although this level of spending was to increase by 21.3% in real terms over the next two decades, it was accompanied by a widening discrepancy in per capita expenditures between the poorer and wealthier provinces. In 1975, the difference in total per capita health expenditures between the four poorer Maritime provinces and the country's three most affluent provinces was 5.3%. By 1994, this gap had widened to 13.5% (Health Canada, 1996a, Table 16b).

Provincial policies have determined whether certain services were included under the rubric of comprehensive coverage. By the early 1990s, for example, insured benefits included care given by Freudian psychoanalysts in three provinces, tubal ligations in eight provinces, and in vitro fertilization and newborn circumcision in two provinces ("How Medicare Can Be Saved," 1995). In contrast to the early days of national health insurance, when virtually all services provided by physicians were covered, some provinces have more recently delisted certain services deemed to be of dubious medical value. In addition, steps have been taken to cap the open-ended coverage of services such as out-of-country care and provincially operated drug plans. These trends became so prevalent that in 1995 the provincial premiers recommended that a common listing of agreed-on essential health services should be developed.

Though raising the level of coverage for all Canadians, the introduction of medical care insurance in Canada has not removed the wide differences that previously existed in the types and dollar value of the medical care received by rural and urban residents. In 1970, for example, Winnipeg residents in contrast to those living in rural Manitoba's Parkland received twice as many general medical examinations, and 2.5 times more specialist consultations and, on average, generated 40% more in medical care expenditures (Manitoba Department of Health, 1972, pp. 26-27; Roch, Evans, & Pascoe, 1985). These differences did not change appreciably during the ensuing two decades, with Winnipeg continuing to have twice as many physicians per 1,000 population than elsewhere in the province and its residents on average incurring 26% more in medical care costs. Compared to people living in Parkland, Winnipeg residents during 1991-92 on average had 19% more ambulatory medical care visits (5,290 versus 4,447 per 1,000), six times as many specialist consultations (1,710 versus 297 per 1,000), and 31.8% more per capita medical care expenditures (Tataryn, Roos, & Black, 1995). Comparable trends occurred in Saskatchewan where the use of medical services rose by about 2% annually between 1976 and 1986 (Saskatchewan Health, 1990, p. 29). At the beginning of this period, the average cost of medical services received by urban residents was 17.3% higher than those of rural residents. By 1986-87, this gap had widened to 23.1%. The available documentation indicates that although direct financial barriers to medical care may have been largely removed, the structure of Canadian society itself as reflected in the differential distribution of health resources and the relative wealth of regions across the country compromises the principle of equitable access to insured health services.

The main intent of national health insurance was to ensure reasonable access to health care for all Canadians, regardless of their health status or ability to pay. The extent to which these goals have been realized depends on the concept of equity adopted and the measures chosen to gauge specific outcomes. Contrasting philosophical and political perspectives about the meaning of equity include equity before the law, equity of access, and equity in benefits received. Before the law and in terms of access, there can be no doubt that all Canadians have benefited from the introduction of national health insurance. The principle of access to health care without economic impediment is now entrenched as a fundamental social right. Despite a growing body of studies, however, the aggregate evidence concerning the relationship between social class and the utilization of health services is somewhat inconclusive. Studies conducted immediately after the introduction of public medical care typically found that there was little change in the use of services by income level. These studies and those undertaken later generally did not distinguish clearly between the benefits gained from this program and those emanating from broader social security measures, and the time frame within which the changes were expected to be realized.

Income disparities between the rich and the poor in Canada have not been appreciably altered since 1951. The top fifth of Canadian households garnered more than 42% of the nation's total income in 1951 and 1990, whereas the share of the bottom fifth hovered between 4.4% and 5.2% during this period. Between 1984 and 1994, the share of the market income of the most affluent rose by 7.7%, whereas that of the poor dropped sharply by 20.5% (Novick & Shillington, 1996, p. 11). That a person's class position still affects how health care is obtained is documented by numerous studies that examine not just the utilization of medical and hospital services but also the actual types and costs of care received. These disparities between rich and poor persons occur in relation to surgical operations, preventive health care, and uninsured out-of-pocket expenses. An extensive review of this body of research undertaken in 1991 suggested that

> in terms of both actual dollar value and as a share of total income, the rich continued to spend more than the poor on health care. The introduction of national health insurance did little to modify this regressive distribution. On the contrary, the benefits provided under this national program may have reinforced this disparity. By providing coverage for middle and upper income groups, a displacement effect appears to have occurred whereby these groups have been given the opportunity to purchase more health benefits and continue in this regard to outstrip the financial capability of the poor. (Badgley & Wolfe, 1992, p. 213; see also Badgley, 1991)

A substantial and growing body of research indicates that despite national health insurance programs, social class differences still persist, with the rich living longer and having less disability than the poor. These conclusions are illustrated by the findings of national health surveys completed over a span of 45 years. According to the Canada Sickness Survey of 1950-51, low-income Canadians had almost twice as many disability days and more illness than those with higher incomes (Dominion Bureau of Statistics, 1960). The poor then received fewer medical consultations and were less often hospitalized than other Canadians. More recent national health surveys (e.g., the 1978-79 National Health Survey, the 1985 and 1991 General Social Surveys, and the 1995 National Population Health Survey) have reached comparable conclusions. The 1985 Canada Health Promotion Survey, for instance, reported that the "health status and quality of life are clearly lowest among the poor" (Wilkins, 1988, p. 8).

Over a dozen studies focusing on longevity have documented an association between income and life expectancy. In one longitudinal study, men in the lowest 5% income group in the two decades before retirement were twice as likely to die before reaching age 70 than were men in the top 5% bracket (Wolfson, Row, Gentleman, & Tomiak, 1990). The aggregate evidence on social class in relation to the utilization of health services and life chances indicates that an equality of opportunity provided by national health insurance has not led to an equality of benefits in terms of the differential health status and levels of disability of individuals.

The Direction of Change

Since its inception in the 1960s, major legislative amendments to the national health insurance program have realigned its co-financing arrangements and reasserted the principles on which it was founded. To control its share of health expenditures and to meet provinces' demands for greater flexibility in the operation of their programs, the federal government changed the financial formula in 1977 from a cost-sharing to a block-funding arrangement. This was followed in 1984 by a consolidation and updating of earlier legislation. The Canada Health Act was intended to reassert the federal presence in the domain of national health insurance and ensure that the standards set by the federal government were adhered to by the provinces.

Despite these important legislative changes, the organization of health care services delivered in Canada was not substantially changed. Canada's national health bill rose to almost 9% of GDP, the supply of health care personnel grew substantially, and the provinces continued to devote a larger share of their budgets to health care. Seeking to curb the rate of growth of these services, provinces also faced pressures to respond to the impact of new technology, a growing elderly population, an entrenched health delivery system, and staunch opposition from strong and influential professional pressure groups. Combined with the split in constitutional authority for health care, these forces precluded the development of a national strategy to deal with health policy issues requiring broad consensus for their resolution. As changes in the financing and administrative roles of both levels of government evolved, Canada developed a loosely coordinated framework for national health planning. The prospect of developing a more centralized approach is not on the horizon, as attested by the continuing divisive debate over constitutional reform proposals.

National health insurance was a necessary first step in removing direct financial barriers to health care—a major public policy achievement. Despite this shift, health services continue to be distributed and used selectively depending on where a person lives, his or her social circumstances, and the supply of health resources. By itself, the program has done little to modify the broader social determinants affecting health. This broader policy framework has only recently been acknowledged as several provinces foster healthy public policies that transcend the confines of the health sector.

Since the 1990s, the political pendulum across Canada has swung sharply to the right, bringing with it considerable political will to cut public expenditures, maximize efficiency, and enhance the powers of local governance bodies. Many of these changes have been long heralded but either have not been introduced or have been introduced on a piecemeal basis in the absence of an overall planning strategy. One of the earliest comprehensive health care plans was prepared by the noted medical historian Henry E. Sigerist of Johns Hopkins University for the socialist Saskatchewan government in 1944. Sigerist set out the principles for the development of a comprehensive public program of hospital and medical care insurance to be enacted within the context of an integrated system of community health services. Local population health needs were to be identified by surveys; "all activities that tend to promote the people's health" (Roemer, 1960, p. 211) were to be emphasized; the services of health centers were to be coordinated with those of hospitals; and, to preclude congestion of acute care hospital beds, long-term care facilities and home care services were to be developed for chronically ill patients and the elderly. Physicians were to be paid salaries with opportunities for continuing education. Although the provincial government would retain responsibility for strategic planning, Sigerist called for the establishment of district health services commissions drawing on "the active participation of the population" (Roemer, 1960, p. 214). Sigerist recognized that "the establishment of a complete network of health services . . . would undoubtedly take considerable time," but he advocated that a beginning should be made "without delay" (Roemer, 1960, pp. 209-210). Sigerist's underlying social democratic philosophy that the machinery of government should be used to plan and direct services ran counter to dominant political and economic interests. Hence, when it was introduced, Canada's national health insurance program was grafted onto a largely unmodified existing health system's framework.

Over the quarter-century of its operation, national health insurance has become Canada's most strongly endorsed public program. Yet ironically, by the mid-1990s, many of the fundamental structural changes to the system that were previously anathema to the health industry and the medical profession were being spearheaded by governments having a neoconservative and populist philosophy. Though at its core the national program is untouchable, its loose network of services, professional standards, and administration is being streamlined in the interests of reducing public expenditures. These changes are facilitated by both a growing belief that Canada's historically well-funded health care system requires restructuring rather than additional revenue and by an erosion of sympathy for the financial plight of physicians, who retain their standing as one of the highest paid fields in the country.

Health care structural reforms are now being undertaken across the country. In early 1996, for example, the Ontario Minister of Health outlined his "solid business plan that affects every area of the health care system" (Ontario Ministry of Health, 1996a, p. 117). Echoing earlier (and largely forgotten) proposals, the Minister asserted that "our new direction will result in seamless and accountable health care for Ontarians. . . . The Ministry will manage and integrate these services to create a coordinated, efficient and effective community health system that promotes health and prevents illness" (p. 117).

As foreshadowed by the business plans for health of both the Alberta and Ontario governments, further changes on the horizon include

- Additional hospital mergers and closures
- "Best values" outcomes for the allocation of resources
- New funding models for physicians that include patient rostering and capitation or mixed-funding systems
- Development of integrated community health care delivery services
- Emphasis on the provincial government's role as a strategic manager of the health care system, with a gradual withdrawal of its role as a direct provider of certain services
- Increased support for limiting public funding to "medically necessary" or "essential" health care services and for expanding the private market to fund other health care services
- Continued devolution of responsibility from provincial governments to regional boards for the allocation of health care funds within specific geographic areas

- More planning emphasis on a population health perspective and on broad determinants of health
- More support for evidence-based clinical decision making and practice guidelines
- Continued decline in the autonomy of physicians under a closed-cap funding system and billing-number restrictions
- Acrimony within medical associations as to how to allocate fee decreases
- Continued high public support for the national health insurance principles

A major challenge facing the Canadian health care system is whether Canada can maintain the national standards in the face of strong counter-vailing trends such as decentralization and growing support for expansion in private sector health care funding. The role of the federal government as the traditional protector of the national standards is critical in this debate. The direction of health policies over the next several years will be critical in steering the Canadian health care system down one of two different paths: further embracing of a two-tiered health care system similar to that in the United States or, alternatively, a reconsolidation and recommitment to what are distinctly Canadian principles of universal access to publicly funded comprehensive health care services on uniform terms and conditions.

References

Again, common sense in Saskatchewan. (1996, March 28). *Globe and Mail [Toronto]*, p. A18.

Alberta Health. (1995). *A three-year business plan: 1995-1996 to 1997-1998—Healthy Albertans living in a healthy Alberta*. Edmonton: Author.

Alberta Hospitals and Medical Care. (1983). *Facts on financing*. Edmonton: Author.

Badgley, R. (1991). Social and economic disparities under Canadian Health Care. *International Journal of Health Services, 21*, 659-671.

Badgley, R., & Wolfe, S. (1967). *Doctors' strike: Medical care and conflict in Saskatchewan*. New York: Macmillan.

Badgley, R., & Wolfe, S. (1992). Equity and health care. In C. D. Naylor (Ed.), *Canadian health care and the state: A century of evolution*. Montreal: McGill-Queen's University Press.

Ball, T. (1991). Hospitals can meet the challenge. *Health Concepts Consultants [Toronto]*, p. 10.

Baltzan, M. (1982, November). *Canada Health Act and health care rationing*. Paper presented at the annual meeting of the Saskatchewan Medical Association, Regina.

Barer, M., Sanmartin, C., & Lomas, J. (1995). *Physician expenditure control in Canada: Re-minding our P's and Q's* (CHEPA Working Paper No. 95-11). Hamilton, Ontario: McMaster University, Centre for Health Economics and Policy Analysis.

Barer, M., & Stoddart, G. (1991). *Toward integrated medical resource policies for Canada: Background document* (CHEPA Working Paper No. 91-7). Hamilton, Ontario: McMaster University, Centre for Health Economics and Policy Analysis.

Bégin, M. (1988). *Medicare: Canada's right to health.* Montreal: Optimum.

Blendon, R. (1989). Three systems: A comparative survey. *Health Management Quarterly, 11,* 2-10.

Blendon, R., & Taylor, H. (1989). Datawatch: Views on health care: Public opinion in three nations. *Health Affairs, 8,* 149-157.

Botz, K., & Singh, C. (1985). Calculating the cost of CMG's in a Canadian hospital. *Health Care, 27,* 53-56.

Canada, House of Commons. (1957a, March 25). Debates, 22nd Parliament, Fifth Session.

Canada, House of Commons. (1957b, April 4). Debates, 22nd Parliament, Fifth Session.

Canada, House of Commons. (1957c, April 8). Debates, 22nd Parliament, Fifth Session.

Canada, House of Commons. (1957d, November 18). Debates, 23rd Parliament, First Session.

Canada, House of Commons. (1957e, November 19). Debates, 23rd Parliament, First Session.

Canada, House of Commons. (1965, April 5). Debates, 26th Parliament, Third Session.

Canada, House of Commons. (1966a, July 12). Debates, 27th Parliament, First Session.

Canada, House of Commons. (1966b, December 6). Debates, 27th Parliament, Fourth Session.

Canada, House of Commons. (1984a, October 14). Minutes of Proceedings and Evidence of the Standing Committee on Health, Welfare and Social Affairs Respecting Bill C-3, Canada Health Act.

Canada, House of Commons (1984b). The Canada Health Act (Bill C-3). Passed by the House of Commons April 9, 1984, 32nd Parliament, 2nd Session, 32-33 Elizabeth II.

Canada, House of Commons. (1989, April 4). Debates, 34th Parliament, 2nd Session.

Canada, House of Commons. (1991a, February 26). Debates, 34th Parliament, Second Session.

Canada, House of Commons. (1991b, March 19). Debates, 34th Parliament, 2nd Session.

Canada, House of Commons. (1991c, October 24). Debates, 34th Parliament, 3rd Session.

Canada, House of Commons. (1995a, March 30). Debates, 35th Parliament, Final Session.

Canada, House of Commons. (1995b, April 27). Debates, 35th Parliament, First Session.

Canada, House of Commons. (1995c, June 1). Debates, 35th Parliament, Final Session.

Canada, House of Commons. (1995d, October 18). Debates, 35th Parliament, 1st Session.

Canadian College of Health Service Executives. (1997). *Health reform update 1996-1997* (4th ed.) Ottawa: Author.

Canadian Healthcare Association. (1996). *Canada's health system under challenge: Comprehensiveness and core insurance benefits in the Canadian health system.* Ottawa: Author.

Canadian Medical Association. (1984a). *Health: A need for redirection. Report of the CMA Task Force on the Allocation of Health Care Resources.* Ottawa: Print Action Ltd.

Canadian Medical Association. (1994b). *Core and comprehensive health care services: A framework for decision-making.* Ottawa: Author.

Canadian Medical Association. (1995, August). *The future of health and health care in Canada: An overview.* Paper presented at the 128th meeting of the General Council of the Canadian Medical Association, Winnipeg, Manitoba.

Carlow, D., & Rea, P. (1988). Physician impact analysis: An imperative for the modern hospital. *Health Care Management Forum, 1,* 22-27.

Carter, G. (1977). Financing health and post-secondary education: A new and complex fiscal arrangement. *Canadian Tax Journal, 25,* 534-550.

Charles, C., Lomas, J., Giacomini, M., Bhatia, V., & Vincent, V. (1997). Medical necessity and Canadian health policy: Four meanings and . . . a funeral? *Milbank Quarterly, 75,* 365-394.

Charles, C., & Roberts, J. (1994). Evaluating physician impact analysis: Methods, results and uses in Ontario hospitals. *Evaluation and the Health Professions, 17,* 96-112.

College of Family Physicians of Canada. (1995, September). *Managing change: The family medicine group practice model: A discussion document on primary health care reform in Canada.* Mississauga, Ontario: Author.

Coutts, J. (1995, October 26). Support for health care principles weaker among well-off. *Globe and Mail [Toronto],* p. A21.

Department of National Health and Welfare. (1984). *Canada health manpower inventory 1983.* Ottawa: Author.

Dominion Bureau of Statistics. (1960). *Canada Sickness Survey, 1950-51: Illness and health care in Canada* (Vol. 1). Ottawa: Queen's Printer.

Evans, R., Lomas, J., & Barer, M. (1989). Controlling health expenditures—The Canadian reality. *New England Journal of Medicine, 320,* 571-577.

Eves, E. (1995). *1995 fiscal and economic statement.* Toronto: Ontario Ministry of Finance.

Federal/Provincial Advisory Committee on Health Manpower. (1984). *Physician manpower in Canada: 1980-2000.* Ottawa: Health & Welfare Canada.

Forster, J., Rosser, W., Hennen, B., McCauley, R., Wilson, R., & Gregan, M. (1994, September). New approach to primary medical care. *Canadian Family Physician,* pp. 1523-1530.

Gibson, T. (1935). *A short account of the early history of the Kingston General Hospital.* Kingston, Ontario: n.p.

Government of Saskatchewan. (1985a, May 22). *Saskatoon Agreement II signed* [Press release]. Regina: Author.

Government of Saskatchewan and the Saskatchewan Medical Association. (1985b, May). *Saskatoon II: Memorandum of agreement* [Press release]. Regina: Author.

Graham, W. (1996). *Primary care reform: A strategy for stability (Draft 6).* Toronto: Ontario Medical Association.

Grauer, A. (1939). *Public assistance and social insurance: A study prepared for the Royal Commission on Dominion-Provincial Relations.* Ottawa: King's Printer.

Gray, C. (1996). Gambling with Medicare. *Saturday Night, 111*(2), 44-50.

Grumbach, K., & Bodenheimer, T. (1990). Reins or fences? A physician's view of cost containment. *Health Affairs, 9*(4), 120-126.

Hall, E. (1980). *Canada's national-provincial health program for the 1980's: A commitment for renewal.* Saskatoon: Craft Litho.

Health Action Lobby. (1994). *Getting to the core of comprehensiveness: A discussion paper.* Ottawa: Author.

Health and Welfare Canada. (1985a, September 20). *Medicare money returned to Manitoba* [Press release]. Ottawa: Author.

Health and Welfare Canada. (1985b, September 20). *Medicare money returned to Saskatchewan* [Press release]. Ottawa: Author.

Health Canada. (1996a). *National health expenditures in Canada: 1975-1994. Full report.* Ottawa: Health Canada, Policy and Consultations Branch.

Health Canada. (1996b). *National health expenditures in Canada: 1975-1994. Summary report.* Ottawa: Health Canada, Policy and Consultations Branch.

Health Services Restructuring Commission. (1997). *Metropolitan Toronto health services restructuring report.* Toronto: Author.

Heiber, S., & Deber, R. (1987). Banning extra-billing in Canada: Just what the doctor didn't order. *Canadian Public Policy, 13,* 62-74.

How many doctors is too many? (1991, December 9). *Globe and Mail [Toronto],* p. A14.

How Medicare can be saved. (1995, September 24). *Toronto Star,* p. F2.

Hurley, J., Bhatia, V., & Markham, B. (1995). Is small really beautiful? Some thoughts on the 1995 federal budget. *Leadership, 4*(3), 12-18.

Katz, S., Charles, C., Lomas, J., & Welch, J. G. (1997). Physician relations in Canada: Shooting inward as the circle closes. *Journal of Health Politics, Policy and Law, 22,* 1413-1431.

Kennedy, C. (1955). *The Kingston General Hospital: A summary of its growth 1835-1954.* Kingston, Ontario: n.p.

Kilshaw, M. F. (1995). *A model for the reorganization of primary care and the introduction of population-based funding.* Victoria: British Columbia Ministry of Health.

King, W. (1973). *Industry and humanity.* Toronto: University of Toronto Press.

Lalonde, M. (1988). Health services managers or managers of health? *Journal of Health Administration Education, 6,* 71-83.

Linton, A., Butts, M. W., & Atkinson, J. W. (1987). New challenges to medical staff organization in hospitals. *Canadian Medical Association Journal, 136,* 804-807.

Linton, A., & Peachey, D. (1989). Utilization management: A medical responsibility. *Canadian Medical Association Journal, 141,* 283-286.

Little, B. (1991, November 5). User fees favoured to pay rising health costs. *Globe and Mail [Toronto],* p. 1.

Lomas, J., Charles, C., & Greb, J. (1992). *The price of peace: The structure and process of physician fee negotiations in Canada* (CHEPA Working Paper No. 92-17). Hamilton, Ontario: McMaster University, Centre for Health Economics and Policy Analysis.

Lomas, J., Woods, J., & Veenstra, G. (1997). Devolving authority for health care in Canadian Provinces: 1. An introduction to the issues. *Canadian Medical Association Journal, 156,* 371-377.

MacEachen, A. J. (1981). *Fiscal arrangements in the eighties: Proposals of the Government of Canada.* Ottawa: Supply and Services Canada.

MacKenzie, I. (1944). Health insurance. *Canadian Journal of Public Health, 35,* 213-233.

MacLeod, W., & Deane, J. (1984.) Impact analysis and medical manpower planning. *Health Management Forum, 5,* 9-16.

Manitoba Department of Health and Social Development. (1972). *White paper on health policy.* Winnipeg: Author.

Markham, B , & Lomas, J. (1995). Review of the multi-hospital arrangements literature: Benefits, disadvantages and lessons for implementation. *Healthcare Management Forum, 8,* 24-35.

Marsh, L., Grant, A., & Blackler, C. (1938). *Health and unemployment: Some studies of their relationships* (McGill Social Research Series No. 7). Montreal: McGill University.

Martin, P. (1985). *A very public life, so many worlds* (Vol. 2). Toronto: Deneau.

McCutcheon, D. (1988). Impact analysis reduces the guesswork in budgeting. *Dimensions, 65,* 24-25.

Medical Care Act of 1966, 14-15, Eliz. II, Ch. 64, R.S.C.

Munro, J., & Inglis, A. (1975). *Mike: The memoirs of the Right Honourable Lester B. Pearson, 1957-1968* (Vol. 3). Toronto: University of Toronto Press.

Murray, V., Jick, T. D., & Bradshaw, P. (1984). Hospital funding constraints: Strategic and tactical decision responses to sustained moderate levels of crisis in six Canadian hospitals. *Social Science and Medicine, 18,* 211-219.

National Forum on Health. (1997). Canada, striking a balance. In *Canada health action: Building on the legacy* (Vol. 2). Ottawa: Author.

National Health & Welfare Canada. (1983). *Preserving universal Medicare.* Ottawa: Author.

Newman, P. (1995). *The Canadian revolution from 1985-1995: From deference to defiance.* Toronto: Viking.

Novick, M., & Shillington, R. (1996). *Crossroads for Canada: A time to invest in children and families* (Discussion Paper). Ottawa: Campaign 2000.

Ontario Hospital Association. (1991). *Guidelines for medical manpower planning and impact analysis in hospitals.* Toronto: Author.

Ontario Legislative Assembly. (1873). *Sessional Papers 1872-73: Fifth Annual Report of the Inspector of Asylums and Prisons for the Province of Ontario, 1871-72.* Toronto: Rose.

Ontario Ministry of Finance. (1995). *1995 Fiscal and economic statement.* Toronto: Government of Ontario.

Ontario Ministry of Health. (1992, January 19). *Working document: Goals and strategic priorities.* Toronto: Author.

Ontario Ministry of Health. (1996a). *Business plan.* Toronto: Author.

Ontario Ministry of Health. (1996b). *Hospital transfer payments for 1996.* Toronto: Government of Ontario.

Organization for Economic Cooperation and Development. (1988). *The future of social protection* (Social Policy Studies No. 6). Paris: Author.

Parfrey, P., Gillespie, M., McManamon, P. J., & Fisher, R. (1986). Audit of the Medical Audit Committee. *Canadian Medical Association Journal, 135,* 205-208.

Parliamentary Task Force on Federal-Provincial Fiscal Arrangements. (1981). *Fiscal federalism in Canada.* Ottawa: Supply and Services Canada.

Pickersgill, J., & Forster, D. (1970). *The Mackenzie King record, 1945-1946* (Vol. 3). Toronto: University of Toronto Press.

Provincial/Territorial Conference of Ministers of Health. (1992, January 28). *Strategic directions for Canadian physician resource management.* Edmonton.

Province of Canada. (1894). *Journals of the Legislative Assembly of the Province of Canada.* Third Provincial Parliament, 2nd Session. Toronto: M. Reynolds.

Rappolt, S. (1997). Clinical guidelines and the fate of medical autonomy in Ontario. *Social Science and Medicine, 44,* 977-987.

Reamy, J. (1995). Health service regionalization in New Brunswick, Canada: A bold move. *International Journal of Health Services, 25,* 271-282.

Roch, D., Evans, R., & Pascoe, D. (1985). *Manitoba and Medicare: 1971 to the present.* Winnipeg: Manitoba Health Services Commission.

Roemer, M. (1960). *Henry E. Sigerist on the sociology of medicine.* New York: MD Publications.

Royal Commission on Dominion-Provincial Relations. (1940). *Report of the Royal Commission on Dominion-Provincial Relations* (Vols. 1-3). Ottawa: King's Printer.

Royal Commission on Health Services. (1964). *Report of the Royal Commission on Health Services.* Ottawa: Queen's Printer.

Royal Commission on the Economic Union and Development Prospects for Canada. (1985). *Report of the Royal Commission on the Economic Union and Development Prospects for Canada* (Vol. 2). Ottawa: Supply and Services Canada.

Saskatchewan Health. (1990). *The growth in the use of health services: 1977/78 to 1985/86.* Regina: Author.

Special Committee on Social Security. (1943). *Health insurance: Report of the Advisory Committee on Health Insurance.* Ottawa: King's Printer.

Stoeckle, J. (1995). The citadel cannot hold: Technologies go outside the hospital, patients and doctors too. *Milbank Quarterly, 73,* 3-17.

Task Force on Program Review. (1985). *Improved program delivery: Health and sports program.* Ottawa: Supply and Services Canada.

Tataryn, D., Roos, N., & Black, C. (1995). Utilization of physician resources for ambulatory care. *Medical Care, 33*(Suppl.), D584-D598.

Taylor, M. (1973). Canadian health insurance programs. *Public Administration Review, 33,* 31-39.

United Nations Development Programme. (1991). *Human development report 1991.* New York: Oxford University Press.

Wilensky, H., & Lebeaux, C. (1965). *Industrial society and social welfare.* New York: Free Press.

Wilkins, R. (1988). *Special study on the socially and economically disadvantaged.* Ottawa: Health and Welfare Canada.

Willard, J. (1959). The Canadian Hospital Insurance Program. *Medical Services Journal, Canada, 15,* 607-621.

Wilson, J. (1996, February 12). *Notes for remarks by the Honourable Jim Wilson, M.P.P., Minister of Health: The new health care vision for ontario* [Press release]. Toronto: Ontario Ministry of Health.

Wilson, R., Rowan, M., & Henderson, J. (1995). Core and comprehensive health care services: I. Introduction to the Canadian Medical Association's decision-making framework. *Canadian Medical Association Journal, 152,* 1063-1066.

Wolfson, M., Row, G., Gentleman, J. F., & Tomiak, M. (1990). *Earnings and death: Effects over a quarter century.* Toronto: Canadian Institute for Advanced Research.

CHAPTER 8

Will Power, Cost Control, and Health Reform in Canada, 1987-1992

CATHERINE FOOKS

> Health care reform is the issue from hell. Tackle it and you tangle with the most powerful lobbies in the country. Ignore it and you may end up on fishing trips with George Bush.
>
> *The Economist*—Advice to President Clinton, 1993

Over the past 5 years, academic journals and the popular press have been full of comparisons of the Canadian and American health care systems. Which is "better," "cheaper," "more efficient," "more popular?" The Canadian health care system is often depicted as a barrier-free, efficiently administered system with health outcomes to be envied by all. Or it is seen as on the verge of collapse, out of resources, with patients waiting years for service from a practitioner not of their choice. Likewise,

AUTHOR'S NOTE: The views expressed in this chapter are solely my own and should not be taken to represent those of the Premier's Councils of Ontario, of which I was Research Director at the time the chapter was written.
EDITORS' NOTE: The analysis presented in this chapter is based on data relative to health care cost control policies initiated in four Canadian provinces during the years 1988 to 1992. The analysis does not take into account events that have taken place since that time.

the American health care system is often depicted as the most modern, high-tech, efficiently run system in the world. Or it is called the most expensive, elitist "white elephant," consuming vast resources and shutting out all but the middle and upper classes. There is probably some truth in all of it, as well as a lot of wishful thinking. Internationally, everyone is unhappy with their health care system, and most countries are talking the language of reform. The trick is not to decide who is right or better. The trick is to match national cultures and preferences to country-specific structures enabling the cost-effective delivery of high-quality health care.

Although the language of cost control has been in the Canadian air for a number of years, real efforts to contain spending at the provincial level are relatively new. What emerges is a picture of governments struggling to convince, cajole, or coopt providers into accepting less and of providers reacting in varying degrees to budget cuts, loss of income, and a restructuring of services. The public has watched with some confusion as the media provide regular horror stories and, once in a while, some useful commentary. We do know that we are in the midst of a long-term process that will eventually enhance governments' ability to manage health care spending, inject some planning principles into delivery decisions, shift some resources away from the hospital and physician sectors into community health services, and make some positive impact on population health.

It is actually difficult to talk about provincial cost control because we have only just started down the road. Therefore, this chapter is less about actual experience and more about the potential ability of the Canadian health care system to contain spending if governments choose to do so. In theory, the design of the Canadian system does allow for the implementation of significant cost control measures. In practice, there is often a political price, which, to date, governments have been reluctant to pay. Thus, the title of the chapter—"Will Power, Cost Control, and Health Reform."

What follows is a brief examination of the expenditure experiences of four Canadian provinces from 1987 to 1992, the period in which cost control became an ongoing and constant theme in the public policy debate; a discussion of the policy levers available for cost control; and some preliminary observations on the experience. Total hospital and medical expenditures are reviewed. Drug plans are not reviewed because only in-hospital drugs are fully covered by provincial plans.

Health Reform in Canada

A detailed description of the Canadian health care system is beyond the scope of this chapter. Suffice it to say that there is no one system. Each

Canadian province funds and administers its own health insurance plan covering hospital and medical services. The federal government does contribute financially on the condition that the provinces meet national eligibility and coverage standards. Although sometimes labeled as "socialized medicine," it is generally recognized that most resources are in the private sector, and the system is often described as publicly funded and privately delivered (U.S. General Accounting Office, 1991). Most physicians work for themselves and earn their incomes on a fee-for-service basis, and most hospitals are private, nonprofit corporations operating on a global budget. The basic tenets of the provincial systems are

- Universal health insurance for all citizens of the province
- Government funding from general tax revenues and government or non-profit administration of the plan[1]
- No point-of-service charges
- No private insurance for universal medical benefits
- Central control of budget levels but discretion for institutions on how to spend within the overall budget
- Central control of dissemination of technology

From the inception of national health insurance in Canada in 1971 to the late 1980s, health care expenditures grew at rates far outpacing population growth. Indeed, in the last 30 years, health care has grown from 5.4% of the gross national product (GNP) in 1960 to 9.9% in 1991. Per capita expenditures have quadrupled from $500 in 1960 to $2,000 in 1986, increasing 50% in the last 10 years (Evans, 1993). Initially, this was expected, for it was assumed that there would be expenditure growth because many in the population had historically not received medical care due to financial impediments. There was some concern beginning in the late 1970s that physicians were extracting further income directly from patients in the form of user fees and extra billing. The Canada Health Act, passed in 1984, made federal financial support conditional on the prohibition of these practices. However, the public debate focused solely on whether physicians should be allowed to charge more than the Medicare rate for a service, not whether the overall amount being spent on Medicare was appropriate. At the time, equity of access to care was more important than cost control as an operating principle for the system.

By the mid-1980s, spending growth attracted the attention of policy makers. In many provinces, the health care budget was approaching one third of overall government spending. For example, in Ontario, health care expenditures amounted to $14 billion in 1989. Tentative discussions about cost control began, largely behind closed Treasury doors, and royal commissions or task forces sprang up across the country. What to do?

Interestingly, but not surprisingly, the conclusions of the various groups were remarkably similar: that the principles of the health care system as espoused in the 1984 Canada Health Act—accessibility, universality, comprehensiveness, portability, and public administration—were sound. Furthermore, there was a clear consensus that the overall level of public resources spent on health care was sufficient—some questioned whether it was too high—and none supported the claim of underfunding or the need for an infusion of private money. There was agreement that spending needed to be controlled and that some resources should be reallocated to other areas of public policy that affected the health of the population. Most made some comment on the need for the evaluation of the services provided to the public due to concerns of appropriateness and effectiveness, and all called for better management of existing resources. Most made some mention of the need to shift the funding of services from a utilization-driven exercise to one based on the health needs of the population (however defined). All discussed the need for better planning and coordination at the local community level rather than leaving all decisions at the central office, and all discussed the need for public participation in decision making both at the micro level of resource allocation and at the macro level of future directions for the system.

By the early 1990s, the debate in Canada had intensified. A number of factors contributed to this. First, the Canadian economy began to experience major structural change, and the pace of economic growth slowed. Provincial ability to sustain spending growth rates of the previous decade was in serious doubt. Concurrently, the size of both federal and provincial government deficits was of concern, and several governments experienced some downgrading of their credit rating. The federal government had recognized the implications for its own treasury in the mid-1980s, and in three consecutive federal budgets, transfers to the provinces were limited. In 1990, entitlements were frozen altogether. If we take Ontario as an example, the federal contribution to provincial health care spending declined from 52% of the total in 1980 to 32% in 1992. The Ontario government calculated the cumulative loss to be $9.6 billion (Graham & Lightman, 1992). Second, although governments generally accepted the idea of better management,[2] they also realized that the extent of reforms needed to bring it about was staggering. It would require tremendous political will and an understanding by the public that what was happening would save the system, not destroy it. Third, there was recognition that no amount of resources would satisfy all needs (or income potential); thus,

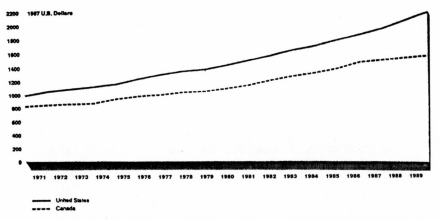

Figure 8.1 Total Health Care: Real Expenditures per Capita (1971-1989)
SOURCE: U.S. General Accounting Office (1991).

NOTE: Expenditures were converted to 1987 constant dollars by dividing health care spending by the gross domestic product implicit price deflators for the United States and Canada. The Organization for Economic Cooperation and Development's purchasing power parity for 1987, $1.24 CAN = $1.00 US, was used to convert Canadian to U.S. dollars.

spending priorities would be required across the whole system, not just within each sector. Finally, there was increased consensus, derived from the work of the royal commissions, that further increases in health care expenditures would not produce commensurate increases in the health status of the population. Reallocation of spending to areas of social and education policy needed to be a long-term goal. So, for a variety of reasons, governments were increasingly clear about the need to rein in health care spending—at least in public discourse.

The Cost Control Experience in Canada

In general, the public funding experiment in Canada created a stabilization of expenditures. Before the implementation of national health insurance, health care spending relative to national income escalated in a pattern similar to that of the United States. After 1971, Canadian expenditures leveled out. Figure 8.1 compares the per capita spending on health care in Canada and in the United States between 1971 and 1989, and Figure 8.2 shows total expenditures as a share of GNP.

Canadian researchers often assert that the keys to cost control in Canada lie in the containment of overall budgets through a single-payer system

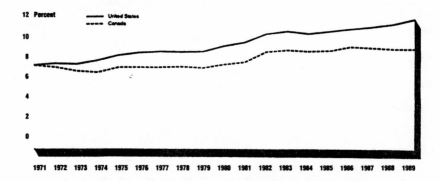

Figure 8.2. Total Health Expenditures as a Share of GNP (1971-1989)
SOURCE: U.S. General Accounting Office (1991).

(without extra payments by patients), containment of technology diffusion, and some control over physician fee increases through central negotiation with providers. The U.S. General Accounting Office, in a 1991 report to the House of Representatives Committee on Government Operations, acknowledged the Canadian record:

> Canada has been much more successful than the United States in containing health care expenditures. In 1971, when Canada fully implemented its system for financing medical service, the two countries spent about the same share of gross national product on health care. In 1989, the US share was 11.6%, whereas Canada's was 8.9%.

However, decision makers are aware that although Canadian growth lines may look good relative to the United States, we are second in per capita spending to all other developed nations—some of which have multipayer systems. In those jurisdictions, however, it is the ability to set common rules for all payers that determines price and overall spending; this is the main element missing in the United States. In a comparative analysis of the American states and Canadian provinces, Kenneth Thorpe (1993) wrote that to a large degree the multipayer and single-payer approaches are similar in that both develop rules guiding transactions between payers and providers and both reflect an underlying political decision to limit the growth in health care spending. We are still left, however, with the duplicative administrative costs, which some analysts argue accounts for a difference of 0.5% of the GNP in the United States (Evans, 1988). Uwe Reinhardt (1988) has described this difference as the

"B Factor"—the costs of bureaucracy that neither provide directly nor support the provision of health care.

There is no doubt that health care costs in Canada have risen over time. However, there is some debate as to why. In recent work, Evans, Barer, and Stoddart (1993) argued that health care costs are not rising faster now than over the past 20 years but that since 1980 the growth of the overall economy has slowed markedly. This is largely due to declines in revenue. Thus, our ability or willingness to pay increasing amounts for health care has lessened.

> This does not mean that there is not a problem of limiting the growth of our health care system to fit within our more limited capacities—there is, and it is a serious problem. But it has not been created by some change in the behavior of the health care system itself, let alone some change resulting from public financing. Health care costs are not exploding, just continuing to rise at the same rate they always have.

Recent Cost Control Experiences in Selected Canadian Provinces

Total health care expenditures are examined for the provinces of Ontario, Quebec, Saskatchewan, and British Columbia from 1987-88 to the 1991-92 fiscal year. Ontario, Quebec, and British Columbia were chosen as the three largest provinces in terms of spending, and Saskatchewan as a smaller province with the largest growth rates in these years. Figure 8.3 shows the annual growth rate for total expenditures (adjusted) for health care over the time period. There is no overall trend; each province has a different story to tell.

Quebec was the only province that showed a steady decline over the period, with spending growth at 3.6% in 1988-89 and at 1.7% in 1991-92. In 1991-92, the growth rate was equal to the growth in population. (This is fairly unusual for Canada.) Ontario's pattern was erratic, with growth in the earlier period, a decline in 1990-91 after a number of years of an imposed fee settlement on physicians and a clampdown on hospital deficits, and a sharp increase in 1991-92 when a physician fee agreement awarded increases above inflation, as well as a onetime retroactive addition to the base for medical services. Saskatchewan showed steady growth as new hospitals came on stream (from almost 0% growth in 1988-89 to 9.3% growth in 1990-91). There was then a sharp decline in 1991-92, with a new government in place facing severe economic constraints.[3] British Columbia also showed a steady growth in

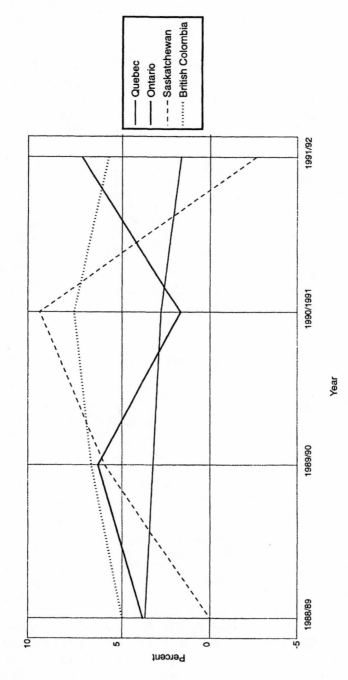

Figure 8.3. Percent Annual Growth in Health Care Expenditures in Real Dollars, by Province, 1987-88 to 1991-92

SOURCE: Health and Welfare Canada.

158

the earlier period until a new government was elected in 1991 and then a subsequent decline in growth for the 1991-92 fiscal year. Growth in adjusted per capita expenditures showed a similar pattern, although it is important to note that Saskatchewan experienced a net decrease in population throughout the period. On average, provinces were spending approximately $1,350 per capita during this time period.

Figures 8.4 and 8.5 provide adjusted growth rates for hospital and medical services in each province. Quebec, Ontario, and British Columbia showed tighter control on the hospital side. Saskatchewan was the exception in that it was actually building new hospitals. On the medical services side, Quebec, Saskatchewan, and British Columbia showed a decline over the period. Ontario was the exception, although the last fiscal year plotted is the year in which there was a fee agreement reached after 2 years of an imposed settlement. Adjusted average per capita spending for the time period ranged from $565 (British Columbia) to $725 (Quebec) for hospital services and from $209 (Saskatchewan) to $356 (Ontario) for medical services.

One has to be careful in drawing conclusions about cost control during this time period. Each province attempted a number of policy reforms aimed in some way at controlling spending. But the jury is still out on their effectiveness. Some did not survive the initial public relations assault but may come back in future years. Some look as if they have been generally accepted as appropriate measures. What is key is that *the levers available to governments have always existed.* They are built into the design of the system. Until recently, governments have not seen the need, or have not been willing politically, to use them. Necessity is now requiring their use.

Policy Levers for Cost Control

Table 8.1 lists the policy levers available to government for cost controls in the hospital and physician sectors. Each is discussed briefly with reference to provincial experiences.

Hospital Sector

Control Over Governance

There is much discussion in Canada at present as to the governance of publicly funded institutions, the need for better accountability for spending of public dollars, and the need for more community input and

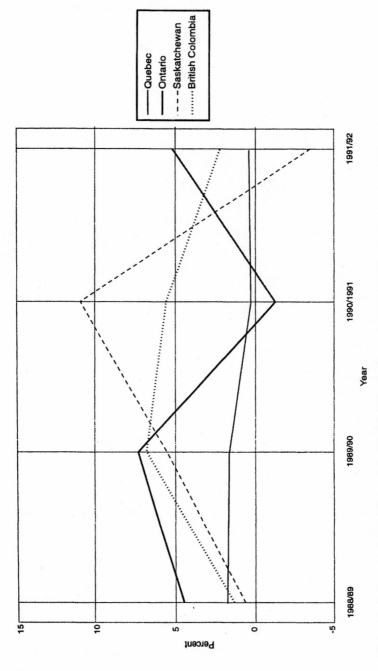

Figure 8.4. Percent Annual Growth in Hospital Expenditures in Real Dollars, by Province, 1987-88 to 1991-92

SOURCE: Health and Welfare Canada.

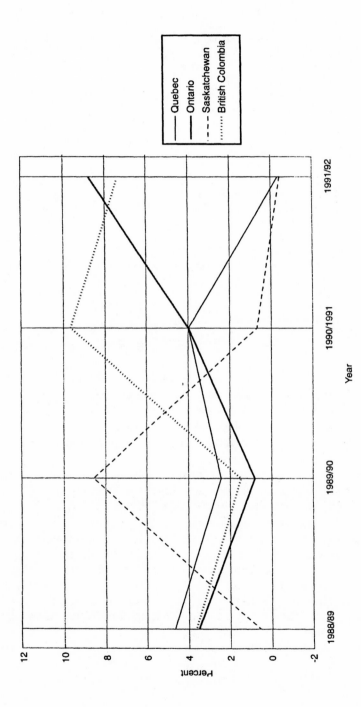

Figure 8.5. Percent Annual Growth in Medical Services Expenditures in Real Dollars, by Province, 1987-88 to 1991-92

SOURCE: Health and Welfare Canada.

161

Table 8.1 Provincial Policy Levers for Cost Control

For the Hospital Sector
- Control over governance
- Control over total budget
- Control over technology dissemination

For the Physician Sector
1. Controls on Fee Schedules
   - Freeze fees
   - Imposed fee increase
   - Thresholds for payments or utilization
   - Cap on global budget or individual billings
   - Deinsurance
   - Resource weights or relative value scales
2. Non-Fee-for-Service Mechanisms
3. Regulation of Supply, Mix, and Distribution of Physicians
   - Restriction of billing numbers
   - Differential fees
   - Restriction of medical school enrollment
   - Restriction of intern and residency positions
   - Use of allied health professionals

control of the decision-making processes of agencies. Hospitals have not escaped the discussion. Most provinces have legislation to govern the funding, management, and operation of publicly funded hospitals. Most of this legislation is in need of revision. Hospitals, as nonprofit corporations, are governed by an elected board of directors, and in most provinces these boards also include government appointees.

The boards tend to see themselves as advocates of the individual institution, not necessarily as representatives of the public interest. Therefore, a number of provinces are attempting to redefine the role of the boards and to facilitate individual institutions working together on behalf of the community in which they reside. British Columbia announced a move to community health authorities that control a budget envelope. Hospitals will be incorporated into the envelope, and there is an expectation that over time individual hospital boards will be phased out or amalgamated into the community board. In theory, the ability to control costs centrally is enhanced by setting up community authorities with clear policy directions and a budget envelope.

Ontario has taken a different approach by redrafting its 60-year-old legislation to remove professional staff from the boards of directors, to mandate community representation on hospital boards and advisory committees, to open up the financial books for community perusal, and to mandate continuous quality improvement processes for all aspects of the hospital's operation. This proposed law was seen as a first step toward community decision making over the individual institution. It would have fostered better understanding of how resources were being spent and the creation of an evaluation climate that, over the long term, would encourage cost savings. However, the draft legislation has not proceeded. Both the Medical Association and the Catholic Church were opposed to the changes and conducted public relations campaigns against the proposed law.

Control Over Total Budget

All provinces have moved from the funding of hospitals on a line-by-line basis to providing a global budget with annual increases. In theory, this allowed the government to control expenditures but gave hospitals more flexibility in determining priorities. In practice, it allowed hospitals to run deficits. Hospitals assumed that government would pick up the extra expenditures at the end of the fiscal year because it was all "necessary spending." They did.

In the last few years, this practice has stopped, and hospitals with deficits must find the resources from within their existing allocation. Governments have also recognized that global budgeting can penalize efficiency and does not allow much sensitivity to changes in patient mix or severity. Provinces are in the early stages of developing funding based on the case mix of hospitals and most have some kind of equity financing to recognize institutional differences.

There was a marked decline in the rate of growth in hospital spending in the early 1990s as governments decreased overall transfers. In Ontario, for example, after averaging growth of 8.5% annually throughout the 1980s, hospitals received a 1% increase during the last fiscal year. Population growth for the same time period was 1.3%. Currently, under "Social Contract" negotiations,[4] hospitals are expected to cut 5% from their base budgets.

Control Over Technology Dissemination

The purchase of high-technology equipment is controlled through central approval processes. Costs of such purchases are not included in global budgets. Therefore, institutions do not have the flexibility to purchase whatever they wish. They must make a case for the release of funds to the Ministry of Health based on needs assessments. This has led to claims that the Canadian health care system does not provide patients with access to "life-saving" technology. It is generally agreed that the rate of technology diffusion is much slower than in the United States; however, there does not seem to be a negative effect when one compares health outcomes for the general population. Furthermore, a policy of conservative technology diffusion, based on paying for new technologies after evaluations, identifies positive health benefits and decreases overall cost.

The Physician Sector

Controls on Fee Schedules

Almost all physicians in Canada are paid by a fee-for-service arrangement based on a fee schedule negotiated between provincial governments and medical associations. Much has been written on the ability of governments to control costs through controlling the fees paid to physicians. In a definitive piece on fee controls in Canada, Barer, Evans, and Labelle (1988) argued that the administrative processes that determine fee levels and fee schedule structures are critical to the success or failure of cost control. In this light, it is important to note that fee negotiations in Canada are moving toward a labor relations model of bargaining. Most provinces now have "framework agreements" that spell out decision rules and procedures, designate the medical association as the official bargaining agent for physicians, require that the RAND formula be applied (payment of union dues), and agree to a process of dispute resolution. Moreover, two provinces have created joint management committees of medical associations and government representatives to oversee decision making. These agreements do have cancellation clauses with proper notification. Within this framework, the focus of physician negotiations has shifted from prices or fees to a combined focus on physician incomes and the overall budget for services (Lomas, Charles, & Greb, 1992).

Freezing of Fees. At first glance, one might assume that the simplest form of control of physician costs would be to freeze the fees paid for the provision of services. This has rarely been done. It is perceived as heavy-handed on the part of the government. Furthermore, without other controls, the government would have no ability to control the amount of service being provided and might not achieve its original policy objective.

Imposition of Fee Awards. Before the signing of framework agreements, a number of provinces imposed fee awards on their provincial medical associations when a consensus could not be reached through bargaining. The longest serving was an imposed 2-year award of 1.75% in Ontario. As in the case of the freezing of fees, an imposition of a fee award was not seen as a useful policy lever. It highlighted the one-sided nature of the negotiation and also provided no ability to control increases in utilization.

Thresholds for Billings or Utilization. The threshold approach to physician fee cost control stems from the belief that there should be a feedback loop between utilization growth and physician billings. This was an important innovation in that it allowed both parties to say that negotiations were not about physician incomes. The threshold that triggered a deduction of dollars billed was based on the quantity of service use. Thus, provincial governments were able to argue that growth in the utilization of services (or growth in physician billings) should not be the entire responsibility of the public purse: Increases should be examined, and a portion of the growth beyond an agreed-on level should be apportioned to physicians. Factors such as population growth, physician supply, natural disasters and other public health problems, and new services or technologies were adjusted for in the accounting process.

Thresholds can be determined prospectively—agreeing in advance what they should be—or retrospectively, after the size of the overrun is known. Thresholds on their own do not appear to have a major impact on physician billings. Individual incomes are not seriously affected, and the total funds available are adjusted only marginally. A 1989 analysis of the effects of thresholds in selected Canadian provinces concluded that their initial impact was discernible but not dramatic. Furthermore, the introduction of other measures might make analysis of the effects of thresholds almost impossible (Lomas, Fooks, Rice, & Labelle, 1989).

Cap on Global Budget or Individual Physician Incomes. The province of Quebec has had a capping system in place since 1976. Ceilings on quarterly billings are in place for general practitioners and specialists. Once the quarterly target is reached, fees are discounted. There is also an overall capped budget for general practitioner and specialist services, which, if overrun, is a factor in discounting the next year's fee increase. Only recently have other provinces—notably British Columbia and Ontario—pledged to implement an overall budget cap.

Analysis of the effect of the capping system in Quebec is difficult because there was also a significant restructuring of the fee schedule.

However, a recent national study of the fee negotiations process in Canada offered the following observation about the Quebec approach. "The major impact has been the extent to which it internalizes to the FMSQ and FMOQ [Federation des Medecins Specialistes du Quebec and Federation des Medecins Omnipraticiens du Quebec] the financial impact of ongoing increases in utilization" (Lomas et al., 1992). Whether the recently announced policies in British Columbia and Ontario will have a similar effect remains to be seen.

Deinsurance. Another potential means of cost control is the ability to "deinsure" items in the provincially negotiated fee schedule: that is, to declare certain items no longer "medically necessary" and therefore no longer covered by public health insurance. To date, this lever has not been used significantly. Alberta deinsured a number of items in 1987, many of which were reinstated after a public outcry.[5] Ontario has recently announced that a number of items will be deinsured: electrolysis, third-party-requested health exams, reversal of sterilization, removal of pimples, repair of the ear lobe, and, most controversially, funding for in vitro fertilization. Although the items selected to date have been fairly minor (with the possible exception of in vitro fertilization), Ontario's action led to public questioning of what is "medically necessary." As part of its agreement with the medical association, the Ontario government has announced a committee to look at the notion of "core services."

Resource Weights. Due to much of the work done for the U.S. Physician Payment Review Commission, there has been interest in Canada in redesigning the fee schedule on the basis of the resource intensity required for fee items. Governments initially hoped that using resource weights might lower overall physician expenditures, and medical associations hoped it might reward certain specialty services. However, the idea faced criticism from the medical community and has not proceeded.

Cost containment for physician services is not as easy as for the hospital sector. Fixed budgets can be imposed on hospitals but have historically been resisted in the physician sector. Because all financial arrangements with physicians are now a negotiated process in Canada, cooperation from the profession is part of the process. Where controls have been "accepted," it would appear that this was based on the wish to avoid a worse outcome. Thus, the shift to the labor relations model for fee negotiations has actually minimized governments' ability to set cost control measures easily in place.

Non-Fee-for-Service Payment Mechanisms

A number of provinces have developed alternatives to the fee-for-service model of service delivery. Quebec has local community services centers (CLSCs; see Chapter 9 of this volume), Ontario has community health centers (CHCs) and health service organizations (HSOs), and British Columbia and Saskatchewan have community clinics. Funding is provided either through a global budget or through an age- and sex-adjusted per capita payment for a roster of patients. Physicians are paid on a salaried basis. However, with the exception of Quebec, these alternate mechanisms employ a very small percentage of physicians—approximately 5% of the total. Comparisons of costs in this sector compared to the fee-for-service sector are few and far between in the Canadian context.[6] Although claims have been made about the efficiencies of these models, there is little rigorous evaluation to support them. Although there is a lot of information on the American models of managed care, the Canadian models are different enough that generalizations are difficult.

Supply, Mix, and Distribution of Physicians

The third major policy lever available to governments in controlling physician expenditures is the control of the supply, mix, and distribution of physicians. As efforts to contain costs through manipulation of the price and quantity of services proved to be difficult, at least in political terms, interest in the supply of physicians increased. Even if the price and quantity of services could be controlled, there was still the question of how many doctors were billing the plan. In a recent study commissioned by the Deputy Ministers of Health from all the provinces, Barer and Stoddart (1991) identified the lack of a national strategy for the management of physician resources. They also identified the following problems associated with this void:

- Increases in physician supply in excess of population growth without any compelling justification
- Numbers and mix of residency training positions—and mix of specialists—that are out of balance with population needs
- Significant geographic variations in physician supply that affect timely and/or convenient access to necessary services
- A nontrivial amount of medical services utilization found to be ineffective, inappropriate, or inefficient

- Conflict between the fee-for-service method of payment and clinical, educational, and public policy objectives
- Deficiencies in both the amount and the quality of basic clinical and management information and incomplete use of the information that does exist

They offered over 50 recommendations to deal with these issues—some of which governments have begun to act on.

Restriction of Physician Billing Numbers. In the mid-1980s, British Columbia attempted to restrict the availability of physician billing numbers. A billing number was required to bill the provincial health insurance plan. The medical profession protested the move and took the government to court, declaring that this restriction was unconstitutional. The court eventually struck down the enabling legislation on procedural grounds. British Columbia is the only province to use this policy lever. (Incidentally, this was not a measure recommended by Barer and Stoddart, 1991.)

Differential Fees. A number of provinces have differential fee schedules to encourage physicians to work in underserviced areas—usually the northern regions of the province. They have been of limited success. For a variety of reasons, contractees usually return south after their contract expires, thus preventing long-term retention for northern communities. Recently in Ontario, as part of the "Social Contract" negotiations, the government proposed a 75% discount on fees for newly graduating physicians if they were unwilling to work in underserviced areas. After a storm of criticism—"The government is eating our young"—the proposal was withdrawn completely. It is unlikely that the idea of discounted fees for newly graduating physicians will be on the policy table for discussion in the near future.

Restricting Medical School Enrollment. Barer and Stoddart (1991) recommended that undergraduate enrollment in medical school be adjusted so as to maintain the current physician/ population ratio. For Canada, this would mean a first-year class size of 1600—a reduction of less than 10%. For the first time, a national consensus on the issue has emerged, and this has been undertaken. Whether the long-term effect is one of cost control remains to be seen.

Restricting Intern and Residency Positions. Barer and Stoddart (1991) also recommended an approximate 10% cut in intern and resident training positions and suggested that capacity be determined by the educational needs of graduates, not the clinical service needs of institutions. Furthermore, they recommended that necessary clinical services provided by residents that are not essential for their specialty training should be provided by other health professionals, including nonphysician personnel. Negotiations are underway to "reduce and realign postgraduate positions to ensure an appropriate mix and number of specialties" (Ontario Ministry of Health, 1993).

Use of Allied Health Professionals. Although there is good evidence that allied health professionals can perform some physician functions at lower cost, publicly funded health insurance has not sanctioned their substitution. Under new legislation in Ontario, 23 health professions are about to be granted self-regulatory status. However, midwifery is the only new group to be given access to public funding. They will be paid on a salaried basis starting at $55,000 (CAN) annually. Some other groups are already in the fee-for-service system with limits on the number of services that may be reimbursed in a given year: chiropractic, optometry, physiotherapy, and in-hospital dental services. However, there has been some discussion as to whether provincial health insurance will continue these payments.

General Observations

In sum, there have been some recent successes in initiating cost control of provincial health care spending. Provinces appear to have broken the historical double-digit growth in hospital spending through a blunt cut in transfer payments. In some provinces, they have broken the automatic assumption that there will always be continuing growth in expenditures. Furthermore, provinces have been very successful in controlling the dissemination of high technology, thereby controlling its associated costs—the purchase price and ongoing billings.

There is an emerging expectation that regional planning and coordination should take place, coupled with more consumer involvement in priority setting and allocation exercises. Almost all provinces, with the exception of Ontario, are looking to devolve some responsibility for planning and allocation to the community level. It is hard to predict what the effect on costs will be, but at a minimum they will be shifted to community authorities.

With respect to physician services, provinces have been successful in breaking the historical refusal to set expenditure targets, to discuss target incomes during fee negotiations, and to discount fees past a certain level of utilization. However, in so doing, they have given away their ultimate ability to impose fee schedules and have slowed decision making through the existence of joint management committees with the profession. There is no indication that governments are ready to tackle seriously alternatives to the fee-for-service system. Early work is under way to link payment to evidence of effectiveness or to clinical practice guidelines, but it is yet to reach the implementation stage. By side-stepping these issues, recent provincial debates have focused more on the applicability of user fees for some services and the necessity of defining core services.

On the human resource question, governments appear to have achieved some early success with a national agreement to restrict medical school enrollment and residency positions. However, this is to be expected, given that these measures do not affect personnel already in the system. The trials of restricting billing numbers and fee discounts for newly graduating physicians did not survive the outcry from the profession, and neither appears to be on the horizon on the near future.

Four general comments can be made about our provincial experience to date. First, although the federal government has been reducing its contribution to the funding of health care for the last decade, provincial governments only recently began cost containment exercises. Therefore, it is early to judge these measures' success or failure. Second, the single-payer nature of our system has allowed provincial governments to move fairly quickly on a variety of measures. Analysts looking back at this time period will probably be able to describe a constriction in health care spending due largely to the blunt instruments available to a single payer: cuts in hospital transfers, some control of physician expenditures through discounting, and a slow reduction of people entering the profession. It should be pointed out, however, that a single-payer system also provides a single target for dart practice—the government. Third, to go much beyond what is now on the policy table would require incredible political will power. Given the uneasiness with which the public is viewing existing cost containment exercises, more reforms are unlikely at present. Fourth, to go further would require major structural change. In particular, changing the funding base for providers (institutions and individuals) is key but is viewed as a major public policy challenge.

To date, provincial governments have opted for better public management of public resources rather than a shift to private, for-profit market forces. Presumably, this choice has been made on the assumption that a foot in the door is better than a closed door. As Barer et al. (1988) have written, controls do beget further controls. We have little real experience and few unilateral policy tools at our disposal. Yet the remarkable Canadian consensus about the value of publicly funded health insurance creates an imperative for governments to learn the required skills. Canada's economic circumstances requires them to learn fast.

One large question remains. Even if we are able to implement successful cost control policy levers, we have yet to understand how we can determine an acceptable level of health care spending. What is acceptable anyway? Like other nations struggling with health reform, Canada does know that it is not a technical exercise but one of societal choice and political decisions.

Notes

1. Recently, the province of New Brunswick has announced that it wishes to turn responsibility for claims processing over to a consortium of private health insurance companies. It is too early to tell whether this will be interpreted as a contravention of national legislation.

2. One provincial Ministry of Health stated that its mission was to be the best health care managers in the world.

3. The federal government had to step in to guarantee the Saskatchewan government's bonds in the 1992-93 fiscal year.

4. The "Social Contract" was a process undertaken in Ontario whereby all public sector transfer partners were asked to participate in a bargaining process to reduce government transfers. It involved spending cuts to avoid large layoffs and was seen as a controversial process.

5. Deinsured items included vasectomies, sterilizations, birth control counseling, and annual eye exams for 19- to 64-year-olds.

6. In Ontario, there is great difficulty in collecting cost data for the CHCs because they only recently became computerized, because they are set up explicitly to serve disadvantaged communities where the health burden is higher, and because they often have a larger number of homeless and transient individuals. In a recent strategic planning exercise for the program, one of the major recommendations was to undertake a careful cost comparison and data collection exercise to better understand the model. In the early years, much was made of the HSOs as a cost-effective alternative to fee for service. However, over time, most of the newer HSOs functioned like a group practice without a community board. Increases in the per capita rates were linked to increases awarded in the fee-for-service sector, thus eliminating any need to demonstrate cost-effectiveness. Furthermore, an extra payment provided to the HSO, originally designed to award HSOs with lower hospitalization rates relative to the peer group, became such a cash cow that some physicians were receiving annual payments of over $100,000. Recently, a moratorium was placed on the growth of the entire program as new ground rules were established. Existing contracts were canceled, and negotiations are under way for a new framework agreement.

References

Barer, M., Evans, R., & Labelle, R. (1988). Fee controls as cost control: Tales from the frozen North. *Milbank Quarterly, 66,* 1-64.

Barer, M., & Stoddart, G. (1991). *Towards integrated resource policies for Canada* (CHEPA Working Paper No. 91-7). Hamilton: McMaster University, Centre for Health Economics and Policy Analysis.

Evans, R. (1988). Split vision: Interpreting cross-border differences in health spending. *Health Affairs, 7,* 17-24.

Evans, R. (1993). Health care reform: The issue from hell. *Policy Options, 14*(8), 35-41.

Evans, R., Barer, M., & Stoddart, G. (1993). The truth about user fees. *Policy Options, 14*(8), 4-9.

Graham, B., & Lightman, E. (1992). *The crunch: Financing Ontario's social programs.* Toronto: Premier's Council on Health, Well-Being and Social Justice.

Lomas, J., Charles, C., & Greb, J. (1992). *The price of peace: The structure and process of physician fee negotiations in Canada* (CHEPA Working Paper No. 92-17). Hamilton: McMaster University, Centre for Health Economics and Policy Analysis.

Lomas, J., Fooks, C., Rice, T., & Labelle, R. (1989). Paying physicians in Canada: Minding our Ps and Qs. *Health Affairs, 8,* 80-102.

Ontario Ministry of Health. (1993). *Managing health care resources.* Toronto: Author.

Reinhardt, U. (1988, August 9). On the B factor in American health care. *Washington Post.*

Thorpe, K. (1993). The American states and Canada: A comparative analysis of health care spending. *Journal of Health Policy, Politics and Law, 18,* 477-489.

U.S. General Accounting Office. (1991). *Canadian health insurance: Lessons for the United States.* Washington, DC: Author.

CHAPTER 9

Preventive and Primary Care Access Systems

CLSCs as Neighborhood and Social Service Centers in Quebec

FRANÇOIS BÉLAND

Over a period of more than 20 years, the province of Quebec has initiated a series of changes in health care services that merit the attention of those concerned with health policy. In a series of official documents and legislative actions, the provincial government of Quebec has put into effect a new approach to health care that combines the resources of traditional medical care and social services with a newer emphasis on health promotion and social and community dimensions of service delivery. This new combined approach is realized through the establishment, over almost 20 years (1972-1990), of a large number of community health and social services agencies (centres locaux de services communautaires—CLSCs) throughout the province. Ideally, these community-based agencies should involve family practice physicians working on a team basis with nonphysician professionals, including nursing, paramedical, and social work personnel, as well as community organizers. Along with traditional medical services, the approach to care involves emphasis on health promotion, the social dimensions of being, and a more active role for patients in the diagnosis and treatment process. The research reported in this chapter indicates that not all objectives of this community approach to health care have been accomplished. However, as a model in process of being tested in action in the province of Quebec, it is well worthy of attention.

The 1971 Castonguay-Neveu Report (Commission d'enquête, 1970), considered by many as the founding act of Medicare in Quebec, introduced changes in the organizational context of health and medical care service delivery. The report proposed new structures and new ways of doing things in the health care system. Among the many organizational innovations proposed in the report, the *centres locaux de santé* (CLSs— neighborhood health centers) were to deliver primary medical and preventive health care (Bélanger, 1992; Bozzini, 1988). This proposition was never enacted. Instead, a dynamic medical profession reorganized the delivery of primary care in the province through physician group practices (Perreault, 1972). These were termed *cliniques* or *polycliniques,* according to the mixture of medical practitioners they included. The *cliniques* have only general practitioners (GPs), whereas the *polycliniques* contain a mixture of GPs and specialists.

The success of the medical profession in this endeavor forced the government to change drastically the conception of the CLSs. They became the CLSCs, with a domain of activities larger than medical and health care (Renaud, Baudoin, & Molinari, 1984-1985). They encompassed community organization as well as social and health services delivery. However, they held only a complementary role in regard to medical care. Their mission included nursing and psychosocial services, comprehensive home care services, services to mothers and children, and care for families with problems of a social nature (Bozzini, 1988). Also, they were to be publicly financed. However, the CLSC implementation process was slow. By 1978, 82 CLSCs had been implemented, whereas physicians had organized more than 400 private clinics (Lemieux & Labrie, 1979). The CLSC network was completed in 1990. Now every Quebec citizen can use a CLSC service; 160 of them are operating (Bélanger, 1992).

A number of policy papers produced in the last 4 years by the Ministry of Health and Social Services of the Province of Quebec assert that primary preventive and community care are responsibilities of the CLSCs. The first in that series of papers, *Pour améliorer la santé et le bien-être au Québec:*

Orientations (Ministère de la santé, 1989), defined four basic strategies
for implementing the ministry's health policies:

1. Health prevention and promotion
2. Reinforcement of individuals' autonomy, including informal social support
   networks and local communities
3. A multisectoral approach to health policy formulation and implementation
4. A strong public sector for services delivery

The two first strategies define the types of actions that the ministry
contemplated; the last two concern the organizational context in which
these actions were to take place.

In the organizational framework of the Quebec health care system,
CLSCs are one of the main components of the Quebec Health and Social
Services Ministry's preventive and primary care policy. Issues raised by this
policy stem from problems with integration of health promotion and
prevention with other activities in the system. Difficulties also arise from
the limited capacity of the CLSCs themselves to implement the ministry's
policy objectives. In this chapter, we refer to both of these difficulties in
describing the problems CLSCs are facing.

Four issues are specifically developed. The first involves the question
as to whether the ministry's preventive and primary care policy objectives
are integrated into a general vision of the Quebec health care system as a
whole. To assess this aspect of the problem, recent policy documents from
the ministry are reviewed. Second, a debate has been raging in the recent
past, and is now being reopened, on the best way to finance medical care
expenditures in Canada in general and in Quebec in particular. In 1991,
the ministry published a document entitled *Un financement équitable à la
mesure de nos moyens* (Ministère de la santé, 1991), in which propositions
to introduce user fees and deinsurance were examined. Are these proposals
in line with policy objectives for health promotion and preventive care,
considering that user fees and deinsurance can have a negative impact on
access to preventive and medical care services (Stoddart, Barer, Evans, &
Bratia, 1990)? A third issue involves the question of whether the Quebec
health care system is adapting itself to a strategy of health promotion and
prevention with a focus on primary and community care. Was there actual
reorientation of expenditures from hospital and medical care toward
CLSC activities? Fourth, it may be difficult to estimate the extent to which
medical practitioners in private clinics are able to integrate preventive and
health promotion activities. But we also need to know to what extent

CLSCs are implementing prevention and health promotion activities. Do physicians in CLSCs have a different practice profile than physicians practicing in other settings? These are the questions addressed in this chapter to assess the importance of prevention and health promotion in the Quebec health care system and the role of CLSCs in fostering these activities.

Health Promotion, Health Policies, and CLSCs in Quebec

In August 1991, a new law on health and social services was created by the Quebec National Assembly (Renaud, Baudoin, & Molinari, 1993-1994). This entailed a vast reform proposed in previously released documents, *Une réforme axée sur le citoyen* (Ministère de la santé, 1990a) and the report of the Rochon Commission (Commission d'enquête, 1988). This reform redefined or confirmed the role of every institution, organization, and service provider in the medical care and social service system in Quebec. The goals of the reform were (a) to correct deficiencies in service delivery, (b) to increase efficacy and efficiency, and (c) to reach an equilibrium between population needs and the ability of Quebec society to pay for health and social services. (For an overview of the reform, see Pineault, Lamarche, Champagne, Contandriopoulos, & Denis, 1993.)

The reform was essentially organizational. Primary care services were to be consolidated; the CLSCs were to be pivotal in this matter. Social services were to be transferred to CLSCs, and their role in the delivery of medical care was to be extended. Primary medical care and family medicine development occurring in hospitals were to be transferred to CLSCs. Also, private primary medical care providers were to be required to work for a specified number of hours each week either in CLSCs or in hospital emergency departments.

The second theme of the reform was decentralization and regionalization. The functions of the Ministry of Health and Social Services were to be limited to orientation and definitions of objectives, program development and evaluation, and distribution of resources to regional bodies. The new *régies régionales* were to have the responsibility of translating into regional goals the objectives of the ministry, including implementing programs and distributing resources to organizations responsible for delivering services. Regionalization was also seen as a way of involving citizens in the decision-making process. Regionalization of health and social services evolved slowly from 1971 on, but the *conseils régionaux,* the predecessors of the *régies régionales* implemented by the 1991-92 Health Care and Social Services Law, increased their jurisdiction over regional activities over the years.

Integration of health and social services was a goal constantly pursued at the governmental level (Turgeon, 1989a, 1989b, 1993). At least, since 1971, both domains have been the responsibility of a single ministry. Also, regional councils have had the responsibility of both sectors. The CLSCs were also conceived as offering both types of services. However, the practical degree of integration of medical care and social activities at all levels of the Quebec system is another matter.

In the reform's third theme, organizations delivering services to the population were redefined. CLSCs were to be consolidated, and the mission of hospitals, nursing homes, physical reeducation centers, and social service centers were refocused. Also, public health departments were totally reorganized. The 32 public health and hospital departments were reduced to 16 and relocated at the sites of the *régies régionales.* Citizens, organizations, and employees were to participate in the administration of the public health and hospital departments. Citizen representatives were to be elected to the executive boards of these organizations.

The fourth theme of the organizational reform concerned the financing of health care and social services. The reform focused on increasing efficacy and efficiency of service delivery rather than on new financing mechanisms. Efficacy and efficiency were to be attained through focusing on objectives defined in terms of results rather than processes. Resources were allocated to each region according to needs and to delivery organizations according to performance. Thus, the organizational reforms also embraced the planning of human resources and the monitoring of the efficacy and efficiency of insured services.

A few months after publication of the reform papers, the ministry published its health and social welfare policy report (Turgeon, 1989b). This document is remarkable from many points of view. First, health and social well-being were considered as being in constant interaction. Second, determinants of health and social problems were identified, and objectives and actions addressing these determinants were defined. Third, services were considered as means to an end rather than as ends in themselves. And fourth, health promotion and prevention, primary medical care, and social services, along with coordination of governmental actions from every ministry, were considered to be at the heart of the ministry's strategies.

Nineteen objectives were proposed involving five domains: social adaptation, physical health, public health, mental health, and social integration. Some objectives addressed specific health or social problems (e.g., cancer, heart disease, violence against women, suicide, and infectious diseases). Other objectives dealt with target groups, such as young offenders, the elderly, and dependent children. The interaction between health and social perspectives was shown in the proposed objective concerning the elderly. It was focused not on services or the costs attributable to elderly persons in health care, but on their social integration.

In summary, whereas some policy documents defined the organizational reform (Ministère de la santé, 1989, 1990a), others were oriented toward health policies (Ministère de la santé, 1992). Policy objectives and strategies gave the main role in the attainment of health and well-being for all to health promotion and prevention programs, community action, and citizen involvement. In that sense, CLSCs and primary care and social services providers were privileged. The foci of CLSCs' action were precisely the promotion of health and well-being and the integration of health and social perspectives in service delivery, and emphasis was also given to community development and citizen participation.

Financing the Health Care System

Strangely enough, the ministry published a document on financing health care before issuing documents on health and social policy objectives. *Un financement équitable à la mesure de nos moyens* (Ministère de la santé, 1991) analyzed health care expenditures in Quebec. Comparisons with other jurisdictions, but mainly with the province of Ontario, were used ambiguously. On the one hand, data showed that Quebec was on the regression line when gross domestic products (GDPs) of the 10 Canadian provinces were regressed on public expenditures on health care. On the other hand, comparisons with Ontario were used to show that Quebec was spending more than it should have on almost every health care item. Essentially, the document used moving targets to give the impression that there was a financial crisis looming ahead if ways to finance Medicare did not change. At the same time, it asserted that overall spending for health care was under control. In 1975, 8.03% of Quebec's GDP was devoted to the health sector; in 1987, health expenditures increased to the level of 8.88%. During the 1982-83 economic downturn, the proportion of health expenditures to GDP reached 9.34%. Thus, during the last decade, the relative share of health expenditures varied inversely with the health of the economy (Evans, 1993).

Overall, use of medical care has increased over the years in Quebec. In 1982, the average number of ambulatory care visits paid on a fee-for-service basis was 5.1 per person insured by the Régie de l'assurance-maladie du Québec (RAMQ), the third-party payer in the Quebec health insurance system (RAMQ, 1983). In 1991, the average was 6.6 (RAMQ, 1993). The percentage of persons using a physician's services increased from 77.8 in 1982 to 81.0 in 1991. During this same period, the population-to-physician ratio decreased from 589 to 554, and the mean number of services provided annually by physicians on a fee-for-service basis increased from 3,235 to 3,638 (Ministère de la santé, 1991; RAMQ, 1983, 1993). Hospital admissions declined slightly (−1.8%) from 1981-82 to 1988-89 (Levasseur, 1992). However, the number of hospital days per 1,000 persons increased 3.1%. Hospital use by children and adults decreased by 7.9% in that period, whereas use by those over 75 years old increased by 21.8%. Thus, during the 1980s there was a small increase in the overall use of medical care and hospital services in Quebec. Patterns of use in Quebec as well as in other Canadian provinces have shifted significantly, with an increase in the utilization by the elderly and a decrease in adult usage (Barer, Evans, Hertzman, & Lomas, 1987; Barer et al., 1989; Evans et al., 1989). Though rates of use of medical care and hospital services did not increase much during this period, the Ministry of Health and Social Services budget increased more rapidly than did total governmental expenditures and at a higher rate than the consumer price index (Ministère de la santé, 1990b, 1993b) (see Figure 9.1).

Provincial governments are only in partial control of the fiscal resources they need to finance Medicare and health expenditures. When Medicare was implemented in Canada, the federal government agreed to share with the provinces more or less half of health care expenditures with little or no control over costs (Ministère des finances, Canada, 1993). This arrangement has been modified a number of times. Lately, the federal government unilaterally limited the growth of its share in expenses for health care. In 1986-87, increases in direct payments were limited to the growth of GNP minus 2%. In 1990, the level of federal contributions were frozen to their 1989-90 fiscal year level. This freeze has been extended through 1995-96 (Conseil national de bien-être social, 1991; Santé et bien-être Canada, 1993). These changes will have dramatic effects on the level of federal direct payments for health care to Quebec (Canadian Hospital Association, 1993).

The 1976 federal-provincial fiscal arrangements divided the direct federal contributions for health care into two parts. A portion was converted into income tax points (shares of income tax receipts). Later,

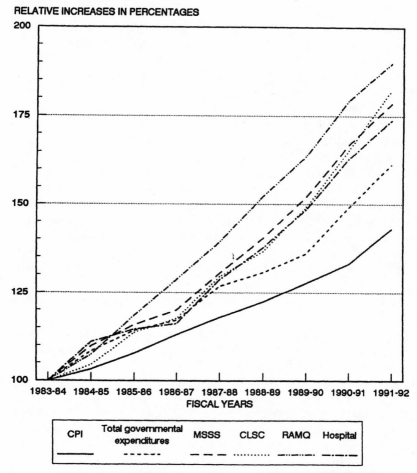

Figure 9.1. Relative Governmental Expenditures, Annual Ministère de la Santé (MSSS) Budgets, and Consumer Price Index (CPI) (1983-84 to 1991-92 Fiscal Years)

SOURCE: Regie de l'assurance-maladie du Québec (1983-1991), *Statistiques annuelles.*

the federal government lowered its share, while the provincial governments were compelled to hike theirs proportionally. The other portion of the federal contribution was made through direct annual payments to the provinces. Figure 9.2 shows how the value of provincial income tax points collected by the federal government for Quebec increased through the years. However, from 1986 to 1990, direct payments were stable, whereas

IN MILLION CANADIAN DOLLARS

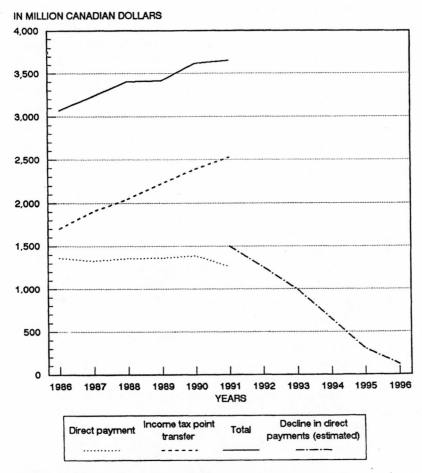

Figure 9.2. Federal Transfers to Quebec for Health Care (Observed 1986-1991; Estimated 1991-1996)

SOURCE: Santé et bien-être Canada (1993).

from 1991 to 1996, they would have come close to zero if the federal contribution to health care and other social program costs had stayed as planned (Conseil national de bien-être social, 1991). The federal government has recently imposed a new fiscal transfer payment scheme on the provinces. All federal transfers are now brought under a single program, with the total sum transferred to be lowered by $5 billion in 1997-98, a sixth of the total federal transfers. Though this new fiscal arrangement maintains the federal government contribution, the integrity of Canadian Medicare may be jeopardized, as the National Forum on Health (NFH) report assessed (NFH, 1997). The principle of the decoupling of medical care use from cost may be abandoned under pressure coming from financially and fiscally strained provinces. *Un financement équitable à la mesure de nos moyens* (Ministère de la santé, 1991) emphasized the federal disengagement from health care financing as one of the major problems confronting the Quebec government. According to this document, problems also stemmed from the disequilibrium of the overall provincial government budget. The argument was made that increases in the health care and social services budget—which are a consequence of changes in the demographic profile of the Quebec population, technologic improvements, and changes in medical practice—could no longer be financed with tax increases. However, the document also maintained that resources already invested in these sectors were sufficient, another example of the document's dubious reasoning. The disequilibrium in the health care and social services budget did, and still does, stem from the reduced federal direct transfer payments to the provinces. The document concluded by asserting the necessity for service recipients to contribute to costs of care either through user fees, de-insurance, or a service tax. Under this tax proposal, users' annual expenditures for services would be added to their income for income tax purposes.

This proposal could not be implemented by the Quebec government without cost. According to the Canadian Health Act of 1984 (Article 20), the federal government would cut direct federal transfer of the amount Quebec would have collected. Allowable exceptions to these cuts in federal transfer are "nonmedically necessary services." Accordingly, the Quebec government deinsured optometric, dental, and pharmaceutical services, amounting to $100 million in fiscal year 1992-93. This move was spectacular in some ways, but the real significance of the document on financing health care lay elsewhere. Since the inception of Medicare in Quebec, the philosophic assumption was that use of health care was to be separated from cost. The document clearly asserted the need to reinstate a link between use and cost through patient charges. However, the aim of Medicare was to abolish the financial barriers to medical care use. Canadian studies have concluded that this program has reached its goal. The effect of Canadian health care policy has been that income is not an impediment to access to medical care (Béland, 1994; Dongois, 1992a; Ministère de la santé, 1994). However, the effect of introducing user fees and deinsurance with regard to access to medical care in general and to CLSCs' health promotion services and preventive care in particular was not analyzed in any of the ministry documents (Ministère de la santé, 1989, 1990a, 1991, 1992). Also, the whole dynamic of financing medical care within an essentially public funded system was not considered. Finally, the organizational reform and health policy reorientation toward health promotion and prevention on the level of financial resources needed was not mentioned in *Un financement équitable à la mesure de nos moyens* (Ministère de la santé, 1991). It was as if the ministry's reflections on financing health care were totally independent of its own actions and planning in the domain of health policy and organization reforms.

Expenditures on CLSCs and on Health Promotion Activities

Where was the money devoted to health and medical care spent in Quebec? How did CLSCs' share in the health care budget evolve over the years? Primary care and health promotion were emphasized in the policy objectives and in the organizational reform documents. Were these commitments also privileged in the budgeting process during the last decade or so? Figure 9.3 shows the relative increase in current dollars with regard to six budget items from fiscal years 1981-82 to 1991-92: health promotion, home health care and homemaker services, day care and day hospital centers, ambulatory family and specialized medical care, laboratory procedures, and physicians' care of hospitalized patients. Health promotion includes activities and programs at the workplace, maternal and child health, bucco-dental health services (mainly for children), and other activities such as inoculation (Ministère de la santé, 1993b). Home health care and homemaker services are delivered in the homes of elderly and handicapped patients by nurses and homemakers. Ambulatory medical care is reimbursed by RAMQ for direct patient care to physicians (on the basis of salary, sessional fee, or fee-for-service schedule). Laboratory procedures include all ancillary procedures processed in hospitals prescribed by physicians to hospitalized and ambulatory patients. Few laboratory tests are processed in the private sector, and such privately processed tests are not reimbursed by the Quebec Medicare system. They are not included here. However, physician services to hospitalized patients are included. Figure 9.3 compares health and medical care activities, not organizational budget allocations. Thus, we have not considered total hospital budgets in this analysis.

RELATIVE INCREASES IN PERCENTAGES

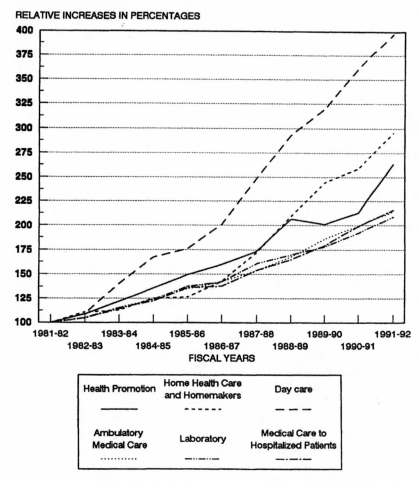

Figure 9.3. Relative Increases in Medical and Health Care Expenditures (Quebec, 1981-82 to 1991-92)
SOURCE: Ministère de la santé (1993b).

Day care and day hospital center activities have increased the most; they nearly quadrupled between fiscal years 1981-82 and 1991-92. The home health care and homemaker expenses increased slowly between 1980 and 1985, but, from 1985 on, their rate of increase was comparable to that of the day care and day hospital budget. Health promotion also increased somewhat more rapidly than the budget share of the three more traditional medical care activities—namely, ambulatory medical care, inpatient medical care, and laboratory procedures. These three items increased at the same steady rate throughout the period.

Budget increases in community-oriented health care were greater than those for the medical care sector. However, in terms of dollars and cents, the two types of activities are not in the same playing field. For example, $18 million was devoted to day care and hospital day centers in fiscal year 1981-82, whereas $340 million was spent on ambulatory medical care. In current dollars, the increase for day care and hospital day centers was $54 million, whereas for ambulatory medical care it was $373 million. Increases in home care and homemaker services when compared with inpatient hospital medical care yielded $168 million in the former case and $668 million in the latter. Thus, though the relative increase in the community health sector budget was almost twice that for the medical care sector, expenditures in this sector increased four to seven times faster than those in the community care sector.

In Figure 9.1, relative increases in expenditures on CLSCs and hospitals are plotted. Increases in hospital expenditure plateaued between fiscal years 1984-85 and 1986-87, whereas those for CLSCs increased somewhat faster during that period. From fiscal year 1986-87 to 1990-91, both budgets increased at the same rate. Only in 1991-92 did CLSCs' budgets grow faster than hospital budgets. Recent data show that this trend continued in fiscal year 1992-93 (Ministère de la santé, 1994).

It is of interest to know how budgets are distributed within CLSCs. What are the shares of different health and medical activities in these organizations? Budgets for health promotion activities, ambulatory medical care, psychosocial services[1] and home health care and homemaker services in CLSCs accounted for 49% of the total budget for CLSCs in 1991-92. Another big item in the CLSC budget is administrative activities; they accounted for 15% of total CLSC budgets.

Figure 9.4 compares expenditures for 1987-88 and 1991-92. Home health care and homemaker service expenses almost doubled in that period. Ambulatory medical care budgets, though a small item on CLSC budgets, also doubled in size. Figure 9.4 shows that health promotion and home care are the two main items on the CLSCs' activities list. They are complemented by social and medical services delivered by professionals, mainly social workers and physicians. The chart also shows that clinical medical services almost reached the level of social case work in 1991.

A variety of CLSC observers (Bélanger, 1992; Bozzini, 1988; Dongois, 1992a) concluded that the 160 Quebec CLSCs, though sharing a philosophy and model of health and social services delivery, were very different in the program packages they offered. CLSCs are supposed to adapt

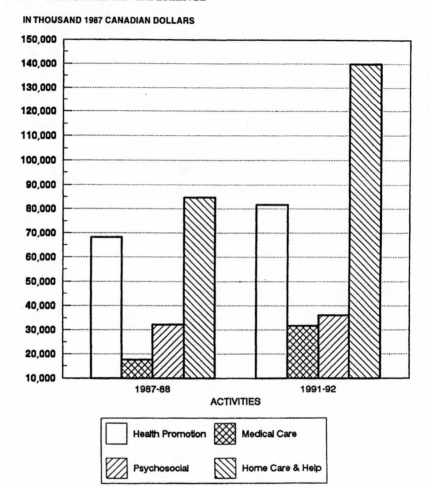

IN THOUSAND 1987 CANADIAN DOLLARS

Figure 9.4. Trends in CLSCs' Activities (1987-88 and 1991-92)
SOURCE: Ministère de la santé (1993b).

themselves to the needs of their population. Thus, there should be
variations in the CLSCs' role in delivering medical care services throughout the province of Quebec. Access to medical care in remote regions can
be assessed through a comparison of the proportions of people using
medical care services. Quebec is divided into 16 health and social services
regions (excluding the far north). Remote regions are Nord du Québec,
Côte-Nord, Gaspésie, Abitibi, and Bas-Saint-Laurent (BSL). The
Saguenay region is a mixed rural and urban region, as are Appalaches,

PERCENTAGES

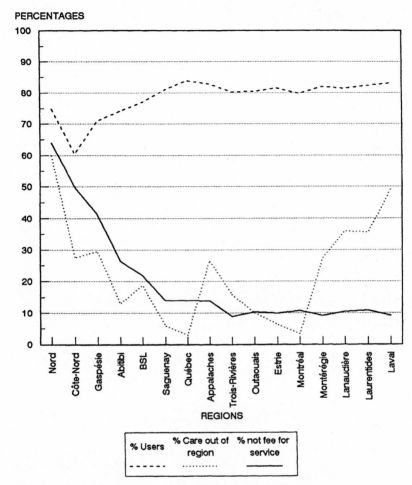

Figure 9.5. Regional Access to Medical Care (Quebec, 1991)
SOURCE: Regie de l'assurance-maladie du Québec (1992).

Estrie, and Outaouais. The Montérégie, Lanaudière, Laurentides, and Laval regions surround the Montreal metropolitan region. Finally, the Quebec City metropolitan area is a region by itself. Figure 9.5 shows that the proportion of users was lower in remote regions (the first four regions on the left) than in other regions. Also, physicians not paid on a fee-for-service basis are concentrated in these four areas. The Quebec Ministry of Health and Social Services has used other payment mechanisms to attract physicians to these areas. Despite this, a higher proportion of people

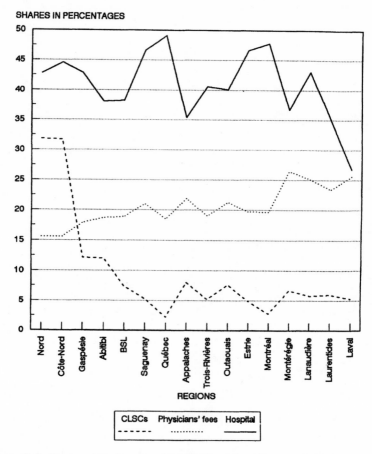

SHARES IN PERCENTAGES

Figure 9.6. Regional Budgets on CLSCs, Physicians' Fees, and Hospitals
SOURCE: Ministère de la santé (1993b).

receive medical services outside of their regions in the nonmetropolitan areas. Finally, Figure 9.5 shows that specialist services are less available outside of the Quebec City and Montreal metropolitan areas. Availability of general practitioners is more uniform across regions.

Do the CLSCs in different regions deliver different packages of services because of regional variations in medical care accessibility? Figure 9.6 shows that in remote regions the CLSCs' budget share was more substantial than in other regions. In Nord du Québec and in the Côte-Nord, CLSCs were important players in the field, accounting for approximately a third of the total regional health and social services budget. Elsewhere, however, they were quite small players compared with hospitals. In these other regions, about 5% of regional budgets was spent on CLSCs, whereas 40% was expended on hospitals. In 1993, general practitioners working in the CLSCs were a significant proportion of all GPs. In the Nord du Québec and Côte-Nord regions they accounted for more than 30% of GPs; in the Quebec and Montreal regions, they were 9.5% and 13.5% respectively.

Activities of CLSCs also differed by regions. Only in remote regions did CLSCs provide any inpatient services (Figure 9.7). These CLSCs were in fact operating some hospital beds. Accordingly, other activity shares in the total CLSCs budget were lowered. But data in Figure 9.7 also show regional variations in other CLSCs' activities that are difficult to explain except by the fact that CLSCs are adapting themselves to local realities. Home health care and homemaker services are the main source of CLSC expenditures. Outside of remote regions, these activities account for at least 25% of their budgets. Health promotion activities are at the level of 15% to 20%. However, ambulatory medical care is shown to be a relatively unimportant CLSC activity, accounting for less than 5% of their budget in most of the regions. Delivery of medical care is thus a marginal CLSC activity at the present time. Except in remote regions, its significance is small.

Physician Practice Pattern in the CLSC

Approximately 15% of general practitioners in Quebec are working in a CLSC in one capacity or another. The total number of CLSC physicians was 1,037 in 1991, with some of them working part-time. Few CLSCs do not hire general practitioners, but not all have developed their medical services to the same degree. For example, in the Côte-Nord region, out of the 39 physicians working in a CLSC, 18 are concentrated in just two settings. In Montreal, out of a total of 174 physicians working in 19 CLSCs, 119 are practicing in 11 of the clinics (Dongois, 1992a).

Among medical services offered by CLSCs, 85% involve physician visits during the day, although 50% of clinics are also open in the evening (Féderation des CLSC du Québec [FCLSCQ], 1991). At CLSC walk-in clinics, physician visits constitute 54% of medical care during the day and 33% of services offered in the evening. A physician is on call 21% of the time during evening hours. In 22% of the CLSCs, physicians are available on weekends. The work of general practitioners in CLSCs is not devoted

PERCENTAGES

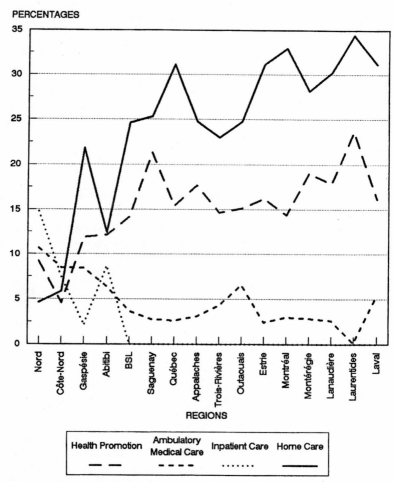

Figure 9.7. Regional CLSCs' Budgets for Four Health Care Activities (Fiscal Year 1990-91)

SOURCE: Ministère de la santé (1993b).

exclusively to clinical practice; out of their 35-hour work week, 25 hours are devoted to clinical work (Dongois, 1992a). Other activities include administrative responsibilities, meeting with the multidisciplinary team, and planning and programming CLSC activities. Responsibilities also involve the training of family medicine residents, research, and other duties. The provision of preventive care accounts for 18% of the CLSC physician's workday (FCLSCQ, 1986).

This diversity of physician activities is planned within the CLSC model of health care practice. But this model is also defined in terms of a different practice style oriented toward a holistic approach, involving multidisciplinary work and community participation and the integration of preventive and curative aspects of medical care. Moreover, the individual and collective dimensions of health care are both embraced in this medical practice model (Bélanger, 1992; FCLSCQ, 1986; Poupart, Simard, & Ouellette, 1986). Have physicians in CLSCs been successful in dealing with these multiple aspects of their medical practice? A number of studies are available to provide a partial answer to this question.

Physicians' self-reported practices in clinics were compared among diverse clinical settings: fee-for-service practitioners in rural and urban settings; CLSC physicians with salaried reimbursement; physicians practicing in hospitals; and physicians in family medicine centres (FMCs) paid on a session basis (Battista & Spitzer, 1982). The research found that CLSC physicians and FMC physicians prescribed preventive services[2] more often than their colleagues in fee-for-service practice. Physicians in fee-for-service practice tended to use inappropriate screening procedures at a higher rate than did CLSC and FMC physicians. Another study (Renaud, Beauchemin, Lalonde, Poirier, & Berthiaume, 1980) showed that CLSC physicians prescribed anxiolytics at a lower rate and for a shorter time period to patients suffering from tension headaches. Clinical encounters with CLSC physicians lasted more than 20 minutes on average but lasted less than 10 minutes with fee-for-service physicians. Also, CLSC physicians more often suggested alternatives to drugs as treatment for patient problems.

In a series of papers, Maheux and colleagues (Maheux, Dufort, Lambert, & Berthiaume, 1988; Maheux, Lambert, Pineault, Beaudoin, & Berthiaume, 1988; Maheux et al., 1989; Maheux, Pineault, Lambert, Béland, & Lévesque, 1990; Pineault, Champagne, Maheux, Legault, & Paré, 1989; Pineault, Maheux, Lambert, Béland, & Lévesque, 1991) studied support among Quebec physicians for aspects of the biopsychosocial model of medical practice. They investigated physicians' attitudes and behavior, patient participation in the diagnosis and treatment procedure, importance of social factors in the clinical process, multidisciplinary teamwork, and significance of illness as a life experience for patients. CLSC physicians were more favorable toward multidisciplinary teamwork and patient involvement in the medical care process than fee-for-service physicians. Female physicians practicing in the CLSC emphasized the importance of social factors in clinical work more strongly than female physicians in other settings. Male physicians in CLSCs think that illness may be a worthwhile life experience more than their male counterparts in fee-for-service private clinics. However, when behavior rather than attitudes was examined, differences between physicians in CLSCs and in private clinics lost statistical significance.

Differences between CLSC and private clinic physicians may stem from confounding factors such as medical training, gender differences, and pre-CLSC preferences for nontraditional medical care models. CLSC physicians are younger than colleagues practicing in other settings. Of CLSC physicians, 55.9% are women, compared to 16.7% of private clinic physicians paid on a fee-for-service schedule. Finally, 32.2% of the former are trained in family medicine, whereas only 11.0% of physicians in private practice have received this training.[3] Though prior conditioning factors may be influential in orienting CLSC physicians toward the biopsychosocial model in medicine, when these factors are taken into account, the differences between CLSC physicians and their counterparts in private practice still remain.

CLSC physicians differ from other physicians not only in sociodemographic background and attitudes and behavior in the clinical encounter (Pineault et al., 1991) but in their pattern of activities. More CLSC physicians practice in rural milieux than do physicians working in other clinical settings. Also, over 80% of them are engaged in group practice. However, they are less involved with hospitalized patients than their colleagues. They also devote less time to hospital emergency departments and tend to visit patients at home less often. Medical training activities are as important for CLSC practitioners as for their colleagues in private clinics, and CLSC practitioners are slightly more involved in administrative work. However, the big difference between CLSC physicians and other practitioners is their involvement in community health: 31.8% of the men and 44.5% of the women among CLSC physicians are working in this field, as compared to less than 10% for other physicians.

Physicians have a special status in the CLSC. They are the only professionals who typically assume responsibility for the administrative aspects of the practice. Also, a medical council must be set up in every CLSC. CLSCs have had difficulties in coming to terms with this administrative status for physicians. It may appear to contradict the ideology of multidisciplinarity, in which every professional is conceived as having a similar status. Recently, a policy statement from FCLSCQ, the representative organization for CLSCs, has expressed its approval for this arrangement (FCLSCQ, 1991). Physicians are in the CLSCs to stay, and CLSCs are clearly and openly promoting a specific model of medical care. It is their claim that this model is markedly different from the private practice fee-for-service model.

Significance of the CLSCs for the Quebec Health Care System

Four issues in the domain of health promotion and preventive care confronting CLSCs have been considered:

1. Are the Ministry of Health and Social Services preventive and primary care policy objectives integrated into an overall vision of the Quebec health care system?
2. Are financial issues in the health care system defined in terms of system objectives in the domain of health promotion and preventive care?
3. Are health care expenditures directed toward health promotion, preventive care, and the CLSCs?
4. Do CLSC physicians promote and practice a model of care different from that of their colleagues in the private clinics?

Examination of data to answer these four questions allowed us to make a tour of the Quebec health care system from policy formulation to implementation of objectives and, finally, to the level of actual day-to-day medical practice in the CLSC, the front-door organizations providing health promotion programs to local communities and preventive medical and social care to citizens. Results of this review have been mixed. Health promotion and preventive care are at the very heart of grand policy statements and thinking about organizational reform. These policy statements constitute the source of recent changes in the Quebec health care system. The CLSCs are the organizations targeted for implementing health promotion and preventive care programs. Furthermore, within the CLSCs, these programs are to be coordinated with social services and community actions. However, the 1993 debate on financing health care gave some indications as to the line of argument used by the ministry: Health policy objectives were totally ignored, and the federal-provincial fiscal arrangements and the policy toward the public debt were the only lines of discussion permitted.

Observation of shares for health care and health promotion activities provided hints as to the ability of the Quebec Ministry of Health and Social Services to implement its policies. Health promotion, community health, and social services were developed at a higher rate than hospital or ambulatory medical care. It thus seems that Quebec was putting money where its policy objectives were. Moreover, financial resources devoted to CLSCs began to increase faster than other budget items in recent years. Also, medical care, though still a small part of CLSC activities, increased between 1987-88 and 1991-92; its budget allocation more than doubled in constant dollars.

In addressing the fourth question, we showed that the CLSCs' role in medical care varies widely according to area. In remote regions, they are major players; they provide medical services to the population. In other regions, their role seems to be to offer an alternative model of medical care. Physicians are encouraged to assume responsibilities for community programs rather than to confine themselves strictly to usual clinical work. Physicians in the CLSC appear to be successful in promoting a new model of clinical practice and in involving themselves in activities other than traditional clinical work. However, research results on their behavioral patterns have been mixed.

CLSC physicians are now involved in the development of a specific approach to medical services (FCLSCQ, 1991). They are promoting an alternative model of care that they claim differentiates them from other types of clinical practice. CLSCs define themselves as being complementary to private clinics rather than in competition with them.

This is not the perception of fee-for-service physicians (Dongois, 1992b). Negotiations between the CLSC physicians' organization (the FCLSCQ) and the GPs' union have not really settled the issue of the role of CLSCs in clinical practice. However, the Ministry of Health and Social Services has clearly signaled that it means to develop medical services in the CLSCs. A plan (Ministère de la santé, 1993a) to add 461 full-time equivalent doctors has been approved. According to this plan, CLSCs are expected to have on average a team of 6.6 full-time-equivalent physicians.

CLSCs are here to stay in the Quebec health care system (Bozzini, 1988). Their activities are at the center stage of Quebec health policies. A number of recent moves by the ministry confirm the viability of CLSCs in the Quebec health and social services system: increases in CLSC budgets, transfers of social and health care services from other organizations to CLSCs, policies oriented toward community approaches to health and social services, and promotion of a medical care model appropriate for the CLSC mission.

CLSCs provide the ministry with a means appropriate to its goal, and they are the best selling point for the policy objectives adopted by the Quebec government. At a time when ways are being sought to devolve care from hospital to communities and from the long-term custodial care sector to the patient's home, the availability of a community level organization is priceless. The value of the CLSCs is underlined by the capacity of these organizations to operate throughout the province, both in the more densely populated metropolitan areas and in remote rural regions with scattered populations. Community services can be implemented everywhere in the province, with care being made available to every citizen and readily adapted to local realities.

The CLSCs' history has been bumpy. These health and social services agencies were implemented in an era of social changes, where social innovations originated by the state were deemed acceptable. Are CLSCs so specific to a historical period and a particular political culture—the francophone in North America—that this model cannot be useful elsewhere? This question is not easy to answer. It is indeed difficult to imagine that a modified HMO similar to the CLSC might be successfully implemented in a community such as Beverly Hills, California, or Palm Beach, Florida. However, a matter for useful speculation is whether some more congenial settings for the CLSC might be found elsewhere in the United States.

Notes

1. Psychosocial services include social services (case work) to individuals, families, and other people and social integration programs for physically or mentally handicapped individuals.

2. For example, mammography to women aged 50 to 59 years, occult blood tests for asymptomatic patients aged 45 years and over, and PAP smear tests.

3. This difference in medical training is likely to fade as time passes. Schools of medicine in Quebec recently moved to a 2-year family training program for general practitioners; the traditional 1-year residency program has been abandoned.

References

Barer, M., Evans, R. G., Hertzman, C., & Lomas, J. (1987). Aging and health care utilization: New evidence on old fallacies. *Social Science and Medicine, 24,* 851-862.

Barer, M., Pulanis, I. R., Evans, R. G., Hertzman, C., Lomas, J., & Anderson, G. M. (1989). Trends in use of medical services by the elderly in British-Columbia. *Canadian Medical Association Journal, 141,* 39-45.

Battista, R., & Spitzer, W. (1982). Adult cancer precaution in primary care: Contrasts among primary care practice settings in Québec. *American Journal of Public Health, 73,* 1040-1041.

Béland, F. (1994). L'accès aux services de santé et les régions publiques d'assurance-maladie. In F. Dumont, S. Langlois, & Y. Martin (Eds.), *Traité des problèmes sociaux* (pp. 843-866). Quebec: Institut québécois de recherche sur la culture.

Bélanger, J. (1992). *Le développement des soins primaires au Québec: Le cas des CLSC.* Montreal: Association pour la santé publique du Québec.

Bozzini, L. (1988). Local community services centers (CSLCs) in Québec: Description, evaluation, perspectives. *Journal of Public Health Policy, 9,* 346-375.

Canadian Hospital Association. (1993). *Health care costs. An open future: A shared vision.* Ottawa: CHA Press.

Commission d'enquête sur la santé et le bien-être social. (1970). *La santé* (Vol. 4). Quebec: Government of Canada.

Commission d'enquête sur les services de santé et les services sociaux. (1988). *Rapport.* Quebec: Government of Quebec.

Conseil national de bien-être social. (1991). *Les dangers qui guettent le financement de la santé et de l'enseignement supérieur.* Ottawa: Author.

Dongois, M. (1992a). Services médicaux en CLSC: Divergences de vue entre l'AMOM et l'AMCLSC. *L'Actualité médicale, 13*(23), 2.

Dongois, M. (1992b). Un médecin de CLSC passe 25 heures par semaine en consultation. *L'actualité médicale, 13*(34), 2.

Evans, R. (1993, July-August). Health care reforms: The issue from hell. *Policy Options,* pp. 35-41.

Evans, R. G., Barer, M. L., Hertzman, C., Anderson, G. M., Pulcins, I. R., & Lomas, J. (1989). The long goodbye: The great transformation of the British Columbia hospital system. *Health Services Research, 24,* 435-459.

Fédération des CLSC du Québec. (1986). *Questionnaire portant sur la situation des médecins dans les CLSC et les centres de santé.* Montreal: Author.

Fédération des CLSC du Québec. (1991). *Les services médicaux en CLSC.* Montreal: Author.

Lemieux, V., & Labrie, P. (1979). Le système cybernétique de CLSC. *Recherches socio-graphiques, 20,* 149-173.

Levasseur, M. (1992). *La consommation de soins dans les centres hospitaliers de courte durée par les personnes âgées Québec 1981-1982 à 1988-1989.* Quebec: Ministère de la santé et des services sociaux.

Maheux, B., Dufort, F., Lambert, J., Béland, F., Lévesque, A., & Dedobbeleer, N. (1989). The professional attitudes and clinical practices of men and women generalists. *Canadian Family Physician, 35,* 59-63.

Maheux, B., Dufort, F., Lambert, J., & Berthiaume, M. (1988). Do female general practitioners have a distinctive type of medical practice? *Canadian Medical Association Journal, 139,* 737-740.

Maheux, B., Lambert, J., Pineault, R., Beaudoin, C., & Berthiaume, M. (1988). Generalists trained in family medicine: A distinctive type of medical practice. *Canadian Family Physician, 34,* 1093-1099.

Maheux, B., Pineault, R., Lambert, J., Béland, F., & Lévesque, A. (1990). Les soins de première ligne au Québec : Profil des médecins omnipraticiens pratiquant en cabinet privé et en CLSC. *Revue canadienne de santé publique, 81,* 27-31.

Ministère de la santé et des services sociaux. (1989). *Pour améliorer la santé et le bien-être au Québec.* Quebec: Government of Quebec.

Ministère de la santé et des services sociaux. (1990a). *Une réforme axée sur le citoyen.* Quebec: Government of Quebec.

Ministère de la santé et des services sociaux. (1990b). *SIFO. Système d'information financière et opérationnelle. Synthèse statistiques: 1981-1982 à 1987-1988.* Quebec: MSSS, Planification-évaluation Santé services sociaux.

Ministère de la santé et des services sociaux. (1991). *Un financement équitable à la mesure de nos moyens.* Quebec: Government of Quebec.

Ministère de la santé et des services sociaux. (1992). *La politique de la santé et du bien-être.* Quebec: Government of Quebec.

Ministère de la santé et des services sociaux. (1993a). *L'organisation des services médicaux en CLSC.* Quebec: Government of Quebec.

Ministère de la santé et des services sociaux. (1993b). *SIFO. Système d'information financière et opérationnelle. Statistiques: 1985-1986 à 1991-1992.* Quebec: Author.

Ministère de la santé et des services sociaux. (1994). *INFO-SIFO.* Gouvernement du Quebec: Author.

Ministère des Finances, Canada. (1993). *Transferts fédéraux aux provinces.* Ottawa: Author.

National Forum on Health. (1997). *La santé au Canada: Un héritage à faire fructifier* (Vol. 3). Ottawa: Ministère des travaux publics et services gouvernementaux.

Perreault, N. (1972). L'affrontement semble inévitable entre les omnipraticiens et le gouvernement. *Médecin du Québec, 7*(8-9), 52.

Pineault, R., Champagne, F., Maheux, B., Legault, C., & Paré, M. (1989). Determinants of health counseling practices in hospitals: The patients' perspective. *American Journal of Preventive Medicine, 5,* 257-265.

Pineault, R., Lamarche, P. A., Champagne, F., Contandriopoulos, A. P., & Denis, J. L. (1993). The reform of the Québec health care system: Potential for innovations? *Journal of Public Health Policy, 14,* 198-210.

Pineault, R., Maheux, B., Lambert, J., Béland, F., & Lévesque, A. (1991). Characteristics of physicians practicing in alternative primary care settings: A Québec study of local community service center physicians. *International Journal of Health Services, 21,* 49-58.

Poupart, R., Simard, J., & Ouellette, J. (1986). *La création d'une culture organisationnelle: Le cas des CLSC.* Montreal: Fédération des CLSC du Québec.

Régie de l'assurance-maladie du Québec. (1983). *Statistiques annuelles 1982.* Quebec: Author.

Régie de l'assurance-maladie du Québec. (1992). *Statistiques annuelles 1991.* Quebec: Author.

Régie de l'assurance-maladie du Québec. (1993). *Statistiques annuelles 1992.* Quebec: Author.

Renaud, M., Beauchemin, J., Lalonde, C., Poirier, H., & Berthiaume, S. (1980). Practice settings and prescribing profiles: The simulation of tension headaches to general practitioners working in different practice settings in the Montreal area. *American Journal of Public Health, 70,* 1068-1073.

Renaud, Y., Baudoin, J., & Molinari, P. (1984-1985). *Services de santé et services sociaux. Loi sur les services de santé et les services sociaux, art. 1, paragraphe 9.* Montreal: Judico.

Renaud, Y., Baudoin, J., & Molinari, P. (1993-1994). *Services de santé et services sociaux. Loi sur les services de santé et les services sociaux et modifiant diverses dispositions législatives.* Montreal: Judico.

Santé et bien-être Canada. (1993). *Loi canadienne sur la santé, rapport annuel 1991-1992.* Ottawa: Health and Welfare Canada.

Stoddart, G. L., Barer, M. L., Evans, R. G., & Bratia, V. (1990). *Why not use charges? The real issues.* Toronto: Premier's Council on Health, Well-Being and Social Justice, Government of Ontario.

Turgeon, J. (1989a). *Une analyse structurale d'un processus de régionalisation: Les conseils de la santé et des services sociaux du Québec (1971-1988).* Unpublished doctoral dissertation, Université Laval, Quebec.

Turgeon, J. (1989b). Bientôt vingt ans de régionalisation: Qu'ont donc à en faire les CRSSS? *Service social, 38,* 220-245.

Turgeon, J. (1993, May). *Second debut for the third level: Health and social services regions in Québec.* Paper presented at the Sixth Annual Health Policy Conference of the Centre for Health Economics and Policy Analysis, McMaster University, Hamilton.

PART IV

The Swedish Experience

CHAPTER 10

Historical and Institutional Foundations of the Swedish Health Care System

ELLEN IMMERGUT

This chapter argues that the Swedish health care system developed within the context of Sweden's "politics of compromise." This was not based on a preexisting consensus or absence of conflict, however. Rather, compromise was forged by political institutions that did not provide opportunities for minority interests to override the executive-level consensus. The result of the pattern of executive-induced conciliation was a health system that represents the public extreme of government financing and delivery of health services. The Swedish government introduced national health insurance and controls on doctors' fees and finally placed all doctors on full-time salary in conjunction with severe restrictions on the ability of doctors to practice privately, thereby converting the system to a de facto national health service. Because health reforms were not

EDITORS' NOTE: This chapter is reprinted in abridged form from *Health Politics: Interests and Institutions in Western Europe* (Chapter 5), by Ellen Immergut, 1992, Cambridge, UK: Cambridge University Press. Copyright 1992 by Cambridge University Press. Reprinted with the permission of Cambridge University Press.

blocked by institutional brakes to change, the Swedish case provides a particularly interesting example of the use of monopsony payment to regulate the health system by changing market incentives to patients and doctors.

Institutional Design

Political bargains worked out in the transition from monarchical rule in 1866 and in the subsequent extensions of the franchise in 1907 and 1918 established a system with some of the same institutional checks as in many other parliamentary democracies. Parliament was to balance the power of the executive, and the indirectly elected First Chamber of the bicameral parliament was to restrain the effects of the expansion of the franchise. Whereas elsewhere—as in France and Switzerland, for example—such institutions provided effective veto opportunities, in Sweden, mechanisms were developed to overcome these jurisdictional conflicts.

In reaction to the opposition between monarch and parliament and between the two chambers of the parliament, Swedish politicians increasingly relied on the institutions of royal committees (*Kungliga Kommité-väsendet*), consultative bodies of interest group and political representatives appointed by the executive to draft legislative proposals. Interested parties were further invited to comment on the committee proposals through written statements, called *remiss*. The committee and *remiss* system isolated policy making from the problem of conflicts between executive and parliament and from unstable majorities in the parliament. Policy preparations continued despite frequent changes in the governing coalitions and vetoes from the First Chamber.

When the Social Democrats effected a stable parliamentary majority by forming a coalition with the Farmers' Party in the 1930s and obtained a majority in the First Chamber, the process was accelerated. The veto points were in a sense closed off because they were filled with representatives of the party that governed the executive. The combination of constitutional rules and the electoral victories of the Social Democrats resulted in an institutional context for policy making that allowed the smooth passage of legislation. The lack of opportunities for abrupt interruption of executive decisions ushered in a period that we could call "executive dominance." This ability of the executive to introduce policies is the key to the Swedish pattern of cooperation among political parties and policy actors and to the specific set of health policies that both Social Democratic and non-Social Democratic governments introduced between 1931 and 1969.

Political Development

These political and institutional features were established by a series of unrelated steps. The Parliament Act of 1866 replaced representation based on four estates (nobles, clergy, burghers, farmers) with a bicameral parliament, whose powers vis-à-vis the monarch were expanded. The king would appoint the cabinet ministers but was dependent on parliamentary approval of legislation. The upper house, or First Chamber, was indirectly elected; the lower house, or Second Chamber, was elected by direct suffrage, but with a limited franchise. Between 1866 and 1917, parliament gradually increased in importance, as a post of prime minister was added and as slowly the cabinet ministers came to be held responsible to parliament rather than to the king. Until 1917, the king chose the prime minister (initially an autonomous selection) on the basis of party standings in one of the two chambers. But the appointment of a Social Democratic-Liberal coalition government in 1917 based on majorities in both chambers marks the final transition to a parliamentary system (Verney, 1957).

The functioning of this institutional design in practice can be understood in terms of three different aspects of the system: the formal institutions, the distribution of political representatives within these institutions, and institutional practices that developed to overcome some of the weaknesses of these institutions. Formal constitutional changes established the bicameral parliament. The difference in methods for election of parliamentary representatives and the property qualifications, however, resulted in a class divide between the two chambers: The First Chamber was filled initially with nobles, industrialists, and landlords, and the Second Chamber by farmers. Thus, parliament reform maintained the clear link between socioeconomic groupings and political representation, although in a different form.

Royal Committees and *Remiss*

To overcome these cleavages, however, institutional practices were developed to mediate these political and social conflicts. Policy making was increasingly delegated to royal committees and the associated *remiss* system. As Hesslén (1927) noted, these committees, as well as the *remiss* system, were established to submit the bureaucracy to greater parliamentary supervision and to reduce the royal administration. Parliamentary representatives regarded the committees as a substitute for the monarchical bureaucracy and hence as a means to reduce royal power, whereas, from the point of view of the monarch, the committees could be used to avoid the parliament and perhaps minimize opposition to royal initiatives.[1]

By removing policy making to an arena partially independent of both executive and parliament, the committee and *remiss* system protected decision making from conflicts between executive and parliament and from conflicts within the parliament. As a result, agreements on policies could be reached despite the class divisions between the two chambers and between the political parties, and also despite the unstable parliamentary majorities and consequent frequent shifts in government that characterized the period from 1866 to 1932, and particularly the 1920s. Even after the achievement of stable majorities, practices developed in this period continued and promoted multipartisan collaboration on Swedish health legislation and conciliation among interest groups.

The County Councils

The same conflicts over democratic political representation were responsible for a second institutional feature that was to influence health policy. Provincial-level government bodies, the county councils, were introduced as a counterweight to monarchical rule. They were to serve as an organ of self-government at the provincial level in order to balance the power of the provincial governors, who were appointed by the king. In addition, the county councils were given the responsibility of providing health care through hospitals.

The delegation of health care responsibilities to these new bodies appears merely coincidental to their political role, however. Odin Anderson (1972) referred to a Swedish government report that discussed the county councils' assumption of responsibility for hospital care:

> Recalling that the creation of the counties was really a method of distributing political power, aside from services to the people, the counties moved into a vacuum by assuming responsibilities in which other governmental units did not already have vested interests. (p. 42, fn. 10)

Later, the county councils became the basis for indirect election to the First Chamber of parliament. This special political role allowed county council politicians to shape health care reforms, not only in their capacity as hospital administrators but especially in their capacities as an informal interest group within the political parties. Moreover, although the county councils were introduced in opposition to the executive, when the executive and county councils were in agreement, they proved to be a virtually insurmountable coalition.

The Electoral Laws

These two contrary tendencies—a politics of class conflict and a politics of conciliation—were further strengthened during the struggles over voting rights. Just as the negotiations for the transformation of the Estates Parliament into a bicameral parliament openly considered the effects of the rules of representation on nobles, farmers, and priests, so too do we observe a pattern of explicit class bargaining as working-class mobilization provoked gradual extensions of the franchise. Extensions of the franchise in 1866, 1907, and 1918 resulted in immediate political gains to the political parties representing the newly incorporated groups (other than women).

In the negotiations over these reforms, hoping to preserve some part of their parliamentary strength, Conservatives and Liberals insisted on provisions in the electoral laws that, ironically, turned out to favor the Social Democrats. The Conservatives insisted on proportional representation, which in fact helped the Social Democrats win seats from the Liberals in the towns, and encouraged the party to moderate its program to attract these voters. The electoral method chosen for the First Chamber was a Liberal idea. Until 1915, the Liberal program called for abolishing the First Chamber entirely to create what they called "lower-house parliamentarism." However, when the Social Democrats' seats in the Second Chamber surpassed those of the Liberals, direct rule by the Second Chamber looked less attractive; the Liberals did not wish to replace Conservative power with Social Democratic power. A Swedish book analyzing the American political system provided a solution. Noting that the U.S. Senate constituted a brake on the House of Representatives through differences in electoral methods rather than property qualifications, the Liberals shifted to support for bicameralism, with indirect election, longer periods of office, and reelection by stages in place of the financial qualifications for the First Chamber. In the end, however, this effort to place constraints on Social Democratic control of parliament was one of the institutional factors that eventually allowed the Social Democrats to control the executive without interruption for 44 years (Verney, 1957, pp. 206-207, 216-217, 226-227).

Class-Based Politics

In sum, the way in which the franchise was extended reconfirmed the class basis of Swedish politics. As political incorporation first of the farmers, then of the workers, resulted in electoral gains to class-based parties—and, as we shall see, in the passage of policies aimed at these constituencies—a logic of politics was established, one premised on transparent relationships between class identities, institutional representation, and public policies. These early experiences encouraged the building of organizations based on these class groupings, the development of ties to the political parties, and the use of parliament to enact social reforms, all of which created a system of interest representation that gave privilege to interests that were class based.

Yet with the clarification of the relationship between economic groupings, political parties, and representative institutions—which might have produced a situation of irreconcilable class conflicts embodied in the institutions themselves—mechanisms were developed to bridge these conflicts. The committee and *remiss* system, which developed from the opposition between the monarch and parliament, was an intended institutional solution. The establishment and maintenance of an institutional veto point, the First Chamber, and the reliance on proportional representation to slow the decline of the Conservatives became, unintentionally, institutions for conciliation as well.

From Minority Rule to Majority Rule

In 1932, the unexpected Social Democratic electoral victory and alliance with the Farmers' Party effected a sea change in the Swedish system that Olle Nyman (1947) has called a shift from minority parliamentarism to majority parliamentarism. The very institutions that were designed to block popular change abruptly switched to favor the Social Democrats. The royal committees, introduced to allow the monarchical bureaucracy to avoid parliamentary opposition, now helped to promote Social Democratic legislation. The upper house of parliament, long a veto point used by Conservatives, suddenly ensured continued Social Democratic rule despite electoral fluctuations.

After this electoral realignment, the system worked as though the veto points had disappeared. Once a decision had been taken in the executive arena, parliament was unlikely to change it, as the executive government rested on stable parliamentary majorities. Only on the very rare occasion of an electoral realignment—or the threat of one—did the electoral arena become significant for specific policy proposals. Consequently, policy making was concentrated in the executive, with interest group representatives under pressure to compromise because the probability was high that executive proposals would pass unscathed through parliamentary deliberations. The only opportunity for affecting political decisions was at this executive stage. For unions and employers, this was an effective route of influence. In fact, executive decision making came to mean, in practice, that if these two groups could agree, a policy was sure to be enacted.

But for doctors, executive decision making was a disadvantage. With political negotiation largely restricted to the committee and *remiss* phases of the policy process, the medical profession was required to present its views in a forum where its opinions were balanced against the demands of the main labor market organizations—the employers (Sveriges Arbetsgivarförening [SAF, Swedish Employers' Federation]) and the unions (Landsorganisationen i Sverige [LO, Trade Union Federation] and Tjänstemännens Centralorganisation [TCO, Federation of Salaried Employees]). Swedish doctors were able to sway members of parliament and gain ample press coverage for their views. They were unable to veto executive decisions through another political arena. This allowed Social Democratic politicians to introduce a number of health policies without obstruction from the medical profession.

Alternative Explanations

This interpretation differs from alternative explanations that have been advanced for the development of the Swedish health system. Swedish health care politics have often been interpreted in terms of a long-standing tradition of public provision of health services. According to this view, an early commitment to public health provision accounts for Sweden's current system of "socialized medicine." Government ownership of hospitals, for example, may be traced to the Reformation, when hospices were appropriated by the state, in the person of Gustav Vasa, along with other church property. Perhaps more important for recent developments, however, were the introduction of a public health officers corps in the 17th century and the creation of the county councils in 1862. The county councils were given responsibility for hospital care, and importantly, the right to tax citizens to pay for these services. Odin Anderson (1972) argued that this "dominant characteristic" of Sweden's health care system resulted in a concentration of resources at these public hospitals that impeded the development of ambulatory care outside of hospitals and explains the "still heavy emphasis on institutional services in Sweden, and the highest bed-to-population ratio in Western countries up to the present time" (pp. 7, 38, 43; cf. Höjer, 1952).

However, early state intervention in health care did not prevent development of private medical practice within the public institutions. Nor did it preclude political conflicts over the role of government in health care provision. Health care politics in the 20th century was far from untroubled and hardly predictable. National health insurance was hotly debated from the 1890s onward but could not be enacted until after the Second World War.

Professional Dominance

Another approach has focused on the preferences of the medical profession. As Dr. Bo Hjern (1976), an official of the Swedish Medical Association, put it, "A Swedish doctor rarely asks himself the question whether he enjoys being a public servant. He is so used to being one that the question is not so emotionally charged as in many other countries" (p. 10). His older colleagues who remember the battles over socialized medicine might not agree, however. Conservative MP Dr. Gunnar Biörck (1977), for example, referred to recent developments in Swedish health care policy as "steps in subjugating a free profession" (p. 815). Many Swedish physicians were opposed to national health insurance and to the restrictions on private medical practice that have since been introduced. In historical terms, Swedish doctors were no more supportive of socialized medicine than were doctors throughout western Europe.[2] Garpenby (1989) has argued that the Swedish process of professionalization was accomplished through the state and that therefore Swedish physicians maintained an orientation to the public sector. It is true that Swedish professionalization was aided by the state; this is, in my view, what made it so successful by the standard measures of professionalization. The first Swedish medical faculties were established at the end of the 17th century, but both a university route and an apprenticeship route to professional credentials (*fältskärare, kirurg,* the Swedish equivalent of the Swiss *Wundearzt* and the French surgeon) were available. The Royal Academy of Medicine (Collegium Medicum) was established in 1663 by four Stockholm doctors, who then received official royal recognition. In 1685, the barbers upgraded themselves to the Surgical Society (Societas Chirurgica), but the Collegium Medicum refused to relinquish its authority to examine the surgeons. Finally, in 1797, the Surgical Society was incorporated into the Collegium Medicum. In 1813, the Collegium Medicum was replaced by the "Health College" (Sundhetskollegiet), which became the National Board of Health (Medicinalstyrelsen) in 1877 (Garpenby, 1989). Thus, university doctors were granted a government agency that they used to control professional licensing. This granting of privilege to the profession was not unlike the situation in Britain, where the Royal College of Physicians was granted a charter to examine physicians by Henry VIII in 1518. However, the Swedish Collegium Medicum was part of the government, whereas the British Royal College (and later the Royal College of Surgeons) was an independent body licensed by the government. The Collegium Medicum was highly successful in limiting the number of licensed physicians, and Sweden still maintains a relatively low physician-to-population ratio. Thus, in terms of establishing a market monopoly and controlling the number of doctors, the Swedish profession was highly successful, but it relied on the absolutist state. At the same time, however, this state took an active role in establishing public forms of health care (public health officers and public hospitals).

Alongside the development of the government bureaucracy for control of licensing, the Swedish Medical Society (Svenskaläkarsällskapet), a scientific society for doctors, was founded in 1808. This society still exists and zealously avoids all involvement with "economic" issues. As measured by government response to its *remiss* statements, the Swedish Medical Society is more successful as a lobbying group than the Swedish Medical Association (Läkarförbundet), although on medical issues, as opposed to economic issues, the association has also been influential (Bjurulf & Swahn, 1980; Twaddle & Hessler, 1986).

The movement for a more economically oriented professional association began at the end of the 19th century. The organizational innovation that produced a permanent association was the development of local medical associations in the 1890s that then federated to form a second national medical association (Allmänna Svenska Läkarföreningen) in 1903. This was reorganized in 1919 into the Swedish Medical Association. From the 1920s on, the association has controlled specialty licensing.

Thus, the Swedish medical profession successfully eliminated competing forms of medical practice, established government control over licensing, and set strict limits on the numbers of doctors. This control was carried out by the state rather than by an independent organization of the profession. But enforcement by the state was essential for medical monopoly throughout Europe.

However, we should recognize the disjuncture between these classical stages in the professionalization process and success at maintaining private medical practice through political means. The technical expertise of the profession was certainly respected. There were no proposals for lay medicine or the elimination of medical monopoly, and medical associations were carefully consulted on medical issues. But Swedish political institutions afforded only limited veto points to the Swedish medical profession. When other interest groups and political actors judged the economic conditions of practice to be political rather than professional matters, the medical profession, unlike its counterparts elsewhere, was not in a veto position, despite its organizational strength and professional resources.

The Social Democratic Model

Yet another argument focuses on the activities of the Swedish Social Democratic Party and the associated LO (Esping-Andersen, 1985; Esping-Andersen & Korpi, 1984). New reforms were introduced following Social Democratic electoral gains, and the content of the reforms roughly parallels other Social Democratic initiatives rather than appearing as highly specific to the health care area. The Social Democratic model "fits" the Swedish case rather well also in terms of the influence of interest groups on health insurance policy making. Although the medical profession was highly visible during debates over health insurance policies, its role pales in comparison with that of more "class-based" groups, such as SAF, LO, and even TCO. In the context of class-based politics, support for health care reforms was widespread. Swedish employers were willing to consider national health insurance at quite an early date; TCO and LO provided a ready source of constituents who could be courted by political parties willing to promote social policies.

Nevertheless, although there is evidence to support the Social Democratic model, the timing of reforms does not exactly coincide with increased Social Democratic electoral strength or increases in union membership. How can we account, for example, for the fact that national health insurance was not enacted until 1946, although the Social Democratic Party was taking the largest share of the electorate as early as 1917 and held the largest number of parliamentary seats in both chambers of the Swedish *Riksdag* by 1921? Or, to draw a cross-national comparison, despite much higher levels of unionization and a larger Social Democratic majority in Sweden, at the same time that Britain enacted its National Health Service such a reform was rejected in Sweden. Moreover, the Swedish Social Democrats rarely enacted legislation based on their parliamentary majority against the wishes of other parties—at least not in the health care area. Most health care policies were supported by the majority, if not all, of the political parties and by a broad array of interest groups, always including SAF, TCO, and LO.

Swedish Health Politics: An Overview

Consensus for political decisions was made possible not only by the "Social Democratic hegemony" but by the fact that the bargains enforced at the executive level could not be overturned in a different political arena. Moreover, as the parties followed party discipline, interest groups needed to convince the party leaderships in order to have an effect. Because the parties had rather stable constituencies, they were not prone to opportunistic shifts.

The lack of veto opportunities made it impossible for groups opposed to executive decisions to overturn these decisions; hence, the effective point of decision was in the executive. This concentrated policy decisions in the royal committees and promoted a pattern of consensual decision making among the large producer organizations. When veto opportunities opened up, however—at times when the First Chamber was still dominated by the Conservatives and when the possibility of electoral realignment threatened the parliamentary coalition—interest groups switched from cooperation to defection and attempted to use these veto opportunities to block policies.

Thus, through a series of unrelated historical events, the Swedish political system came to work according to a rather straightforward political logic. Voters voted according to their class position and joined interest groups with ties to those same political parties. Employees enrolled in the unions—LO and TCO—and voted for the Social Democratic Party; farmers joined the farmers' organizations and voted for the Farmers' Party; employers joined the employers' organization and voted for the Conservative Party; and small employers and craftsmen were represented in a small business organization as well as the employers' organization and voted for the Liberal Party (Elvander, 1966; Särlvik, 1967).

Political decisions were based on agreements worked out in executive procedures between these groups. The commission and *remiss* system constituted a mechanism for reaching consensus within society and between parties that undergirded the Social Democratic approach to power. Further, the emphasis on executive rather than parliamentary or electoral arenas of decision making positioned the county councils to control the agenda of the reform process to an unprecedented degree; county council politicians were able to parlay their political resources into ever-greater administrative control and direction of health care services. Holding this system together, however, was the lack of veto opportunities that encouraged cooperative strategies.

Parliamentary Instability

Although Swedish electoral laws from 1866 to 1918 resulted in the maintenance of a Conservative majority in the First Chamber that could veto legislation, and although stable parliamentary majorities were lacking, the committee system protected Swedish policy making from the vagaries of the shifting parliamentary coalitions. Committees appointed by one government prepared legislative proposals, only to submit them several years later to a new government in a completely different political environment. Nevertheless, the parliamentary practice was to continue the work of the committees, despite the change in government. Reform initiatives came mainly from Liberals, often supported by Social Democrats, but also from Conservatives. Swedish doctors were not inclined toward government support for health insurance, but their main concern was with the effect of health insurance programs on relations between physicians and sickness funds. They were adamant that increased government funding for the ambulatory sector should not interfere with private medical practice.

Efforts to enact national health insurance (or, more correctly, "compulsory health insurance," as these programs were called) failed. In its place, a series of laws providing for government subsidies for voluntary health insurance were passed in 1891, 1910, and 1931. If anything, however, Swedish government programs for health insurance lagged behind those of other European countries. In the Swedish case, national health insurance was blocked not by partisan or interest group conflicts but for financial reasons. Instead of national health insurance, a series of sickness fund laws was introduced. Doctors, sickness funds, and small businessmen opposed an expanded role of government, and they were to some extent successful in using their parliamentary contacts to oppose reforms. But the logic of the Swedish system was already beginning to point to executive-level bargaining that excluded these groups.

Early efforts to enact national health insurance in Sweden did not constitute a purely Conservative response to the "social question," nor did they represent the triumph of the Social Democratic rise to power. The

Sickness Fund Laws of 1891, 1910, and 1931 were all enacted at times of heightened worker unrest and increasing representation of the left in the Swedish parliament. Yet they were not introduced by Social Democratic representatives against the resistance of the center and right. The 1891 law was enacted at a time when both Liberals and Conservatives were interested in promoting "social peace" in the heated atmosphere of the crisis in Swedish-Norwegian relations and as a result of large electoral gains for the left in the Stockholm elections to the Second Chamber. The 1910 law came in the wake of the 1909 general strike and as the effects of the 1907 voting rights reform began to be felt. The 1931 law was enacted in the same month that newspaper headlines were dominated by an event that constituted a watershed in the history of the Swedish labor movement: the killing of two strikers and four spectators by the military at Ådalen.

Although stimulated by working-class mobilization, health insurance legislation was not a top priority of union and Social Democratic leaders. In contrast to the German pattern, in which the funds served as a crucial organizational tool for unions and the Social Democratic Party,[3] in Sweden the sickness fund movement was more closely linked to the temperance movement and to the Liberal Party. Consequently, if any party exerted the leading role in health insurance reform, it was the Liberals, whereas the Social Democrats and LO focused on workmen's compensation, universal suffrage, the 8-hour day, and unemployment measures (Lindeberg, 1949, p. 121).

The Sickness Fund Laws of 1891 and 1910 provided for government subsidies to local "sickness funds" (*sjukkassor*) that provided mainly cash benefits to cover income lost during periods of illness. In some cases, they provided coverage for medical treatment as well, for which they often attempted to hire physicians on a contract basis to provide treatment to members for low flat fees. Despite the subsidies, however, membership in the Swedish voluntary sickness funds had grown relatively slowly. As late as 1925, only 13.3% of the Swedish population was enrolled in sickness funds (or 17.5% of the adult population), as compared with 60% for Denmark. Moreover, very few of these persons were insured for medical treatment: In 1921, only 12% of sickness fund members were covered. In addition, as in other countries, the organization of voluntary insurance was rather haphazard, with funds unevenly distributed throughout Sweden and engaged in highly competitive practices that interfered with adequate provision of social security.[4]

Influenced by international developments, Swedish politicians from a number of parties proposed national health insurance as a remedy. Beginning in 1913, proposals for compulsory health insurance for low-income earners were drawn up by a series of committees appointed by successive Liberal, Conservative, and Social Democratic governments. The most important of these proposals, the 1919 proposal of the Social Insurance Commission, which had been appointed by Conservative Oscar von Sydow, head of the Department of the Interior in a nonpartisan government, called for a combination of compulsory and voluntary insurance that would cover cash benefits, drugs, and medical treatment for an estimated 80% of the population. In contrast to earlier proposals, the committee envisioned a system of public sickness funds that would replace the previously established voluntary funds.

Just as the pressures for national health insurance did not come directly from the Swedish labor movement, opposition to reform did not come from expected quarters. Although the Swedish Medical Association (Sveriges Lakarförbundet) had been founded in 1903, the association did not play an especially important role in these early debates. Nor did business groups attempt to oppose reform. Nevertheless, the proposal was eventually shelved for financial rather than political reasons by both Conservative and Social Democratic governments in 1919, 1921, and 1922. In 1925, the State Budget Cutting Committee (appointed by a Conservative government) urged that plans for national health insurance be abandoned. Instead, a new sickness fund law should be enacted that would rationalize the voluntary health insurance system. State subsidies should be allocated to only one sickness fund per local area, the committee argued. This would allow better coordination between sickness, pension, and workmen's compensation benefits, which would lower administrative costs and eliminate eligibility for pension supplements in some cases. Gustav Möller, Social Democratic Minister of Social Affairs in 1925—who has been called the architect of the Swedish welfare state—agreed with the Conservative committee's assessment, but he favored a transition to national health insurance at a later date.

Although the sickness fund movement was interested in increased government subsidies, the plan for restricting the subsidies to one fund per local area generated opposition. The Swedish situation was complicated by the fact that the sickness fund movement was split into two competing movements, each based on a different approach to health insurance and each represented by a separate association. Founded in 1907, the General Sickness Fund Association represented the smaller funds that were restricted to a local area. In 1916, a second association, the National Sickness Funds' Central Organization, was founded to represent the national funds. The former stressed the importance of membership participation in the sickness funds and its role in political education. It lobbied for national health insurance. The association of national funds, on the other hand, was more bureaucratically inclined. The national funds were responsible for extending the sickness fund movement to the Swedish countryside and were more concerned about pooling risks, for which large funds were needed, than about the democratic character of the funds. It was opposed to national health insurance. Both associations did have ties to the temperance movement and to the Liberal Party, but the links between the national funds—the more conservative group— and the Liberal Party were much stronger, not least because G. K. Ekmann, prime minister for several years in the 1920s and the head of the Radical-Liberal Party, was a former president of the largest national fund.

The fund movement adeptly used its parliamentary contacts to block proposals for a new sickness fund law in 1926-27. By 1928, however, pressured by stagnating membership figures and the possibility of vastly increased government subsidies, the two organizations were able to agree on a reorganization of voluntary health insurance. The law would cover two types of funds, central and local. The local funds would cover smaller territorial areas for short-term risks, and the central funds would serve a larger area, equalizing expenditures by picking up the costs of long-term illnesses. Once the sickness fund organizations agreed to divide their area of operations into local and national jurisdictions, the rift between the two organizations was largely eliminated. This compromise removed one of the main political and administrative impediments to health insurance legislation, and the executive government presented a new sickness fund proposal in 1930.[5]

Now, for the first time, the Swedish medical profession emerged as an important pressure group. The leadership of the Swedish Medical Association was willing to accept a new sickness fund law, but the majority of its members were not. Many doctors perceived the introduction of a new requirement for sickness funds to provide medical benefits as a threat. As elsewhere, relations between the medical profession and the sickness funds were strained. In 1907, the Swedish Medical Association's committee on sickness funds had warned of the threat to physicians posed by the sickness funds. Pointing to the poor working conditions of German and Danish doctors, who were often hired by sickness funds on a contract basis and paid at low rates, referred to by Swedish doctors as "piece rates," the committee argued that Swedish doctors would face the same problems if the funds became more involved in the provision of medical benefits. Much of the early activity of the Medical Association was aimed at eliminating the contract practices of the funds, and one of the problems of the association was preventing doctors in need of employment from signing such contracts.

By requiring the sickness funds to provide medical benefits, the 1930 sickness fund law threatened the private medical market. Medical opponents, in a letter from a local medical association to the central steering committee of the Swedish Medical Association, argued that this was a step toward national health insurance, after which "the free calling of medicine would become only a pretty memory" (Värmlandsföreningen, 1930, p. 1266). Although 21 out of 28 local medical associations objected to compulsory medical benefits, the Central Steering Board of the Swedish Medical Association decided to support the 1930 proposal. Despite open criticism of this decision in the association's journal, *Läkartidningen,* the leadership held its ground, asserting:

> It has been said that the majority of the country's doctors are of a different opinion concerning the proposals put forth in the health insurance question than the National Board of Health [Medicinalstyrelsen] and the Swedish Medical Association's Central Steering Committee [Centralstyrelsen]. This, however appears to have its natural explanation in the circumstance that these Boards have at their disposition a more thorough knowledge of the details of these proposals than what many of the doctors out in the countryside in general have obtained for themselves. (Petrén, 1931, p. 585)

The leadership was accused of ignoring the opinions of its local affiliates, not only by members of the medical profession but also by a group known as the Taxpayers' Association (Skattebetalarnas Förening), which published a Swedish Medical Association survey of local medical associations showing that the majority of local affiliates opposed compulsory medical benefits. Clearly, the Taxpayers' Association cooperated with one or more powerful officials of the Swedish Medical Association, for otherwise it certainly could never have obtained the results of an internal survey.

Given the reactions to health insurance initiatives in other countries, we might expect that employers would constitute a potential source of "tax opposition." Although the Taxpayers' Association played an important role in influencing public opinion, it never participated in *remiss* activities. Although the organization's steering committee was dominated by powerful industrialists such as Jakob Wallenberg, who served as president from 1953 to 1969, SAF stated in 1925 that it opposed plans for rationalization of voluntary health insurance through a new sickness fund law, when only through national health insurance could this rationalization be effectively achieved (*Riksdagens Protokoll,* 1926, p. 24).

Opponents of the 1930 sickness fund law circumvented the more moderate medical association leadership and appealed directly to members of parliament and to the press. And the strategy worked, briefly. The 1930 Sickness Fund Law passed in the Second Chamber but was blocked by a last-minute push from Conservatives in the First Chamber, for which Swedish private practitioners claimed credit.[6] In the long run, however, this was not an effective political strategy in Sweden. For although the doctors and the taxpayers were successful in gaining access to selected conservative MPs, they seemed unable to penetrate the official commission and *remiss* proceedings. Neither the Swedish Medical Association nor SAF—the groups that we might expect to represent the views of these opponents—responded to these attacks. Instead, the National Board of Health (Medicinalstyrelsen), to which the Medical Association submitted its positive reply along with some dissenting comments of the locals, strongly supported the reform, as did the two sickness fund associations, SAF, the Pension Board, the Welfare Inspector, the Federation of County Councils, and the Swedish Welfare Association.

The Swedish policy process was based on executive access, and government officials were the gatekeepers to that access. Swedish medical association leaders were concerned that if they did not cooperate in drafting health insurance legislation, they could be excluded from decision making, as they had been in the past. By analogy, in a political system in which good relations with the executive were at a premium, it is not surprising that employers might choose an independent organization, such as the Taxpayers' Association, to express discontent, rather than damaging the neutral image of SAF. For according to Nils Elvander (1974), this is not where effective political pressure occurs in the Swedish system: "Group influence is expressed mainly in the preparatory stages [of policy making] through representation on investigative commissions and so-called *remiss* comments on commission reports—and at the executive stage in the agencies. The least significant target is parliament" (p. 27).

Swedish procedures for interest representation were not vulnerable to political opposition outside of the official *remiss* proceedings. Although the parliamentary majorities were not stable, the parties were not fractionated and cross-cut by electoral competition. The First Chamber could be used as a veto point, but the Conservatives would be risking their chances of gaining Liberal support by vetoing a policy affecting the Liberal sickness funds, and the reliable constituency of the Conservatives, SAF, was not publicly fighting the law. Thus, it is no wonder that even if the doctors and taxpayers were successful in winning over Conservative MPs to their cause in 1930, the Sickness Fund Law was still approved by the *Riksdag* in May 1931 by majorities so large that no vote was taken.

The 1931 law shaped the future development of the system, as it transformed the sickness fund movement from a randomly scattered group of voluntary associations to a national network of coordinated insurance funds that was later to serve as the basis for national health insurance. As a result of the law, state subsidies more than doubled within 3 years, and medical benefits were greatly increased. Voluntary membership expanded from 1 million in 1930 to 1.5 million in 1940 and 2.5 million in 1945, a shift from 20% of the adult population (persons over 15 years of age) to 48%.

This law was made possible by a long process of political negotiation. Furthermore, it was prepared not by a conflictual process that pitted the Social Democrats against the other parties but by a multiparty process that, as a result of the committee system, continued uninterrupted through 12 different changes in government. Thus, although it was not complete, even in this period before the Social Democratic rise to power, we can observe the beginnings of executive level policy consensus in Sweden.

Majority Parliamentarism and the Postwar Settlement

The agreement between the Social Democrats and the Farmers' Party to exchange farm price supports for employment measures effected a political realignment. From 1932 on, the executive was governed by majority parliamentary coalitions in place of the unstable minority governments of the 1920s and earlier. This shifted the balance of institutional power from parliament to the executive, reversing the previous shift from king to parliament. Once the risk of parliamentary veto was removed, the effective point of decision was more firmly rooted in the executive than ever before. Previously, the commissions had protected policy making from the shifting parliamentary majorities; now, within the context of Social Democratic majorities, they provided an arena for hammering out policy compromises under Social Democratic leadership. This shift in power was buttressed by a reorganization of the political parties and interest groups that was to strengthen the pattern of executive-induced political compromise. The two competing liberal parties regrouped into a single party, representing largely urban, small business interests. Wealthier farmers moved into the Conservative Party, leaving the Farmers' Party to represent farmers proper, rather than large landowners. Interest organizations grew at an unprecedented rate, leading to the coining of the phrase "Organization Sweden."[7] As Douglas Verney (1957) wrote:

> The stability of the Swedish political system in the last twenty years has led some observers to suggest that the liberal period of competing political parties has given way to a settled social order in which Government tends in some ways to adjudicate the claims of various large social groups, none of which can expect to strengthen its position perceptibly. . . . It would be reading too much into this development to regard it as a return to the old order in which social groups, like the Estates, meet together to be administered by a comparatively disinterested government. On the other hand, it may be no accident that in a country which has had so short an experience of liberalism and individualism, these tendencies towards the traditional representation of interests of the realm should be observed and discussed. (p. 229)

Introduction of National Health Insurance

As elsewhere in Europe, the end of the Second World War was viewed as the moment to enlarge the scope of social citizenship. The Swedish welfare state was to be based on the standard set of social insurance programs considered throughout western Europe at that time. In 1946 and 1947 alone, legislation was promulgated on pensions, family allowances, health insurance, and housing subsidies. With a popular mandate to continue the Keynesian policies of the 1930s, the Social Democrats were now able to introduce the main pillars of the Swedish welfare state. Consequently, this period is known as the Social Democratic "Harvest Time." This partisan element is without a doubt a critical factor in the postwar reforms. The reforms had been outlined in *The Postwar Program of the Workers' Movement* or *The 27 Points,* Sweden's version of Britain's Beveridge Plan, published jointly by LO and the Social Democratic Party in 1944. The party now had the electoral strength necessary to implement the reforms. Moreover, it was prodded to take action by Communist gains in the 1944 elections.

With regard to national health insurance, however, support for the program was widespread, extending far beyond the Social Democratic Party and its electoral base, LO. Although the Social Democrats held a sufficient electoral majority to be able to enact the reform on their own, this proved to be unnecessary. All of the political parties supported the national health insurance law of 1947, and it passed by a nearly unanimous vote. Not every interest group was completely in favor of national health insurance. Unable to threaten parliamentary or referendum vetoes, however, each group expressed misgivings but agreed to cooperate.

SAF pointed to the virtues of voluntary insurance and questioned the financial wisdom of immediately introducing national health insurance but essentially agreed to the reform. The white-collar union, TCO, noted that

> the introduction of national health insurance will doubtlessly be viewed by large groups of salaried employees as a rather serious intervention in the freedom of the individual citizen, so much more so as this intervention will appear as of little personal benefit to many employees. Nevertheless, . . . TCO wishes to support this proposal in principle, out of consideration for the valuable step that this reform constitutes in the striving for better social conditions in this country. (TCO, 1946/1944, p. 3)

The Swedish Medical Association stated that it preferred voluntary insurance to compulsory insurance and urged the government to concentrate on more pressing public health needs. It would, however, go along, particularly as the proposal provided for a reimbursement mechanism for payment and for a free choice of doctor.

Small businessmen complained about their exclusion from political decision making. They were not consulted on the matter of national health insurance; at least, there is no record of a *remiss* comment from this group. Complaining that small businessmen were underrepresented in the *Riksdag,* they campaigned to improve their political standing. However, this resulted in the addition of only rather insignificant numbers of small businessmen to the party lists, overwhelmingly concentrated in the Liberal Party.

The 1948 Höjer Proposal

Two years later, however, an opportunity presented itself to these opponents of government expansion. The opposition parties were gearing up for the 1948 electoral campaign and hoped that the 1947 balance-of-payments crisis would erode Social Democratic electoral support. Although enacted into law, national health insurance was delayed by the pending commune reform, which was to consolidate the most local bodies of government—the primary communes—into bigger units, more suitable for social policy implementation, and by disagreements within the labor movement and the Social Democratic party over the cash benefits portion of the law. During this delay, the release of a government report calling for the creation of a national health service provided a focus for a Conservative backlash. This opportunity was seized by political parties · and interest groups that saw a chance to revise the Social Democratic status quo.

The Höjer Commission, chaired by J. Axel Höjer, director of the National Board of Health, had been appointed by the government in 1943 to study the need for reorganization of Swedish ambulatory medical care and to make recommendations that would be used in the final scheme for national health insurance. The report (Statens Offentliga Utredningar [SOU], 1948a, 1948b) included a thorough and lengthy analysis of ambulatory care; an overview of international developments, with particular emphasis on the British National Health Service; and recommendations for the total reorganization of Swedish health services. These recommendations ranged from building local health centers to a reform of medical school curricula. Of more immediate concern were the provisions for the consolidation of all forms of outpatient care into one system under the auspices of the county councils and the eventual transfer of all doctors to full-time salaries. Salary, the report argued, was the only rational and efficient means of physician remuneration and constituted a necessary step in providing affordable medical care to all citizens.

In sum, the Höjer Report was a proposal for a national health service whose ambitions surpassed those of the British National Health Service. Not only would hospital inpatient care be delivered at virtually no cost, but all forms of outpatient care—whether taking place in doctors' private offices, in the government offices of public doctors, or in the hospital outpatient clinics—were to be integrated into this service. Private patients and private fees, which all Swedish doctors—whether hospital or office based, private or public—depended on, would be eliminated.

The Swedish Medical Association dropped its usual conciliatory stance to protest the Höjer reform: "It was not the principle of compulsory health insurance that became the chief issue but methods and amount of payment and professional freedom as the profession defined it. . . . a salaried service was beyond tolerance" (Anderson, 1972, pp. 78-79). The two physicians who sat on the commission, aside from Höjer himself, issued dissenting opinions, criticizing the commission for going far beyond its appointed field of inquiry and disavowing its recommendations for full-time salaries. Immediately on publication of the report, the Medical Association launched a campaign against the proposed reforms, and against J. Axel Höjer personally, in the medical press, in the newspapers, and by appealing to other interest groups.

The newspapers gave front-page coverage to the association's comments on the reform, often adding editorial criticisms of their own. The report was depicted as a doctrinaire call for the immediate socialization of medicine and the downgrading of doctors from free professionals to state civil servants. The Conservative *Svenska Dagbladet* editorialized: "Mr. Höjer's goal emerges with frightening clarity: the profession's total socialization and the economic levelling of physicians, decreasing the quality and increasing the costs of health care for citizens" ("Fri sjukvård," 1948, p. 3). The Liberal *Dagens Nyheter* was equally critical, noting that a national health service might be appropriate for Britain but not for Sweden ("Medicinalchefen Axel Höjer," 1948, p. 3). Only the Social Democratic *Morgontidningen* supported the reform, castigating the other papers for acting as if "not the public health but guild interests should be the guidepost for reform" ("Alla under 16," 1948, p. 4).

The Medical Association's lobbying efforts were successful in convincing other groups to come to their defense. The Conservative Party's Business Group warned of the consequences of socialized medicine, based on its experience of hassles and bureaucracy "that state collectivism brings," and praised the competitive free market for encouraging "individual initiative" among private doctors ("Högerns företagargrupps resolution," 1948, p. 2). In its remiss answer to the Höjer Report, SAF (1954/1948) objected to the high costs of the reform and to this "complete socialization of the medical profession" and concluded that the reform was "completely unacceptable" (p. 6). Even LO, which fully adhered to the goals of the report, suggested that a fuller cost analysis might be advisable, given the discrepancies between Höjer's estimates and those made by the Medical Association (LO, 1954/1949, p. 4).

But interest groups were not the only *remiss* bodies that spoke out against the Höjer reform. The Social Democrats' own bureaucracy and the Federation of County Councils, the local unit of government that owned and administered hospitals, recommended that no legislative action be pursued based on the Höjer Report. The county councils feared that by eliminating private practice within hospitals and by converting hospital doctors to a salary system, the Höjer reform would drive doctors away from hospital practice and into the private sector. Consequently, hospitals would find it more difficult not only to staff their outpatient clinics but to staff their inpatient wards as well. The councils argued that the government should first increase the number of doctors, and that only later, when, it was implied, the market position of doctors would be considerably weakened, should it address the question of jurisdiction over hospital outpatient care.

The debate continued throughout 1948. *Svenska Dagbladet*'s yearbook noted that no other legislative proposal received as much or as critical press coverage in 1948 as the Höjer reform. Höjer himself was attacked both in the bourgeois press and in the medical journals. Heidenheimer (1980a) described the acrimonious tenor of these debates, in which the Medical Association chairman Dag Knutson referred to Höjer as a "dangerous man who must be removed from his post as soon as possible" and Höjer "felt entitled to label the [association director as] pro-Nazi" (p. 122). Debate over the Höjer reform became so heated that it was viewed as politically impossible to draft a legislative proposal or to take up the question in the *Riksdag*—a highly unusual end to a Swedish royal committee study. But the pattern was the same for economic and tax policy as well: The nonsocialist parties relied on the press to carry out an electoral campaign that has been singled out as being unusually aggressive and ideological in tone.

Fearing a potential breakdown of future prospects for Farmer-Labor coalition governments as well as electoral losses, the Social Democratic government backed down completely, not only on the Höjer reform but also on a controversial proposal for a new inheritance tax and on other elements of its economic program.

The defeat of the Höjer reform has been viewed as a victory for the Swedish Medical Association. And it was. Private medical practice was preserved both in public hospitals and in private offices. No local health centers would compete with private office practice. Doctors would be paid on a fee-for-service basis, and they would be paid by patients and the insurance funds rather than by a salary from the state, as proposed by Höjer. Thus, in place of a national health service, a new national health insurance law was introduced in 1953 and went into effect in 1955. The program covered the entire population for medical and cash benefits, which would be provided through the preexisting sickness funds and paid for by payroll tax contributions from employers and employees, as well as subsidies from the government.[8]

In 1945 and 1946, the Social Democratic Party was perceived as having a mandate to establish a Swedish welfare state; no party dared to voice opposition to these reforms. As in many other countries, however, the climate of public opinion shifted rather quickly after the war. Particularly as the party moved from enacting social policies to introducing new taxes to pay for them—as well as toward a planned economy—the consensus for social democracy began to erode. Reactions to the Höjer reform fit very neatly into this general backlash against the welfare state. SAF, for example, used its defense of professional freedom as an opportunity to criticize the government, charging that monetary stabilization would be impossible as long as the government continued to introduce expansionary social policies. These exchanges came to a head in the 1948 election campaign, one that has been singled out as being unusually vicious and ideological in tone, with a general attack on socialism led by the nonsocialist parties.

The Social Democrats' share of the popular vote decreased by only 0.6%—from 46.7% of the popular vote in 1944 to 46.1% in 1948, compared with a decline of several percentage points for the Conservatives (from 15.9% to 12.3%) and the Communists (10.3% to 6.3%), while the Liberal Party nearly doubled its share of the electorate (from 12.9% to 22.8%) through a 10% increase in voter participation. Yet this was sufficient for the Social Democrats to lose three seats in the Second Chamber, narrowing its majority there to 112 seats to 110 held by the Conservatives, Farmers, and Liberals. Not only was the margin small, but the continued downward trend from 134 seats in the 1941 elections, despite the large number of social reforms, was worrisome. However, Social Democratic control of the executive was saved by its absolute majority in the First Chamber, where its representation had increased from 75 seats in 1941 to 83 in 1945, 86 in 1947, and 84 in 1949. Thus, the First Chamber had been transformed from a veto point to a guarantor of Social Democratic control of the government. Indeed, this led to a discussion of the abolition of the First Chamber in 1953, but the Social Democrats refused (Hadenius et al., 1978, pp. 306-307; Verney, 1957, p. 217; von Sydow, 1989, pp. 43, 51). The 1948 election thus exposed the vulnerability of the party to small electoral shifts, but the First Chamber provided a counterbalance. This election marks the definitive end to the postwar "Harvest Time" and the beginning of a period of Social Democratic pragmatism.

Harpsund Democracy: The 1950s and 1960s

The defeat of the Höjer reform preserved a number of forms of private practice that were of significance to the medical profession. It was not long, however, before the economic autonomy of doctors was threatened once again. After the setback of the late 1940s, the Social Democratic government went ahead with a number of health policies, often without consulting the Medical Association. The overall direction of these policies was to reduce the market power of doctors by increasing their numbers and reducing the scope of private practice. In health and in other policy areas, the pattern was the same: incremental policy making introduced through executive negotiations, with an emphasis on technical preparation of reform rather than partisan conflict.

Indeed, in the 1950s and 1960s, so much decision making was removed from the parliamentary arena to tripartite agreements between the Social Democratic Party, SAF, and LO that this is the era famed for "Harpsund" democracy, a reference to the retreat where labor and employer leaders met with government officials to decide on policy. The notable institutional feature is the absence rather than the presence of institutional constraints. The Social Democratic majority in the First Chamber stabilized the executive rather than providing a point of veto. The narrowness of the Second Chamber majority and the knowledge that proportional representation would allow for sudden electoral shifts encouraged the Social Democrats to obtain nonsocialist support for policies and to reach out for a broader, white-collar constituency. But party discipline and the stable majority governments, some in coalition with the Farmers' Party, prevented parliamentary stalemate. At no time was the medical profession able to avail itself of a strategic opening similar to that of 1948.

As enacted, the National Health Insurance Law allowed for a variety of forms of private medical practice. Within public hospitals, senior doctors could receive private patients as inpatients in "private beds" or during private ambulatory consultations. Outside the hospitals, a small number of private clinics were in existence; private ambulatory consultations took place in private doctors' offices, as well as at the offices of district and provincial doctors. The district and provincial doctors were subsidized by the government and were paid a part-time salary, in return for which they agreed to treat low-income patients at fixed rates but were free to treat private patients.

Swedish national health insurance covered doctors' fees for all of these forms of private practice. Patients paid doctors directly and were later reimbursed by the insurance agencies for a percentage of an official fee schedule (75%), and doctors were free to extra-bill for all patients coming to their private offices or clinics.[9]

In the big cities, where the bulk of Sweden's population is concentrated, the extent of this private medical sector was considerable. Private inpatient care—that is, private beds in public hospitals and private clinics—was never extensive.[10] But private outpatient care was widespread in Stockholm, Göteborg, and Malmö. In Stockholm, as much as 70% of outpatient consultations in September 1968 took place in the private sector, 62% at the offices of private practitioners. In the rest of the country, private practitioners were responsible for only 22% of outpatient consultations in the same month.

Step by step, Social Democratic governments reorganized the health system and eliminated opportunities for private medical practice. They aimed to increase government planning and to achieve a better distribution of hospital resources through the regionalization policies of the 1950s. At the same time, they took steps to reduce the market power of doctors by increasing their numbers and reducing the scope of private practice—that is, the exit opportunities for doctors. Each of these reforms was prepared in the executive and easily ratified in parliament. Over the opposition of the Medical Association, the government expanded the number of physicians through the building of three new medical schools and an increase in class size. As a result, the number of doctors licensed each year increased by a factor of seven between 1947 and 1972. These increases began in the early 1950s. The first step was in fact the importation of 100 Austrian doctors, which had been suggested by Höjer in the early 1940s and was repeated in the Höjer Report of 1948. The fact that the government could oppose the Swedish Medical Association so soon after the defeat of the Höjer reform lends further support to the thesis that the profession triumphed in 1948 because political opportunities for opposition to government policies presented themselves rather than because it could, by itself, threaten to sabotage the health care system. The profession's control over the number of doctors was further eroded when the government took over specialty accreditation from the Swedish Medical Association in 1960.

Through the 1959 Hospital Law, the state began to take direct steps to restrict private medical practice. It eliminated private hospital beds and private fees for hospital inpatient care and also required hospitals to provide hospital outpatient care, thereby competing with the private office hours of the hospital doctors and with the private office-based practitioners. Consequently, hospital outpatient visits increased from 7.4 million in 1952 to 18.4 million in 1963, or more than 40% of medical consultations.[11] In response to the law, some doctors tried to revive the private clinics. But this movement suffered a failure of nerve when the National Board of Health and Welfare announced plans to build local health centers in the mid-1960s.

Absolute Majority:
The 1969 Seven Crowns Reform

The most dramatic threat to the private sector came in 1969 with the introduction of the "Seven Crowns" reform. This reform eliminated private practice from public hospitals entirely and replaced fee-for-service payments to hospital doctors with full-time salaries.

The Seven Crowns reform was motivated by political as well as health policy factors. It was part of a package of policies in the areas of health care, taxation, and economic policy that aimed to solidify the party's electoral standing at a time when it was at the peak of its power, but when its future control of the government was in jeopardy. The Social Democrats had finally agreed to abandon the First Chamber, and in 1970 new elections would be held for the shift from a bicameral to a unicameral parliament. This constitutional change would make the Social Democratic Party more vulnerable to electoral swings and would reduce the political influence of the county councils (Carder & Klingeberg, 1980, p. 150). Although the future looked uncertain, the Social Democrats had won a landslide victory in the 1968 elections, winning an absolute majority for the first time since 1940. With such a margin, they could undertake fairly bold policy initiatives, and they were under pressure to do so quickly, before the 1970 elections. Moreover, they viewed social policy expansion as the route to electoral success. The struggles over superannuated pensions had shown that the public was ready for increased social reform. When the Liberal Party lost nearly half of its voters as a result of its negative stance on pensions, the parties began to outbid one another in the social policy area: "The opposition understood that they had burned their fingers in the ATP conflict [superannuated pensions conflict]" (Sven Aspling, former Social Minister, personal communication, June 1980). The 1968 electoral success seemed to be a result of Social Democratic training and employment programs (the "Active Manpower Policy"). At the same time, the party was under fire because the recently released Low-Income Commission Study showed that 20 years of Social Democratic rule had failed to eradicate poverty in Sweden.

Provisions of the Seven Crowns Reform

The Seven Crowns reform was prepared and introduced in three steps. First, in executive proceedings, the government prepared the proposal, minimizing interest group comment as much as possible. Second, the proposal was debated in parliament, where it was enacted into law by the Social Democrats' absolute majority; however, Center and Liberal MPs also voted for the law. Third, after passage of the law, negotiations between the Federation of County Councils and the Swedish Medical Association completed the reform. The legislative portion of the reform transformed the payment mechanism for hospital outpatient care. Patients would no longer pay doctors directly and then wait for reimbursement from national health insurance. Instead, they would pay the hospital a uniform flat fee of 7 crowns (hence the name of the reform), which was worth about $1.40 at the time. National health insurance would pay 31 crowns for each visit directly to the county councils. At the same time, the private office hours of senior physicians were eliminated; no private practice was to be carried out within the walls of public hospitals.

Once the reform had been approved by the *Riksdag*, the Swedish Medical Association and the Federation of County Councils held negotiations to decide how to pay doctors for hospital outpatient work, now that they would no longer be paid on a fee-for-service basis by patients. In these negotiations, it was decided to pay all hospital doctors a salary that would cover both outpatient and inpatient duties at the public hospitals. Initially, it had been intended to extend the flat-rate "Seven Crowns" system to public district doctors and private office-based practitioners. Negotiations over the exact details of the plan for the private practitioners broke down, however. Nevertheless, this failure aided the government.

Because the private practitioners were left out of the reform, patients would have an economic incentive to seek care at hospital outpatient clinics, where they would pay 7 crowns, rather than at private offices, where they would pay full fees, later receiving only a partial reimbursement if the doctors extra-billed. This would hurt the office-based practitioners and at the same time close off an "exit" option for hospital doctors dissatisfied with the reform. Senior doctors would not easily be able to transfer their private hours to private offices outside the hospitals, and complete exit into full-time practice would also be made more difficult by the new incentive structure.[12]

Together, the Seven Crowns reform and the related negotiations introduced several of the more controversial points of the Höjer reform. The county councils would have sole jurisdiction over outpatient care within public hospitals, and service within the outpatient clinics (*polikliniks*) would become a mandatory part of hospital duties. Furthermore, hospital doctors would in future be paid a full-time salary. Had the Federation of County Councils and the Swedish Medical Association been able to agree on extending the reform to private practitioners, Höjer's program would have been complete: All private office-based practitioners would have been placed under the jurisdiction of the county councils, thereby establishing a fully integrated national health service for ambulatory care, completely under the control of one government body, the county councils.

The Seven Crowns reform was intended as a rationalizing measure. In eliminating the reimbursement system for hospital outpatient care, the direct costs to patients of each visit would be comparable to the costs for hospital inpatient care, which had been set at a flat rate since 1955. It was hoped that the reform would remove the economic incentives to choose the more costly inpatient care.[13] The reform was intended to rationalize the behavior of physicians as well as patients. If private medical practice was removed from public hospitals, senior physicians would no longer prefer to spend time in their private office hours, leaving the *polikliniks* to be staffed by the junior physicians. Removing the lucrative private practice available to senior hospital doctors in the cities would, in addition, reduce one of the differences between city and rural hospital practice; this might encourage more doctors to move into rural areas. It would also make doctors' incomes more subject to tax scrutiny, a topic of concern because a recent tax investigation had revealed substantial unreported income among doctors. Although the Swedish Medical Association criticized the Seven Crowns reform—in particular, the elimination of private practice from public hospitals and the neglect of the private practitioners—the association eventually accepted the reform when it was enacted by the *Riksdag* and pursued a moderate course in subsequent salary negotiations with the Federation of County Councils.

There were advantages for the leadership in accepting a salary form of payment. With an increased number of physicians, which not only weakened the market position of doctors but also brought in a large cohort of younger doctors, the leadership could improve the situation of its members more effectively by pursuing a hard line in salary negotiations than by clinging to private practice privileges. In addition, inequalities caused by the reimbursement system, as well as differences in access to private patients, were creating friction among the association's membership that would be mitigated through the more rational distribution of a salary system. At the same time, as Heidenheimer (1980a) pointed out, the position of the county councils, and especially their federation, had been strengthened by an increased reliance on centralized planning through the regionalization of the health system, the delegation of several new responsibilities to the councils, and the fact that negotiations with the medical profession now took place on a national level, between the Federation of County Councils and the Swedish Medical Association.

With the absolute Social Democratic majority in the parliament, passage of the Seven Crowns law was a *fait accompli*. This explains the conciliatory stance of the Swedish Medical Association leadership both during the preparatory stage preceding the parliamentary debate and in the negotiation stage that followed the passage of the law by parliament. The constraints imposed on the leadership by this political context, and not professional interest, led the leadership to cooperate rather than protest.

Younger hospital doctors and rural practitioners were not affected by the removal of private practice from the hospitals or the competitive pressures against private office practice and extra billing. The younger doctors would benefit from the more even distribution of hospital work; rural practitioners would be hurt by the competition from the hospital outpatient clinics, but this private practice was less widespread than in the cities, and these doctors did not tend to override the fee schedule to the same extent as the urban practitioners. Thus, professional interests were divided. Restrictions on private practice were of concern to senior hospital physicians and urban private practitioners but not to younger doctors and rural practitioners.

Although moderate in its presentation, the Swedish Medical Association did indeed voice objections to the Seven Crowns reform. When its lobbying efforts at the executive stage failed, however, cooperation made sense, even though the leadership was faced with membership protests. For although the association had the organizational resources to mount a strike or other protest activity, collective action was not effective against a united executive government. Thus, the weak position of the Swedish medical profession was fundamentally political rather than economic or organizational. Even though the increases in medical school admissions would be expected to weaken the market position, the number of inhabitants per doctor remained lower in Sweden than in other countries, where the medical profession was more successful in defending its access to a private market. Furthermore, the Medical Association had successfully carried out several economic actions, such as a strike in 1957 in which doctors organized an alternative private health service, the building of private clinics in the early 1960s, and a strike threat in 1965 that resulted in substantial increases in the reimbursement schedule. Each time, however, the government had reacted by taking a *political* step that constrained the private market. The defeat of the Höjer reform was met with the increases in medical school admissions in the 1950s; the 1957 strike was followed by the 1959 Hospital Law; the private clinics were combated by announcements that the government planned to build local health centers in the mid-1960s; and the increases in the fee reimbursement schedule in the late 1960s resulted in the Seven Crowns reform.

In 1969, as with the 1931 Sickness Fund Law and with the 1947 National Health Insurance Law, the Medical Association was faced with unified support for an expanded government role in health care. SAF, in sharp contrast to its opposition to the Höjer reform, now supported restrictions on private practice and the elimination of the reimbursement mechanism as a means of controlling health care costs. It stated in its *remiss* paper that the reform would lead to a more rational organization of health care and that doctors would be able to devote themselves more fully to the care of patients if they were removed from financial matters. LO and TCO were strongly in favor of the reform, as was the Federation of County Councils.

Not only was there widespread support for the reform from a number of central political actors, but use of the executive arena allowed the Social Democratic government to accelerate the reform process and to discourage lengthy discussions over the reform's more controversial points. From a procedural point of view, the Seven Crowns reform was highly unusual in that it was essentially worked out between the Federation of County Councils, the Social Department, and the National Health Insurance Office without the presence of representatives of the Swedish Medical Association. The restriction of the preparatory stages to high levels of the bureaucracy was of strategic importance, for it helped to ensure the passage of the reform within a year. There was less time for opposition to the reform to develop within the medical profession or for the profession to launch an opposition campaign among potential allies (Carder & Klingeberg, 1980, p. 143).

This pressing time frame for the reform and the attempts to minimize interest group input, however, were related to the overall electoral strategy of the Social Democratic Party. Indeed, that strategy was not limited to the health area. A 1970 tax reform was passed through the same kind of process: Preparation was not carried out through a royal committee, the Social Democrats were accused of precluding public discussion of the reform, and the reform process was controlled completely from within the government with little input from the political parties. For the officials of the Social Department and the Social Minister Sven Aspling, the absolute parliamentary majority won by the Social Democrats in the 1968 election provided an opportunity to introduce reforms that had been in the works for a number of years and to push things through more quickly than usual.

Despite this rather extraordinary position, the party did not impose reforms based on its electoral majority; it relied on consensus among certain key parties and interest groups, but a consensus that was aided by the structure of Swedish interest representation. Here the role of the county councils was crucial. During the postwar period, nearly 50% of MPs held posts on county councils; within the Center Party, the proportion ranged from 67% to 85%. As an informal political coalition, known as the "County Council Party," or Landstingspartiet, members of the county councils were essential in convincing their fellow party members to vote for health reforms. Thus, a certain multipartisan aspect lay beneath the surface of the Social Democratic initiatives, causing some doctors to complain bitterly that the socialization of the medical profession was accomplished with the help of nonsocialist politicians.

A second source of conciliation was provided by the continuing negotiations between the main labor market organizations. Brought into nearly constant contact with one another and with the government, SAF, LO, and TCO had a strong interest in not disrupting collective bargaining agreements by turning national health insurance policies into symbolic ideological issues. SAF was willing to accept national health insurance and restrictions on private practice. LO was willing to discuss cost containment and to weigh benefit increases against their financial implications. TCO was willing to give up special fringe benefit schemes in the name of solidarity with all wage earners.

The same procedures that brought together a limited number of central political actors and encouraged cooperative bargaining shut out potential sources of particularistic vetoes of government policies. Groups such as the medical profession were not privileged with the same kind of access to political decision making as were the county councils or the labor market organizations. In the context of royal committees and bureaucratic politics, the medical profession was only one of several interest groups that had to be polled. Morever, if the labor market organizations agreed, it was not necessary to represent the profession in a royal committee or even to set up a committee. As Conservative MP and physician Kaijser protested, "The Parliamentary decision is a mere formality. . . . The real decision has taken place over the heads of the MPs" (*Riksdagens Protokoll,* 1969, p. 72). Dissident views were expressed in the press, as well. One economically liberal newspaper stated, "It is not too much to demand that Parliament and the Swedish people be given the opportunity to discuss and examine thoroughly a reform proposal which can be said to entail the 'socialization' of the majority of the medical profession" ("Pressgrannar," 1969, p. 2). Another liberal paper (*Göteborgs Handels & Sjöfartstidning* (December 10, 1969) ran the headline "Health Care Reform Resembles Coup" and later in the month (December 31, 1969) warned that "this secret socialization will surely cause a rapid emigration of doctors from Sweden to countries with freer working conditions" (p. 3). But with the support of the Liberal and Center parties, the Social Democratic majority held firm. The Seven Crowns reform became law on December 3, 1969.

After passage of the law, the conflict passed to the collective bargaining arena, where the Swedish Medical Association agreed—despite strong criticisms from some of its members—to a salary system of payment. The leadership was attacked for not informing the membership about the full implications of the reform and for not pursuing a hard line in the negotiations with the Federation of County Councils. The leadership defended itself on the grounds that it was "stuck" in a situation where it was hard to bargain with resolution and strength. Once again, when politically isolated, the association pursued a moderate course of action, despite membership criticisms.

Results of the Seven Crowns Reform

With the enactment of the Seven Crowns reform, the Swedish health system moved a decisive step toward becoming a national health service. The vast majority of doctors worked as salaried employees of the government. Patients paid only a small sum at the time of treatment, with the rest of costs being paid for through national health insurance and local taxes. At private office-based practitioners, on the other hand, patients continued to pay full fees with subsequent reimbursement from the insurance funds. Consequently, the percentage of full-time practitioners dropped from 15% in 1964 to 6% in 1979, and the average age of private practitioners rose to 57 years, compared with an average of 39 years for the profession as a whole.

In 1975, however, the private practitioners were given the option of registering with the insurance funds in return for adhering to a fee schedule. Thus, virtually all forms of private practice were incorporated into the government scheme. From this time on, visits to unregistered doctors would not be covered by national health insurance. As the private practitioners had "found it hard to compete with the public sector . . . the reform in 1975 and the new system of reimbursement was an improvement for the private practitioners. It was clear, however, that the social democratic government was aiming at limiting private practice" (Smedby, 1978, p. 250). Hospital doctors were required to have the permission of the county council for which they worked before opening up a part-time practice. The hospital's need for overtime was required to be fulfilled before doctors could go into overtime private practice.

Post-1976 Changes

When the nonsocialist government came to power in 1976, the restrictions on spare-time private practice for hospital doctors were lifted, and, at the initiative of the Conservative Party, a study was made of the need for private practitioners. At the same time, however, plans for putting all private practitioners under the jurisdiction of the county councils for planning purposes only resulted in protests by private practitioners in 1979 (Serner, 1980, p. 112; Socialdepartementet, 1982).

In 1982, the Social Democrats were returned to power and reintroduced restrictions on private practice. Previous limits on private practice had reduced the number of full-time private practitioners, and the numbers had continued to decrease under the nonsocialist government. In 1975, there were 800 full-time practitioners; in 1984, only 600. But during the early 1980s, the number of spare-time private practitioners increased dramatically—from 233,000 patient visits to such physicians in 1981 to more than 600,000 in 1983. The number of spare-time private practitioners may have increased as a result of a hospital doctors' strike in January 1982. In addition, many doctors signed up when the Social Democrats returned to power in the fall of 1982, anticipating that the Social Democrats might move to curtail spare-time private practice in the future.[14]

Repeating the pattern of the past, the Social Democratic government countered doctors' efforts to exit from the public sector by imposing new restrictions on private practice. The controversial Dagmar reform of 1986, like the Seven Crowns reform, was worked out largely between the Social Department and the Federation of County Councils. Under this reform, government subsidies to hospitals would no longer be paid for each patient visit but would be distributed according to the number of inhabitants. This change was meant to ensure that funding for health care would be evenly distributed and would not reward overuse of the system, as generally occurred in the better-funded areas such as the cities. In addition, the law changed the possibilities for doctors to sign up for private practice. Doctors who had previously signed up could continue their private practice, but hospital doctors would no longer be required to sign contracts with county councils. Full-time private practitioners, as well, would be required to sign contracts with the county councils for their patients to be covered by national health insurance. At the same time that Social Democratic policies increased the control of the county councils over the private sector, more authority was delegated to the individual county councils, and the oversight powers of the National Board of Health and Welfare were lessened. Thus, Social Democratic health policy of the 1980s continued to restrict private practice; nevertheless, private medical practice increased at the margins, and the health system became more decentralized.

An End to the Social Democratic Model?

The enactment of the Seven Crowns reform was both the culmination of a long period of Social Democratic rule and the start of a new era. The elimination of the First Chamber has destabilized the Swedish system, allowing for more frequent shifts in government during the 1970s and 1980s and undermining the certainty of continuous Social Democratic rule that provided the political framework for the period of Harpsund democracy. With this destabilization, more conflicts within Swedish society have become apparent. The old, class-based politics has not captured the young or professional groups; the strategy of national economic management with generous social policies is not adapted to the global environment. Indeed, the shifts between Conservative governments trying to expand the private sector and Social Democratic governments trying to cut it back are representative of more general changes in the Swedish model since 1976. Not only has the emphasis on a nationally planned public health system come to be questioned, but key features of the Swedish post-Second World War settlement—such as centralized collective bargaining and wage agreements, the class-based party system, and the ability of SAF, TCO, and LO to represent divergent interests— have come under debate.   •

As this analysis of the piecing together of the Social Democratic model shows, however, these conflicts are not new; they were always part of Swedish society. The difference is the lessened ability of the system of political representation to make some conflicts less politically relevant and to find ways of adjudicating among the others. Whereas previously the Social Democrats could weather a storm such as the 1948 election, slowing down their policy agenda but maintaining their position as the governing party, the increased instability of a unicameral system based on proportional representation is reversing the Swedish pattern of radical policies achieved through institutions meant to impede change.

Conclusion

The Swedish state was able to take steps to control the medical market because its actions could not be vetoed in alternative arenas. This was not simply a matter of Social Democratic electoral victories. The Swedish executive was able to attain its goals because the initial policy changes were not blocked; rather, they led to further interventions.

Nor were these policy changes a result of peculiar preferences on the part of the medical profession or a result of any inherent economic or organizational weaknesses. Swedish private practitioners viewed market autonomy as the key to professional freedom. They promoted a liberal model of medicine, protesting mandatory medical benefits under the 1930 Sickness Fund Law, begrudgingly accepting national health insurance but insisting on a reimbursement payment system, blocking the Höjer plan for a national health service, and attacking the medical association leadership for not protesting more forcefully the Seven Crowns reform. Thus, Swedish medical opinion did not differ radically from that in other countries, nor did the medical association seem incapable of collective action.

The striking difference between the Swedish medical profession and the others lay in its strategic political position. Although strikes had indeed been effective in the past—for example, in increasing doctors' fees—these victories were short-lived. After each successful strike, the government took a *political* step to constrain the private market, such as removing private beds from public hospitals or eliminating the fee system entirely, as under the Seven Crowns reform. Not only did the Social Democratic government hold the parliamentary votes that would ensure passage of the legislation, but it buttressed its reform by changing market incentives to both doctors and patients. The Seven Crowns reform made private office practice less attractive to patients because hospital outpatient care was now virtually free, whereas in private offices patients were required to pay the full fee and were later reimbursed for a portion of the fee. This made it difficult for doctors wishing to protest the Seven Crowns reform to flee to the private sector.

Thus, the idea that doctors can block any reform by going on strike appears to be a myth. In economic conflicts, the government can use political means to change the terms of the conflict. The Social Democratic government was able to convert its electoral gains into concrete policy decisions because political bargains worked out within royal committees were enforced by stable parliamentary majorities that closed off veto opportunities for dissident groups. Only when electoral realignments provided a strategic opportunity for veto did interest groups defect from this game of cooperative bargaining.

The Swedish pattern of executive-induced compromise was built up in a series of steps through a combination of constitutional rules, electoral results, and historical accident. Policies were made by consensus, but in a process that increased the probability of agreement by concentrating decisions at a single point with a group of actors that met repeatedly. The forging of consensus does not mean that conflicts or disagreements were nonexistent, but the conditions for conciliating conflict were helped by the lack of decision points where single actors could unilaterally overturn the executive-level consensus. The framework for this process was a double framework: the long period of political control by the Social Democrats of the executive, and the committee and *remiss* procedures that moved decision making to a protected arena, even when the First Chamber and parliament could be used as veto points.

These institutional features did not determine that Social Democrats would be so successful in getting out the popular vote or that union organizers would be able to consolidate such a large variety of workers' interests into a single confederation. But what the institutions did accomplish was to eliminate sources of political blockage and interest group veto. The Swedish case is an example of what can happen when the executive can enact its program without risk of legislative or electoral vetoes.

Notes

1. Royal committees are appointed by the government to investigate specific policy problems and to draft legislative proposals. Originally divided into "expert" committees and "political" committees (*sakkunniga* and *politiska kommittéer*), the two functions are now virtually merged, with both technical and political experts appointed to the same committees. Proposals formulated by government departments and/or the royal committees are sent to interest group and government representatives for comment. Their written responses are called *remiss* statements. See Hesslén (1927) and also Kelman (1981, pp. 131-132), Anton (1969), Meijer (1969), Heclo (1974), and Heclo and Madsen (1987).

2. This is the view of Marmor and Thomas (1972).

3. Heidenheimer (1980b) pointed out the significance of union-sickness fund linkages for the formation of government programs in health. When unions used the sickness funds as an organizational tool, as in Germany, government-administered health programs were impeded.

4. Ito (1980) listed the 1925 figures as 13.3% for Sweden, 42.5% for Denmark, and 32% for Germany. Flora and Alber (1981, p. 75) listed the 1925 figures in terms of members as a percentage of the active labor force: Sweden, 29%; France, 21%; Switzerland, 50%; Germany, 57%; and Denmark, 99%. There are, of course, problems with this type of comparison. Swedish children, for example, are not counted as members, even though they are insured by their parents. The Swiss figures are inflated because so much double-counting occurs.

5. In 1934, the two organizations merged to become the Swedish Sickness Fund Association (Svenska Sjukkasseförbundet).

6. For those interested in the public image of the profession, it is of note that during the parliamentary debate, Dr. Järte, a Conservative MP and physician, was forced to defend the motives of opponents to the reform: "The majority of Sweden's office practitioners criticize the reform for reasons that honor the corps, as one can easily calculate what doctors would come to earn from social insurance. But they say with their foreign colleagues in mind: lead us not into temptation" (*Riksdagens Protokoll*, 1931, p. 45).

7. Between 1930 and 1945, LO's membership increased from 553,456 to 1,106,917, SAF's from 2,969 to 8,645 (covering 306,520 and 530,161 employees, respectively), and TCO's from 20,000 in 1931 (DACO) to 204,653 in 1945. SACO was founded in 1947 with about 15,000 members, SR (government employees) was founded in 1946 with about 18,100 members, and RLF (an agricultural organization) increased from 19,237 members in 1930 to 154,339 in 1945 (Hadenius, Molin, & Wieslander, 1978, p. 336). On the shift in parties, see Nyman (1947). On the labor movement, see Esping-Andersen (1985) and Korpi (1983).

8. Although sickness fund membership had continued to grow after the war, the national health insurance law expanded coverage considerably, from 3.17 million in 1954 to 5.4 million in 1955, or from 48% of the adult population in 1945 and 60% in 1954, to 78% of the population in 1955. With family members, 100% of the population was insured. With the introduction of national health insurance, the voluntary contributions were eliminated, and contributions were shared between the national government (29%), employers (27%), and the insured (44%). According to Uhr (1966, cited in Broberg, 1973, pp. 45, 194, 206), financing in 1962 was 19% by the insured, 11% from employer contributions, and 70.4% from national and local government revenues; the figures for 1955 are about the same.

9. Even within public hospitals, for patients defined as public patients, hospital doctors were paid for outpatient visits on a fee-for-service basis by patients, but these charges were restricted by the official fee schedule.

10. In 1960, 50 doctors were attached to the private clinics known as *Läkarhus*. By 1978, the number had grown to 390, compared with over 10,000 active physicians. These private clinics have been much more successful for dentists, whose number grew from 30 affiliated dentists in 1966 to 1,720 in 1978 (figures from Praktikertjänst AB [the company that organizes the clinics], personal communication, 1978). Recently, there have been new (and controversial) attempts to start private clinics, and they have had more success, notably Stockholm Akuten, an emergency care service.

11. Younger doctors, interested in better relations with the government, were important for the passage of the 1959 Hospital Law. This does not mean that enactment of the law came free of disputes. The Medical Association insisted that the hospital outpatient clinics be limited to specialist care. Later, these restrictions were lifted by the 1963 and 1972 Hospital Laws. See Carder and Klingeberg (1980), Heidenheimer (1980a), Serner (1980), and SOU (1978, p. 27).

12. Patients at the hospital *polikliniks* and at district doctors would pay 7 crowns, whereas at private practitioners' offices they would pay the full fee, with reimbursement for 75% of the official fee as under the fee schedule. Because private doctors—or public doctors in their private hours—charged above officially recognized rates, the actual rates of reimbursement to patients were significantly lower than those guaranteed by law. This overcharging, as well as the theory that these increases in fees created a market pressure to increase the fee schedule for all doctors, was part of the motivation for the Seven Crowns reform.

13. In addition, the reform was triggered by the county councils' plan to raise the cost of inpatient care from 5 to 10 crowns per day; the introduction of the 7 crowns flat fee for outpatient care would compensate patients for this increase. Pensioners, the group most likely

to be hurt by the increased inpatient fees, were placated by doubling the number of free hospital days available to them, from 180 days to a full year. The shift in outpatient care financing from reimbursement to flat fee was estimated to cost 250 million crowns annually, 200 million of which would be financed through an increase in the employer contribution to health insurance from 2.5% to 2.9% of the wage bill.

14. On growth of private practice, see also Rosenthal (1986).

References

Alla under 16 år får fri läkare. (1948, March 10). *Morgontidningen*, pp. 1, 4.

Anderson, O. (1972). *Health care: Can there be equity? The United States, Sweden and England.* New York: John Wiley.

Anton, T. (1969). Policy-making and political culture in Sweden. *Scandinavian Political Studies, 4,* 88-102.

Biörck, G. (1977). How to be a clinician in a socialist country. *Annals of Internal Medicine, 86,* 815-816.

Bjurulf, B., & Swahn, U. (1980). Health policy recommendations and what happened to them: Sampling the twentieth century record. In A. Heidenheimer & N. Elvander (Eds.), *The shaping of the Swedish health system* (pp. 75-98). London: Croom Helm.

Broberg, R. (1973). *Så formades tryggheten: Socialförsäkringenshistoria 1946-1972.* Stockholm: Försäkringskasseförbundet.

Carder, M., & Klingeberg, B. (1980). Towards a salaried medical profession: How "Swedish" was the Seven Crowns reform? In A. Heidenheimer & N. Elvander (Eds.), *The shaping of the Swedish health system* (pp. 143-172). London: Croom Helm.

Elvander, N. (1966). *Intresseorganisationerna i dagens Sverige.* Lund: CWK Gleerup.

Elvander, N. (1974). Interest groups in Sweden. *Annals of the American Academy of Political and Social Science, 41*(3), 27-43.

Esping-Andersen, G. (1985). *Politics against markets: The social democratic road to power.* Princeton, NJ: Princeton University Press.

Esping-Andersen, G., & Korpi, W. (1984). Social policy as class politics in post-war capitalism. In J. Goldthorpe (Ed.), *Crisis and order in contemporary capitalism* (pp. 179-208). Oxford, UK: Oxford University Press.

Flora, P., & Alber, J. (1981). Modernization, democratization, and the development of welfare states. In P. Flora & A. Heidenheimer (Eds.), *The development of welfare states in Europe and America.* New Brunswick, NJ: Transaction.

Fri sjukvård, inga privatläkare, oenighet redan i utredningen. (1948, March 10). *Svenska Dagbladet,* p. 3.

Garpenby, P. (1989). *The state and the medical profession: A cross-national comparison of the health policy arena in the United Kingdom and Sweden 1945-1985.* Linköping, Sweden: Linköping Studies in Arts and Sciences.

Hadenius, S., Molin, B., & Wieslander, H. (1978). *Sverige efter 1900: En modern politisk historia* (8th ed.). Stockholm: Aldus/Bonniers.

Heclo, H. (1974). *Modern social politics in Britain and Sweden.* New Haven, CT: Yale University Press.

Heclo, H., & Madsen, H. (1987). *Policy and politics in Sweden: Principled pragmatism.* Philadelphia: Temple University Press.

Heidenheimer, A. J. (1980a) Conflict and compromise between professional and bureaucratic health interests, 1947-1971. In A. J. Heidenheimer & N. Elvander (Eds.), *The shaping of the Swedish health system* (pp. 119-142). London: Croom Helm.

Heidenheimer, A. J. (1980b). *Unions and welfare state development in Britian and Germany: An interpretation of metamorphoses in the period 1910-1950* (International Institute for Comparative Social Research SP-II Discussion Paper, IIVG/dp/80-209). Berlin: Wissenschaftszentrum.

Hesslén, G. (1927). *Det Svenska Kommittéväsendet intill år 1905: Dess uppkomst, ställning och betydelse.* Unpublished dissertation, Uppsala University.

Hjern, B. (1976, April). *The Swedish health services from the standpoint of the profession: Negotiating and bargaining.* Unpublished paper.

Högerns företagargrupps resolution. (1948, March 12). *Svenska Dagbladet,* p. 2.

Höjer, K. (1952). *Svensk socialpolitisk historia.* Stockholm: P. A. Norstedt & Söners.

Ito, H. (1980). Health insurance and medical services in Sweden and Denmark, 1850-1950. In A. Heidenheimer & N. Elvander (Eds.), *The shaping of the Swedish health system* (pp. 44-67). London: Croom Helm.

Kelman, S. (1981). *Regulating America, regulating Sweden: A comparative study of occupational safety and health policy.* Cambridge, MA: MIT Press.

Korpi, W. (1983). *The democratic class struggle.* London: Routledge & Kegan Paul.

Landsorganisationen i Sverige [LO]. (1954, April 30). *LO-remiss, betänkande angående den öppna läkarvården i riket (SOU 1948:14) och bilagor (SOU 1948:24)* [LO position paper, January 10, 1949). In Riksarkivet [Swedish National Archive], Inrikeskonseljakt [Department of the Interior's File], No. 82.

Lindeberg, G. (1949). *Den Svenska sjukkasserörelsens historia.* Lund, Sweden: Svenska Sjukkasseförbundet/Carl Bloms Boktryckeri.

Marmor, T., & Thomas, D. (1972). Doctors, politics and pay disputes: "Pressure group politics" revisited. *British Journal of Political Science, 2,* 436-437.

Medicinalchefen Axel Höjer visar två ansikten. (1948, March 10). *Dagens Nyheter,* p. 3.

Meijer, H. (1969). Bureaucracy and policy formulation in Sweden. *Scandinavian Political Studies, 4,* 103-116.

Nyman, O. (1947). *Svensk Parlamentarism 1932-1936: Från minoritetsparlamentarism till majoritetskoalition* (No. 27, Skrifter Utgivna av Statsvetenskapliga Föreningen i Uppsala genom Axel Brusewitz). Uppsala: Almqvist & Wicksell.

Petrén, A. (1931, April 27). Letter. *Läkartidningen,* p. 585.

Pressgrannar. (1969, November 25). *Dagens Nyheter,* p. 2. [Originally printed in newspaper *Handelstidningen*]

Riksdagens Protokoll [Parliamentary Minutes]. (1926). Proposition 1926:117, p. 24.

Riksdagens Protokoll [Parliamentary Minutes]. (1931). Andra Kammaren [Debates of the Second Chamber], Collection 6, Vol. 35, p. 45.

Riksdagens Protokoll [Parliamentary Minutes]. (1969). Första Kammaren [Debates of the First Chamber], Vol. 39.

Rosenthal, M. (1986). Beyond equity: Swedish health policy and the private sector. *Milbank Quarterly, 64,* 592-621.

Särlvik, B. (1967). Party politics and electoral opinion formation. *Scandinavian Political Studies, 2,* 167-202.

Serner, U. (1980). Swedish health legislation: Milestones in re-organization since 1945. In A. Heidenheimer & N. Elvander (Eds.), *The shaping of the Swedish health system* (pp. 99-116). London: Croom Helm.

Smedby, B. (1978). Primary care financing in Sweden. *Annals of the New York Academy of Sciences, 310,* 247-251.

Socialdepartementet. (1982). *Promemoria om nyrekrytering av privatpraktiserande läkare* (Ds S 1982:9). Stockholm: Author.

Statens Offentliga Utredningar. (1948a). *Bilagor till medicinalstyrelsens utredning om den öppna läkarvården i riket* (No. 1948:24). Stockholm: Inrikesdepartementet.

Statens Offentliga Utredningar. (1948b). *Den öppna läkarvården i riket: Utredning och förslag av medicinalstyrelsen* (No. 1948:14). Stockholm: Inrikesdepartementet.

Statens Offentliga Utredningar (SOU) (1978, p. 74); *Husläkare—en enklare och tryggare sjukvärd. Betänkande av kontinuitetsutredningen.* Stockholm: Socialdepartmentet.

Sveriges Arbetsgivarförening [SAF]. (1954, April 30). *SAF-remiss, betänkande angående den öppna läkarvården i riket (SOU 1948:14) och bilagor (SOU 1948:24)* [SAF position paper, December 30, 1948]. In Riksarkivet [Swedish National Archive], Inrikeskonseljakt [Department of the Interior's File], No. 82.

Tjänstemännens Centralorganisation [TCO]. (1946, September 27). *TCO-remiss, prop. 312 del. I. Remiss betr. SOU 1944:15, 16 (ang. Lag om allmänn sjukför säkring), Dnr 2038/44, Stockholm 19 Maj 1944* [TCO position paper on legislative proposal 312, part I. Position papers regarding government report SOU 1944:15,16 (concerning the Law on Universal Health Insurance), file no. 2038/44, Stockholm, May 19, 1944]. In Riksarkivet [Swedish National Archive], Socialdepartementet Konseljakt [Social Department's File], No. 123.

Twaddle, A., & Hessler, R. (1986). Power and change: The case of the Swedish Commission of Inquiry on Health and Sickness Care. *Journal of Health Politics, Policy and Law, 11,* 14-40.

Värmlandsföreningen. (1930, October). Letter to Sveriges Läkarförbunds fullmäktige [Swedish Medical Association, Central Steering Committee]. *Läkartidningen, 27,* 1266.

Verney, D. (1957). *Parliamentary reform in Sweden, 1866-1921.* Oxford, UK: Clarendon.

von Sydow, B. (1989). *Vägen till Enkammarriksdagen Demokratisk författningspolitik i Sverige 1944-1968.* Stockholm: Tidens.

CHAPTER 11

Evolving Roles of the National and Regional Governments in the Swedish Health Care System

RICHARD B. SALTMAN

The unitary structure of the Swedish state is often taken to imply that its national government is all-powerful. Though this is in fact the case in some unitary states, such as the United Kingdom, Sweden has a long history of shared governmental responsibilities among national, regional, and municipal governments (Scott, 1977). Typically, these shared responsibilities have involved a mix of what is termed "frame legislation" (*ramlag*) at the national level, setting broad policy objectives and standards, with a varying degree of administrative discretion at the regional or local level with regard to the operating mechanisms by which the stipulated outcomes are to be achieved.

In the recent past, the setting of national standards was often felt to be intrusive and restrictive by lower levels of government, particularly in human service sectors such as health and social services. For instance, in the 1950s and 1960s, the National Board of Health (now the National Board of Health and Welfare) issued strict criteria about medical staffing qualifications, personnel ratios, and the like (Serner, 1980). Similar regulations on municipal activities stipulated such things as the number and purpose of local administrative boards, their composition, and other administrative details.

In the early 1980s, however, a concerted effort began to reduce national controls on county and municipal administrations. One example of this effort was the "Free Municipality" (*freikommuner*) experiment, in which a small number of municipal governments undertook demonstration projects in which a substantial number of national regulations were temporarily waived. One key area of experimentation involved the transfer of certain primary care services from county to municipal jurisdiction— working on the theory that because the municipalities were already responsible for social and home care services, combining primary care and social and home care services within one administrative body would enhance coordination and efficiency, especially for services to the elderly. In any event, these efforts were undone by the unwillingness of physicians and nurses to shift from county employment (where medical personnel were the majority and had strong unions) to municipal employment (where most personnel were nonmedical). This experiment did, however, subsequently serve as one basis for the 1992 Ädel reform, of which more will be said shortly, as well as for a current experiment along similar lines in five municipalities.

At the county level, the reduction of the burden of national controls was considerably more thoroughgoing. As a preface to these early 1980s changes, however, and the series of events that followed over the next decade, it may be useful to briefly review the complex and evolving structure of regional government in Sweden.

The Changing Role of Regional Government in Health

Formally, there are two levels of regional government in Sweden. One, *länsstyrelsen* (county administration), is a provincial system that serves as the representative of the national government. These bodies are headed by an appointed governor (designated originally by the king, now by the national government). Earlier in Sweden's history, this provincial system played an important health care role in that it supervised those general practitioners appointed by the Crown who, in return for a government post, provided care to the indigent. In contemporary Sweden, however, the county administrations have little direct health sector responsibility.

The second and far more important level of regional government is the elected county councils (*läns landsting*). Sweden's 26 elected counties became responsible for operating a network of general hospitals in 1864.[1] In the mid- and later 20th century, the counties have taken on an increasingly important health sector role (Saltman, 1988). The national government decentralized ownership and management of state mental hospitals and university teaching hospitals to those counties in which they were situated. In addition, in the 1970s and 1980s, the counties developed a network of primary health centers, becoming the source for more than 90% of all primary care visits in Sweden (SPRI, 1992).

By the passage of the Health Services Act in 1982, the counties had become the predominant actors in the Swedish health sector: More than two thirds of health care expenditures were raised through direct county taxes on personal income, and the counties provided almost all inpatient and outpatient hospital, mental health, primary care, and nursing home services. The counties also had become concerned almost entirely with health care; although they retained some residual responsibilities in education, transportation, and industrial planning, these had been reduced to well below 20% of county activities.

The 1982 Health Services Act, followed by the Dagmar reform of 1983-85, introduced two major changes that further strengthened the independence and authority of the county councils. The 1982 act established the broad "frame" policies under which Swedish health care was to be delivered. The most important of these was arguably the requirement that the county was to ensure that each patient received treatment "under equal conditions" (*lika villkor*) to all other Swedish citizens. Although this phrase did not require the county to provide all possible services, it did stipulate that all citizens across the country with the same clinical indications were expected to have access to an equivalent standard of medical service.

The Dagmar reform of 1983-85 (designated for the name-day on which a crucial meeting about the reform was held) redirected the flow of revenue from the national sickness insurance fund (*försäkringskassan*) for office-based physician visits. Previously, these revenues were paid directly by the fund on a per-visit basis to either the county (for publicly employed physicians) or the individual private physician. Once fully implemented, the reform shifted the way in which the payment was calculated to an annual capitated amount for each citizen and paid these funds directly to the county on a prorated periodic basis. This reform, in practice, established a national cap on the total amount of funds available (at least from the national health insurance fund) for primary care services (Calltorp, 1996). Equally important, it paid all funds directly to the counties, enabling them to plan the availability of all primary care services, both public and private. In practice, this required physicians in private practice (estimated at approximately 5% of all physicians at that time) to obtain explicit contracts from the counties for the volume and value of the services that they would be allowed to provide with public funds (Saltman & von Otter, 1992).

To complete this picture of regional government in the health sector, however, it is necessary to mention a third element. In addition to the *länsstyrelsen* and the county councils, there are regional planning agencies (*planneringsnämnden*). These agencies are based upon voluntary agreements among adjacent county councils to develop cross-county cooperation in one section of the country. In the health sector, the regional planning agency in western Sweden has been perhaps the most visible, helping its five counties (Göteborg, Bohuslän, Halland, Älvsborg, Skäraborg) to develop closer operating connections. The western Sweden regional planning office was instrumental, for example, in a 1985 agreement that allowed residents of the five counties to seek care in any of the other counties—this 6 years before the entire country adopted a "free choice" (*valfrihet*) stance. This pressure for more integrated regional health service provision across current county lines also could be observed in the Malmö region of southern Sweden.

Thus, by the end of the 1980s, there were three closely related forces at work concerning subnational responsibilities in the health sector. The first was the strongly felt desire by both the counties and the municipalities to reduce the degree of national direction and control over their day-to-day administrative operations. The second was, for counties, the reality of decentralization of increased decision-making authority from the national government—or, for municipalities, the desire for increased responsibilities. The third was a need for increased regional cooperation among the counties, particularly in the Göteborg and Malmö metropolitan regions.

In the 1990s, these three pressures—less national regulation, greater decentralization, and more regional cooperation—helped shape the health system reforms that occurred. Efforts in various counties to establish either patient choice-based or "buy-sell" models of health care provision resulted in health providers being restructured into "public firms," with revenues tied to performance, and with growing managerial independence from both county and national controls (Anell, 1995). The previously mentioned Ädel reform, implemented in January 1992, was the result of national legislation that consolidated responsibility for all residential services for the elderly, including what were previously county-run nursing homes, at the municipal level. This reform also required municipal social services to accept "finished" hospital patients within 5 days or to pay the full cost of their continued hospital stay (Johansson, 1997). The success of the Ädel reform is considered by many observers to lay the groundwork for the eventual transfer of most primary care services from the counties to the municipalities.

Last, a national commission was established in 1992 to explore ways to rationalize the roles of the three existing regional levels of government. In its final report in March 1995, this commission recommended incorporating *länsstyrelsen,* the county councils, and the regional planning agencies into from six to eight new "regional parliaments" (*länsparliamentets*), which would take responsibility for running the health care system (Statens Offentliga Utredningar [SOU], 1995). This new model fits well with the Reformed County Council option, discussed in the Expert Panel's Report to the National Commission on Funding and Organization of Health Services and Medical Care (HSU 2000) (SOU, 1993). The five county councils in western Sweden anticipated the regional commission's likely report by appealing to the national government in 1994 for permission to establish a regional parliament in western Sweden as soon as feasible. This body is now scheduled to be established after the next county-level election in 1998. In addition, two other regions—in Skåne in southern Sweden and in Jämtland in the north—have indicated their desire to establish regional parliaments.

Thus, by the mid-1990s, the county councils had become the most important regional bodies in Sweden's health sector. Yet in the foreseeable future, their roles may well be diminished by the transfer of additional primary care services downward to the municipalities, and they will be eliminated entirely in some sections of the country by new regional parliaments that may be responsible only for the hospital subsector. In important respects, the rise and probable decline of the county councils reflect the evolving nature of regional government in Sweden.

The reforms of the 1990s are the most recent expression of this long-term process of devolution of authority in the Swedish health system. Beginning with state-initiated changes in the 1960s, operational decision making had been shifted from national to county government. With the 1982 Health Services Act, this shift of administrative authority away from the national government was formally recognized and consolidated in law. As noted above, this 1982 legislation, in combination with the subsequent Dagmar reform in the flow of physician visit payments, further enhanced the independence of the county councils in the health sphere.

The logic behind devolution in the health sector was similar to the reasoning prominent in other areas of Swedish public life. There was, first, the belief that it was both more democratic and more economically efficient to place decision making "closer to the people." This reflected the fact that the average Swedish county had a population of only 250,000 to 350,000 people. Second, there was a growing awareness that human services such as health should be less uniform and more responsive to the preferences of individual citizens. A third factor was the recognition that lower-level governments had become administratively "mature" and were competent to handle health sector administration. Last, some commentators believe that as resources in the health sector have become squeezed and as decision making has become more difficult, there has been an inclination on the part of national politicians to pass off some of the harder choices to politicians at lower levels of government. As one well-respected analyst observed of national decision makers, "There's little likely benefit here for them, but potential for considerable harm" (C. von Otter, personal communication, December 1994).

This independence set the stage for what was largely a county-generated process of health system restructuring in the late 1980s and early 1990s. Beginning in Stockholm County in January 1988, but shortly thereafter in most other counties, county councils experimented with different reform models to push operational decision making down to the individual hospitals and health centers.

In Stockholm County, a Conservative-led administration sought to make the hospital sector more efficient through a variety of organizational initiatives. Out of 10 hospitals in the county, one was transformed into an eye surgery facility to handle the increased demand for corneal lens implants. A second—after considerable controversy—became a much smaller outpatient unit. The county sought to place a third hospital— St. Görans—under private management. After extended efforts, the idea was dropped once negotiations with bidders made it clear that a private for-profit management firm would require a guaranteed revenue stream and profit margin.

A central part of the restructuring process in Stockholm County was the development of nine district boards that had responsibility both for operating primary health centers and for negotiating contracts for patient care with their districts' hospitals. Although the contracting role of these boards was formally limited by patients' ability to choose their health provider and facility, some district boards sought to convince patients to utilize contracted hospitals by offering more desirable or higher-quality services there. The Western District Board, for example, developed contracts that sought to integrate hospital services with primary and community care services for chronic medical conditions, creating what would be a higher-quality as well as lower-cost package of care (T. Malm, personal communication, June 10, 1994).

Dalarna County, a rural area in the center of Sweden, developed a reform model that expanded the role of primary care even further. Fifteen subcounty district boards were created, each composed of elected county council members from a specific municipality, and each was made responsible for running the primary health center that served that municipality. These district boards also held the entire hospital-level budget for their inhabitants, and this allowed them to enter into indicative (noncompulsory) contracts with the four county hospitals. Although the overall managerial and financial performance of the "Dalamodel" has been somewhat mixed (Bergman & Dahlbäck, 1995), this reform represents an ingenious effort by a county council to decentralize its activities as close as possible to the municipal level.

Both the Dalamodel and, in a more constrained manner, the Stockholm reforms place hospital budgets in the hands of primary care boards. This aspect of the reforms represents one of their most far-reaching initiatives in that it provides direct financial reinforcement to the goal of creating a primary-care-driven delivery system first enunciated in the Höjer Report in 1948 (Serner, 1980). Much as in the United Kingdom (general practitioner fundholders) and Finland (municipal health and social service boards), giving hospital budgets to primary care also was seen as an effective way to require hospitals to transform themselves into self-managing public firms, to be judged and paid not by a fixed budget but on the basis of their medical and organizational performance (Saltman & von Otter, 1995). This particular budgetary reform can thus be viewed as one that can generate a thoroughgoing strategic realignment of curative care services within the county-based delivery system.

It is important to note that neither Dalarna nor Stockholm privatized its hospitals or health centers—all remained publicly owned institutions. In behavior broadly consistent with the theory of public competition (Saltman & von Otter, 1992), the central county administrations continued to determine strategic policy and to design and monitor these new arrangements, as well as to retain control over capital expenditures and new service development.

Freed from rigid national controls, however, some more aggressive county officials set in train some activities that were of dubious value. One particularly egregious example was the contracting out of laboratory analyses for primary care in the Northeast District of Stockholm County to a privately owned firm under less than effective safeguards. A major scandal ensued when it became public knowledge that this private laboratory had fabricated test results in order to meet the lab's internal productivity standards ("Medanalys personal mådde mycket dålight," 1995). The aftermath of this episode generated calls to strengthen national supervisory authority over private sector health providers of all types.

The Changing Role of the National Government in Health

As the counties have taken on—and then passed along—increased decision-making authority, the national government has found itself grappling with the new parameters for its health sector role. In some quarters of the national government in the early 1990s, it was not uncommon to hear national civil servants, worried that certain Conservative-led counties appeared to be pushing the boundaries of socially responsible experimentation in their own internal devolution, argue that the national government had given up too much control over county behavior in the 1982 Health Services Act. Thus, as the county-led reforms generated an increasingly pluralistic delivery structure, with a growing number of independent decision-making nodes, the national government began to develop a new oversight framework for the health system. This new framework combined existing levers with new measures, each of which will be discussed in turn.

Despite the impact of the 1982 Health Services Act and the Dagmar reform, the national government retained a number of supervisory mechanisms over county actions. Among the most important was, first, the frame legislation itself, and with it the clear statement that broad health policy issues were to be decided nationally and were to apply equally to all Swedish citizens. Perhaps the most interesting—and controversial— manifestation of this national role came with the efforts of the 1991-94 Conservative-led national government to impose its own programmatic initiatives on the counties. One measure required the counties to replace their primary health centers with a system of personal doctors (*husläkare*), and another would have allowed medical specialists to establish practices wherever they might like and to be reimbursed by the counties for any patients they saw. Though both measures lost majority parliamentary support even before the Conservative-led coalition was voted out of office in September 1994, they demonstrate the continued national role in setting broad health sector policy.

A related area concerns the national government's authority to set macroeconomic policy. Though this normally deals with such matters as monetary and fiscal policy, in recent years the Swedish government has been particularly concerned about the size of public sector expenditures and the overall proportion of the gross domestic product (GDP) being absorbed through taxation (Einhorn & Logue, 1989; Rothstein, 1994). Both Social Democratic and Conservative-led governments sought to minimize growth in county and municipal revenues by freezing their taxation rates in the early 1990s (*skattestop*). Thus, much as current legislation enables the national government to determine broad health policy, macroeconomic policy has led the national government to modify health care financing activities.

A second area of national authority continues to be accreditation of medical professionals and facilities. Though the National Board of Health and Welfare no longer stipulates specific working procedures for individual personnel, it sets the qualifications for professional licenses, and it must grant operating permits to new medical facilities. This accreditation role, though of only marginal overall importance, ensures that practicing personnel and facilities meet a clear set of national standards.

A third area of national responsibility is in the area of malpractice and medical discipline. The National Board of Health and Welfare administers both a no-fault patient compensation system and a disciplinary program to deal with negligent or inappropriate medical providers (Rosenthal, 1988). Each Swedish hospital also has a chief physician who is required to report any act with possible criminal implications to the National Board.

A fourth national lever is special grants and payments. Although a number of dedicated grants were eliminated by the Conservative-led government (von Otter, 1994), the state continues to make equalization grants to those counties with below-average tax bases and to contribute to the cost of education and research in university hospitals. These grants and payments ensure that citizens in rural counties have access to the same standard of medical services and that, conversely, citizens in counties with university hospitals are not required to provide undue support for programs of national value.

A fifth area of national standard setting concerns research. Among other units, the national government maintains a technology evaluation center (SBU), which provides data on appropriate usage of new technologies. It also shares ownership (with the Federation of County Councils) of SPRI, a health services research center.

A sixth, indirect but crucially important factor in the state's role concerns medical education. In Sweden, as in most developed countries, medical schools are nationally funded, with student numbers, training residencies for specialists, and curriculum approved by the Ministry of Education. Thus, the size of the medical profession, its specialist composition, and its clinical knowledge base all reflect national government decisions. This is a long-term lever of influence, but it nonetheless highlights a key structural facet of national government authority over the development of the Swedish health sector.

Although these six levers indirectly help set national standards for service quality and delivery, national policymakers have keenly felt the importance of enhancing the standard-setting process with a series of specific measures to monitor and evaluate the performance of county-level provider institutions. A key role in this monitoring and evaluation process has been taken by the National Board of Health and Welfare (which lost its prior assignment of setting tight staffing and operating standards for health providers). The National Board has established six regional units to continuously monitor population-based data regarding the health delivery process in the counties. Once every 3 years, each county would have a week-long on-site evaluation, which would generate a published report comparing its service delivery with national norms. This Swedish process of monitoring and evaluation focuses explicitly on both preventive and curative health service delivery and outcomes, making it quite different from the newly introduced British system of "outposts," which focuses exclusively on financial matters and reports directly to the Treasury.

As this last National Board initiative indicates, national policymakers in Sweden are intensely concerned that increasingly autonomous service providers must be held accountable for their health-related as well as their financially related performance.

Conclusion

The relative roles of national and county government in Sweden are in a continuous process of development. Although political power at both national and county levels has swung back and forth since the mid-1970s, the relationship between the state and the counties has evolved along more or less consistent lines throughout this period of time. The overall direction has been to push operating authority to an increasingly lower level in the public sector, down to the individual provider units in many instances. Simultaneously, the national government has retained responsibility for establishing the broad health policy parameters and setting standards, as well as staking out a newly developing role in the monitoring and evaluation of health-related outcomes.

As the discussion above suggests, these relationships are by no means final. Rather, as the roles of the county and potentially of other regional bodies as well as the municipalities evolve, it is likely that the national government will also adjust its own activities. One also can point to the tax freeze imposed on the counties in the early 1990s, part of a broader macroeconomic strategy to reduce the level of taxation, as the type of extra-health-system event that can affect overall sector relationships. Thus both intra- and extra-health-system developments can be expected to influence the emerging balance.

Perhaps the most important issue in this process is whether the emerging balance between national, county, regional, and municipal responsibility will be able to ensure that the reformed Swedish health system will be not only more financially efficient but also able to satisfy the health service expectations of the Swedish citizenry. This balance has again come into question in 1996 and 1997 due to two concurrent factors. On the one hand, there is the continued decline in aggregate economic resources that Sweden spends on the health sector—to an estimated 7.1% of GDP in 1996. On the other hand, there is the reemergence of patient queues and personnel "burnout" as important policy issues. Indeed, some health sector analysts have begun to wonder if cost containment has not, in effect, been too successful in Sweden. Moreover, additional cost-generated changes in health sector organization, such as the scheduled January 1998 transfer of financial responsibility for all outpatient pharmaceutical costs from the national government to the county councils, can be expected to further complicate the picture. Ultimately, the impact of the current allocation of public sector responsibility among the respective levels of government must not only be evaluated by scholars but stand the electoral test applied by the Swedish citizenry. So far, that assessment has been a positive one.

Note

1. Sweden has 23 counties and three municipalities—Malmö, Göteborg, and Gotland—that have health sector responsibilities. These three municipalities are members of the Federation of County Councils and thus, though not formally counties, are included among the county councils for most health-related purposes.

References

Anell, A. (1995). Implementing planned markets in health services: The Swedish case. In R. B. Saltman & C. von Otter (Eds.), *Implementing planned markets in health care:*

Balancing social and economic responsibility (pp. 209-226). Philadelphia: Open University Press.

Bergman, S.-E., & Dahlbäck, U. (1995). *Att beställa häls -och sjukvård: Erfarenheter från landsting med beställarstyrning.* Stockholm: Lanstingsförbundet.

Calltorp, J. (1996). Swedish experience with fixed regional budgets. In F.-W. Schwartz, H. Glennerster, & R. B. Saltman (Eds.), *Fixing health budgets: Experience from Europe and North America.* New York: John Wiley.

Einhorn, E., & Logue, J. (1989). *Modern welfare states.* New York: Praeger.

Johansson, L. (1997). Decentralization from acute to home care settings in Sweden. In R. B. Saltman & N. M. Kane (Eds.), *Comparative experience in pharmaceutical and home care policy. Health Policy, 41*(Suppl.), S131-S144.

Medanalys personal mädde mycket dåligt. (1995, March 5). *Dagens Nyheter.*

Rosenthal, M. (1988). *Dealing with medical malpractice: The British and Swedish experience.* Durham, NC: Duke University Press.

Rothstein, B. (1994). *Vad bör Staten göra? Om Välfärdsstatens moraliska och politiska logik.* Stockholm: SNS.

Saltman, R. B. (1988). Health care in Sweden. In R. B. Saltman (Ed.), *International handbook of health care systems* (pp. 285-294). Westport, CT: Greenwood.

Saltman, R. B., & von Otter, C. (1992). *Planned markets and public competition: Strategic reform in northern European health systems.* Philadelphia: Open University Press.

Saltman, R. B., & von Otter, C. (1995). *Implementing planned markets in health care: Balancing social and economic responsibility.* Philadelphia: Open University Press.

Scott, F. D. (1977). *Sweden: The nation's history.* Minneapolis: University of Minnesota Press.

Serner, U. (1980). Swedish health legislation: Milestones in reorganization since 1945. In A. J. Heidenheimer & N. Elvander (Eds.), *The shaping of the Swedish health system.* New York: St. Martin's.

SPRI. (1992). *The reform of health care in Sweden* (SPRI-Rapport 339). Stockholm: Author.

Statens Offentliga Utredningar. (1993). *Three models for health care reform in Sweden: A report from the Expert Group to the Committee on Funding and Organization of Health Services and Medical Care (HSU 2000)* (No. 1993:38). Stockholm: Ministry of Health and Social Affairs.

Statens Offentliga Utredningar. (1995). *Regional future: A report from the Swedish Commission on Regional Administration* (No. 1995:27). Stockholm: Ministry of Health and Social Affairs.

von Otter, C. (1994). Reform strategies in the Swedish public sector. In F. Naschold & M. Pröhl (Eds.), *Produktivität öffentlicher Dienstleistungen.* Gutersloh, Germany: Bertelsmann Stiftung.

CHAPTER 12

Cost Control in the Swedish Health Sector

CASTEN VON OTTER

The year 1982 stands out in Swedish social history as the year the country lost its position as the world leader in health care expenditures to the United States. At the time, a top rank was seen with some pride as an indicator of advanced social development and wealth. Today, Sweden ranks in the same statistics in 14th place among the Organization for Economic Cooperation and Development (OECD) countries, and ironically, this too is a source of some satisfaction. Sweden is one of only two OECD countries that is year by year reducing the share of gross domestic product (GDP) spent on health (the other being Ireland).

After Swedish national health care expenditures peaked in 1980 at 9.4% of GDP, correction of the national statistics for improved international comparability reduced this rate by around 1.5% by transferring institutions for the mentally retarded and long-term elderly care to the social welfare budget. Although the remaining "genuine" reduction of the share of GDP to 7.0% is not too dramatic, it is significant that this happened during a very severe recession with falling GDP and with an aging population.[1] During the very last few years, when efforts at reducing costs accelerated, personnel in the health sector decreased by 12%, and productivity increased by 2% to 3% per year (Landstingsförbundet, 1995). The quality of care is by most estimates very good, with an internationally very low infant mortality rate, very high life expectancy, and very good rankings on the "avoidable mortality" index (Westerling et al., 1994). However, in the last year or so, there has been a growing concern that the retrenchment policies, reflecting the sad state of the national budget deficit, are finally not just reducing slack but undermining essential qualities.

In virtually all countries in Europe and North America, control of public health care expenditures has moved up on the political agenda. Historically, European governments have tried to obtain economic control by regulatory interventions on the supply side rather than on the demand side. However, in the last 5 or 10 years, the dominant approach has been to use market mechanisms more actively in allocating resources at the micro level. This has created uncertainty about whether regulatory arrangements are needed to moderate supply.

Thus, some radically divergent opinions about the roles of institutions and market mechanisms in cost control have emerged. Though it would be quite unfair to claim that the public debate about health economics has been totally based on mainstream neoclassical theory (in which change occurs through perfectly operating markets), most people—at least those living within public systems—still feel that the recent debate has stressed too much the frictionless ideal world of market theory. Many see monopsonistic power as the key to economic control (Abel-Smith, 1992), and others have argued for more institutionally mixed models (Saltman & von Otter, 1992). According to health policy institutionalists (a theoretically rather diverse bunch), social structure and cooperation are what really count in understanding and changing a health system. They might want to second Nobel laureate Douglas North's opinion (1981) that the purely marginalist world "begs all the interesting questions."

Governance and Finance

Swedish counties are responsible for planning and operating health care services. Each county is governed by the politically elected members of its council, which formally exercises full administrative and managerial powers. However, in practice, county councils delegate a fair amount of the executive functions to public managers and professionals. Since 1982, according to the Health Services Act, the counties have been responsible for all health-related planning. However, for more advanced health care as well as for research and training, the country is subdivided into six regions, each with one or more university hospitals.

Of all county health service costs in 1992, state grants accounted for approximately 7%, National Social Insurance added another 6%, patients' payments contributed around 2%, and the rest was paid by county taxes. The county tax base is defined by the national government, but the level of taxation is decided by each county (under varying government pressures to keep the rates down). The national government finances research and development and medical education and contributes to the budget of six regional and university hospitals. In addition, a system of tax equalization is in place to even out regional income differences. Patient copayments have almost doubled in the last few years. Given the universalistic principles associated with the welfare state, North Americans are often surprised by the substantial user charges and by the fact that they are levied with the multiple purposes of discouraging demand and guiding patient flows, as well as raising funds.

Studies have shown a considerable variation among OECD countries in levels of health expenditure and in the volume of care that this money can buy. In international comparisons using ordinary exchange rates, the Swedish volume is underestimated, for measures based on purchasing-power parities show that in Sweden, relative prices for health services in 1985 were quite low—0.54, well below the overall Swedish price level of 0.95 (U.S. = 1.0). This might indicate that the reason health care costs are low in Sweden does not necessarily reflect greater effectiveness but rather stricter control of costs and prices, resulting in lower relative salaries and prices of relevant resources (Gertham & Jonsson, 1991).

Pharmaceuticals are paid for by the state unless for inpatient use, when they are paid by the county. Patient copayments cover about a quarter of these costs, which are controlled by a "positive list" of approved drugs, the prices of which are negotiated by the National Insurance Board. A reference price system, aimed at controlling costs of drugs with generic alternatives, was recently introduced, with strong positive initial effects. There are at present only 1,900 drugs on the pharmaceuticals list. Pharmaceuticals are distributed by a state monopoly of pharmacies, which also owns the major wholesale corporation. The whole system is quite cost-effective by international standards: Swedish prices for prescribed drugs are about 40% below those of the United States. The share represented by drugs of all health service expenditures is the lowest in the OECD (Andersson, Gunnarsson, & Ljungkvist, 1995).

The Swedish case is singled out in comparative health policy discussions for certain reasons. Even though the science and technology applied is the same, the "game" of practicing medicine in Sweden is, in several respects, distinctly different from that in the United States or the countries of continental Europe. One difference is the high level of system integration, with regulation, financing, and provision of services all occurring within the public sector.[2] Another aspect, in seeming contrast to integration, is pluralism. Responsibility is shared by many parties, with medical services dispersed among the counties, so that Sweden has one of the most decentralized health systems, public or private, anywhere in the industrialized world. Finally, the combination of integration and pluralism offers a unique opportunity to see how control mechanisms are grafted onto existing structures in theoretically heterodox combinations.

In accounting for the relative success of cost control in Sweden, one set of explanations can be dismissed from the start. No "wonder technology" is at work—no spectacular administrative tricks, not even advanced information technology. In a system that had full control, constantly recurring budget crises like those in Sweden—such that spending must be adjusted under dramatic circumstances to balance the budget—would not take place. What counts is not so much ex ante cleverness as ex post determination. What is interesting is how the principals of the health services are able to maintain a tight budget constraint while eliciting the positive and active support of most parties. The answers are clearly not all to be found within the framework of economic analysis.

The 26 more or less different county health systems, undergoing change within the framework of one national environment, offer a unique test site for health service models and policies. Adding to its relevance for policy discussion is the Swedish experience with quasi-market reforms during the 1990s. Half of the counties have developed various planned-market experiments; others have focused change on new management systems, process reengineering, and similar concepts; and still others have thus far chosen to sit on the fence (Anell, 1995). In public health systems, this might be as close as one can expect to get to the conditions of a controlled experiment.

Sweden has already moved from an initial enthusiastic endorsement of market-inspired systems to a stage of dialectical clashes with the existing policy framework and institutional culture. Evaluations show impressive increases in productivity, reduced waiting lists, and trimmed-up technologies. However, the same studies have failed to establish meaningful relationships between the insertion of market mechanisms and cost control (Bergman & Dahlbäck, 1995; Svalander & Åhgren, 1995). Counties that have adopted strategies other than market reform are doing as well, sometimes even better. Most seriously, several counties and institutions that have spearheaded productivity-based payments have lost a firm grip over their budgets and have run into severe financial problems. Already they are modifying their newly adopted market systems.

In 1994, Social Democratic regimes took office nationally and in all but one county. The new minority government, which replaced a Conservative-Liberal coalition from 1991, is searching for an advanced synthesis that includes elements of both "markets" and "hierarchies" in a more balanced way than hitherto, and with more respect for what the outgoing government liked to call "Swedish idiosyncrasies."

Advantages and Disadvantages of Public Systems

Universal public systems, such as the Swedish, have a few things going for them that are too often played down. There are fewer complicated and interest-bound transactions. The whole apparatus that competing insurers or providers use to enroll clients is not needed. Systemwide bargaining and rule making make administration simpler, and providers need to confront only one set of rules. The cost control methods used in a system of universal coverage are more cost-effective because incentives for shirking and gaming are less strong. Opportunities for "cost shifting" can be more easily controlled or radically reduced. There is no need for detailed billing per case or procedure, and thus more can be spent on necessary medical care and less on administration.[3] Further, a universal system has an advantage in its ability to plan systematically the capacity of the health care system as a whole, thus making sure that investments are cost-effective and allocated to units where they are of the best use. Costly duplication of services can be avoided, and each institution can be assured a sufficient flow of patients to maintain professional qualifications (Goldberg, Marmor, & White, 1995).

To be sure, there are also certain drawbacks, mostly in terms of a lower level of dynamic innovations, fewer opportunities for varied choices, and, perhaps, more inconvenience for patients. The weakness of a system with many tight public controls and rather few personal incentives built in is, of course, the risk that the services will be offered in a rigid and inflexible manner, so that patients may experience health institutions as paternalistic and self-serving. However, international comparative studies indicate a high degree of patient satisfaction with most public systems. Moreover, the fact that all citizens are covered by the same offerings and rules makes for political pressure to ensure that good care is provided (*Vetenskap & Praxis*, 1995).

Effects of the Social System on Economic Behavior

In this discussion, some theoretically based arguments from the literature of institutional economics should be considered. Market forces can do much to invigorate health services but are not a panacea for all health policy ills. Even in ideally competitive health care markets, opportunistic behavior can prevail because of information impactedness and bounded rationality (Williamson, 1985). Moreover, in the presence of information asymmetries there can be no ideal incentive system (Miller, 1992).[4] Any formal incentive system leaves room for self-interested behavior, leading to persistent efficiency losses due to opportunism. Consequently, a health service organization that can induce the right kind of cooperation—defined as voluntary deviations from self-interested behavior to serve the good of the health system—will have an important edge over others. Social institutions that condition the choices of individuals favorably have a greater chance of motivating such behavior than do short-term economic rewards (North, 1990).

Some organizations have developed ways of institutionalizing the long-term mutual commitments that markets lack. This makes it possible to accumulate and trade off social acceptance and esteem against other valued rewards (e.g., income and/or career development) at a later stage, thus making "good moral choices" not only gratifying on altruistic grounds but materially supported as well. The obvious difference between an exchange relationship with someone you trust compared to one with a total stranger is also demonstrated in a more sociologically informed discussion of the embeddedness of complex transactions in a political and administrative culture and in professional norms.

Governing the public health system is a complex matter because of third-party financing and the preeminence of ensuring what is called equity in access, which in reality is allocation as a matter of social rights according to complicated needs-based medical and social formulas. In principle, in a public health service system, the government internalizes all the financial and production-related risks, unlike in other systems where a degree of risk sharing takes place between insurers and individuals. As a monopolist in the finance, purchase, and/or provision of services, the state keeps maximum control over transaction costs and future contingencies.

However, total power does not necessarily translate into full control, and the exercise of power is not without cost. If power is disproportionately distributed between agents, the first casualty is the game itself. Those who lack trust and feel deprived of influence will not want to enter into a long-term venture with a monopolist, except at a very high price. There are very obvious reasons why highly qualified professionals and health care producers should distrust the government and the long-term viability of the terms it offers. For example, for constitutional reasons there are narrow limits to how much a sitting government can make commitments on behalf of future governments. The problem for state-run health services is how they, as monopolists, can establish compliance with their objectives and achieve credibility for their future-oriented commitments without surrendering essential sovereignty. Designing an effective power base for a monopolist that will achieve cost control and medical priorities is a challenge that involves minimizing losses in efficiency, client satisfaction, and (perhaps) productivity.

Strategic Crossroads in Swedish Health Care Policy

The strategic crossroads that the Swedish health policy regime has encountered includes four major issues. Their resolution has gone far to determine the structure of the Swedish system:

1. *Integration and monopoly power:* Dealing with the "market-or-hierarchy choice" by establishing strategic control over financing and delivery through administrative corporatism
2. *Pressures of the workplace:* organizing the work process and division of labor in ways that can reconcile managerial accountability with professional autonomy
3. *Commitment and incentives:* encouraging personal drives that can foster public-oriented professionalism, intrasystem cooperation, and compliance with health policy objectives "beyond any contracted function" (to use the celebrated phrase of Talcott Parsons; Parsons & Smelser, 1956)
4. *Legitimation of policy:* making the political process accountable and transparent to the public so that the people will accept it

Integration and Monopoly Power

As noted above, the Swedish system has concentrated authority for area health services in the hands of the county councils. Given the priority accorded to cost control and distributional targets in the Swedish system, a fairly strong theoretical case can be made for vertical integration within an operational area such as a county. Transaction cost analysis provides a rationale for a tightly knit institutional system of policy making, financing, and service delivery. Theory suggests that contracts in the health care area may always be complex and legally incomplete. At least some people are prone to adverse selection, to offering biased information, and to erecting entry barriers. Rather than trying to make contracts ever more perfect at high administrative cost, a policy that warrants trust and good faith and is supported by long-term commitments is likely to stimulate more effective transactions (Williamson, 1985). The relatively small size of a county and the limited scope of adversarial interests support this kind of policy.

Separation of finance and provision of services may expose transactions more openly to opportunism. When competitive (large numbers) exchange relations obtain, guile and dishonesty pose relatively little risk to the contracting partners. However, there are rarely large numbers of competitors for long, especially in the health sector—and in sparsely populated Sweden—because the relationship between buyers and sellers is transformed in the process of the transaction. Therefore, unsuccessful bidders find it difficult to come again a second time, and the incumbent may accrue cost advantages from economies of scale, learning by doing and sunk cost investments. The result is that a small-numbers supply condition is likely to obtain at the time of contract renewal. This is a costly and risky position to be in unless the relationship is protected by a broader and more long-term commitment.

Opportunism does not pose the same difficulties for internal, sequential supply relations in an integrated county health administration as it does when negotiations take place across a market. This is because its internal divisions act under common ownership and supervision to maximize joint profits (Williamson, 1985). Moreover, the internal incentives and controls can be much more extensive and refined than those that obtain in market exchanges. An integrated county system should therefore be better able to take a long view of investments and to adjust to changing market circumstances in an adaptive, sequential manner.

Though "market or hierarchy" is often seen as a clear-cut and simple dichotomy, possible variations within each category must not be neglected. Lately, several studies have been made of alternative styles of planned markets (Saltman & von Otter, 1995). Others have commented on the vast differences among "hierarchies," in which variations go from a military command model to popular movements under democratic and participative forms of leadership (Thompson, Frances, Levacic, & Mitchell, 1993). A system broadly viewed might also consist of plural combinations of organizations: hierarchies (firms) operating within a market, hierarchies operating within hierarchies, and so on. In the Swedish case, one needs to distinguish at least two levels—the national health care system hierarchy, with ministries, national organizations, and unions, and the individual counties. Neither is strictly a command-and-control managerial hierarchy but involves participation and other measures to harmonize interests.

County health services are prevented from becoming a monolithic structure by the numerous public actors, with overlapping responsibilities for policy—at least in practice, if not formally. Though from the point of view of providers, there is a single source of funding—the county budget—it is actually funded from various official sources. This gives each contributor some weight in negotiations and informal talks. With little or no jurisdiction over the counties, a number of national agencies can make their views heard by the counties because they can back up their arguments with some economic clout. Significant actors on the national scene in addition to the ministry include the National Board of Health, the National Board of Insurance, the Council on Technology Assessment in Health Care (SBU), the Federation of County Councils, and the Swedish Medical Association. Each organization can make its independent analysis based on its own sources of information.

In many countries, public health policy is based on a grand compromise between the political authorities and the medical profession. An appropriate term for the Swedish case could be *administrative corporatism* because of its similarity to the kind of consensus-building process between industry and labor that characterizes the corporatist economic system in Scandinavia.

Pressures of the Workplace

Most individual decisions occur within the context set by various collectivities. Though "ethics" and "professional attitudes" have been used by sociologists to explain why other than self-interested behaviors occur, there is little evidence that these concepts explain important elements of professional performance as well as does the organization of the immediate work environment and the pressures of the situation (Freidson, 1988).

The Swedish medical workplace is different in several ways from others. The whole system is biased toward secondary and tertiary care; institutional spending is 25% above the OECD average. Primary care is organized in fairly large centers and equipped with advanced technology and appropriate technical personnel. Solo practice is a rare exception. Thus, the work process for most Swedish health employees takes place within a functional bureaucracy, whereas in many other countries doctors and paramedical personnel are organized in small entrepreneurial groups or network arrangements. This functional organization makes the application of modern industrial managerial technologies and control strategies (such as those associated with managed care in the United States) easy to carry out. Though this kind of organization may deprive professionals of some job control and economic rewards, it offers them interesting opportunities in research and management and alternative rewards in different nonclinical careers.

Whereas professionalism in many countries is basically enacted in individual meetings with patients, in Sweden there is also a strong collective and public aspect. Interpreted in a Durkheimian mode, a kind of organic solidarity based on a *conscience collective* has established moral restraints on individualism. Values strongly embedded in the policies of the health system are equity, equal access, and fair treatment for all. There are few strongly held views about individual rights, either of patients or of professionals. Economic rights of physicians to establish a practice or those associated with freedom of trade are not significant parts of the discussion. The employment structure decides the power balance within the profession and determines the formation and reproduction of the medical elite.

With an advantage not only in status and proximity to medical science but also in numbers (approximately 65%), hospital doctors dominate the professional organizations. They can act to preserve the ideology of the hospital-factory system rather than that of the private practice cottage industry.

A crucial role in establishing treatment protocols, with strong implications for cost containment, is taken by the 60 to 70 national associations for medical specialties. These associations are meeting grounds for doctors in different positions and with various connections to science, practice, and policy. Though their function is easily overlooked because they lack formal status, they play a key role in analyzing and recommending "best practice" even though the final decision about which protocols to adopt remains with each clinic. Furthermore, the pluralist county structure is well suited for benchmarking, yardstick competition, and other similar arrangements; these methods are regularly used by health managers to question high costs.

The establishment of a policy to help clinicians make rational decisions about clinical techniques has been rather noncontroversial in Sweden.

Involvement of doctors in clinical evaluation studies is an important means of socialization, demonstrating and questioning the standards held by professional seniors.[5] Membership on national committees is also an important part of the professional reward system. The power and the status is attractive in itself and indirectly can be financially rewarding. The reason this works so relatively well is probably related to the homogeneity of the medical profession. All doctors are trained in one of a handful of state universities, and the academic community in medicine is small enough for all within a specialty to be at least vaguely acquainted.

Certain aspects of professional autonomy are more circumscribed in Sweden than elsewhere. Some have found the degree of reliance on state patronage to be "staggering" (Keams et al., quoted in Erichsen, 1992), whereas others believe the close relationship between the state and the medical establishment may "constitute the very conditions within which occupational autonomy is possible" (T. Johnson, quoted in Erichsen, 1992). In many ways, how medicine is practiced today still reflects the fact that Sweden was once a rural, poor, and very sparsely populated country, with about a tenth or less of the population density of Germany or England. Few urban centers were able to sustain private medical practices. The profession grew from its base in public health, along with the opportunities that public employment gave to receive private patients on the side.

Commitment and Incentives

A frequently voiced anxiety is that policies based on narrow self-interest will destroy the very ties that make public health service organizations effective. Health policy texts abound with warnings that economic incentives related to personal income will create cross-pressures that will cause suboptimal choices (Dahlgren, 1994). Economic incentives in health systems can clearly be like the spirits in Pandora's box.

When fee-for-service systems have been replaced by either salary or capitation fees, physicians are far more likely to provide good-quality care for the most needy and to accept peer control.[6] When income is stabilized as a fixed salary, professional incentives play a larger role in the way work is performed, and the cooperative behavior essential to effective peer review is facilitated. This is, generally speaking, the accepted view in Sweden. Outside the circle of macroeconomists, there are few proponents of direct productivity-based salaries. Following recent negative experiences with production-based budgets in hospitals, which led to sharp increases both in productivity and in nonessential care (Gustafsson, 1994), all varieties of productivity-based payments have come into disrepute.

One of the problems most often highlighted in health economics concerns the mode of third-party payment. Fee-for-service leaves providers and users of the service with weak incentives to restrict use. On the other hand, prospective methods of payment (e.g., fixed annual budget) provide no incentives for productivity. Within the Swedish system, strong economic incentives have been rarely used. Instead, budgets have been population based, involve capitation, or involve special negotiated contracts that include negotiated standards for production and service levels. Initial experience in counties with fee-for-service or diagnosis-related group (DRG)-based reimbursements found it difficult to reconcile these systems with a tight budget constraint. Therefore, production targets were added, beyond which compensation was reduced. For example, DRG-based payments have been used up to a predefined level of production, and then for extra volumes radical reductions of from 25% to 100% have been imposed (Bergman & Dahlbäck, 1995). Apart from the small niche of private medicine, all conflicting interests affecting profit flows are tightly controlled.

Though Swedish physicians are not likely to be ethically superior to their colleagues in other countries in responding to economic opportunities,[7] they are less often presented with economic temptations. Since 1970, all direct bonuses for personal productivity have been excluded from the public health care field. The 90% of physicians who are in public employment are fully salaried and are no longer allowed to receive private patients in the hospital or to collect fees from patients. Step by step, the (nationally negotiated) employment contract for physicians has become "normalized." Recently, the Swedish Medical Association had to accept that doctors will be subject to scheduling, like other personnel, to make interdisciplinary work teams possible and to adjust working hours to better reflect patient flows.

However, under the new payment systems implemented since 1991, an individual productivity-related salary is set for each person. (Previously, during the 1970s and 1980s, payment moved along scales that reflected little else than position and seniority.) Now a doctor can benefit from good productive work as part of an overall assessment of his or her job performance. These new incentive systems, which vary between counties in specific details, are mostly applied at the organizational level. Efficient clinics are likely to get more resources and prestige than less prolific units and to be less threatened by retrenchment. Economic independence of provider units might also make it possible for a clinic to translate some of its surplus into attractive features, such as research or training and a nonsalary bonus at the year's end. An ineffective clinic will lose control over strategic organizational features, and the people in responsible managerial positions will risk losing their jobs. Incentive systems such as these are found in most counties, not only in those that have used planned-market techniques.

Ensuring Public and Professional Acceptance of Public Policy

No condition for effective cost control is more important than mobilizing the profession's active and positive commitment. Studies of the retrenchment policies of the last decade in Sweden show clearly that the medical profession's participation in planning such policies as well as complying with them is essential for their success (Sarv & Carlsson, 1994). To elicit support, it is essential that the experience of the government's economic management be seen as "legitimate," not only in the common meaning of "lawful" and "proper," but also in the sense of being "true to its role" as this is commonly understood (Habermas, 1976).

The legitimation process is linked to appropriate accountability procedures that make the implementation of health policy responsive to basic norms. Performance in keeping with particular expectations is ascertained through three traditional and two more recently introduced mechanisms: (a) democratic electoral and participatory civil processes, (b) a formal process of legal control, and (c) professional self-regulation. In Sweden, these are all well-established institutions. Though all three remain important, two additions from the market repertory have been recently added: (a) contestability, a weaker form of competition, and (b) patient choice. According to the surveyed views of health care employees, the latter two mechanisms have contributed positively to revitalizing public accountability (Saltman & von Otter, 1995; see also SOU, 1993).

A high standard of public transparency is a prerequisite for a high degree of trust in the system. According to a leading constitutional principle of Swedish government, all official and administrative documents that originate from or enter a public agency must be registered and made accessible to the media and to the public. Only in special cases where confidentiality is felt to be important (as, for example, with patients' files) may documents be withheld. Equally important is that the public discussion not be impaired by restrictions on the right of personnel to speak out. Conflicting interests between the principle of free public access to information and what has been claimed to be business interests have been identified in the new provider organizations (both public and private), but it is significant that complaints so far mostly have been decided in favor of freedom of information and speech. However, difficulties in establishing fair market deals without impairing the traditional openness of the Swedish public sector cannot be dismissed. Indeed, this is one reason that has carried weight in decisions against applying regular market relationships in health services. The one big case of suspected fraud (*Medanalys AB,* recently under police investigation), could not have gone on as long as it did if private ownership had not protected the records held by the company and restricted free speech of its employees.

Reforming Structure and Payment Mechanisms

An illustration of how the theory of the "game" is enacted in specific situations is provided by more recent health policy developments. As noted above, during the 1980s, a set of structural reforms were carried through to solidify financing and budget controls. The later years of this period saw a radically new stage of development, with the introduction of planned-market elements. This experience is relevant both to understand the basic parameters of Swedish policy, as well as the differences in approach taken by various counties (Saltman & von Otter, 1992).

Vertical and Horizontal Integration

In the 1980s, the health sector was rearranged by a few main integrative changes to straighten out some contradictions in finance and management of the services. The different initiatives illustrate how policy implementation is achieved under administrative corporatism. Negotiating mechanisms are often built into the authority structure. No party has full "exchange autonomy," and the shadow of other control mechanisms is always visible. The initiatives were linked to a new Health Policy Act (1982) and led to complete integration of all publicly financed health care under one planning structure within each county and a tight budget constraint.

The first initiative (*Dagmar,* 1983-1985) developed from negotiations between the government and the Federation of County Councils (an organization of great importance but dubious constitutional status). Its objectives were to regulate the relationship between public financing and private care and to simplify complicated financial arrangements through a combination of state grants and county tax-based budgets. The fee-for-service system by which private providers had been compensated (directly by the state) was replaced by population-based global grants from the state directly to the counties. This enabled the counties to assume full control of primary care and to plan and pay for the provision of all public and private primary care services on the basis of a single fixed annual budget. Long-term policy objectives were consolidated within the publicly operated system, turning a soft budget constraint into a much harder one.

Another interface, which had inspired some "cost shifting," was that between counties and municipalities in caring for the elderly. Improvement of coordination of medical and community care for the aged between the 26 counties and the 288 municipalities was necessary because spending for the elderly was growing beyond control: Patients over 75 years accounted for nearly 85% of the total increase in Swedish health care spending while per capita costs were actually falling for other age groups. Demographic changes partly explained this increase—the population was the oldest in the world, with 1 in 10 over 75—but medicalization of old age, shown by the doubling of per capita costs for the elderly over 10 years, was an even larger part of the problem.

Under the supervision of the government, the federations of counties and municipalities sat down to negotiate. A deal materialized in a new act by which all residential home care and care in nursing homes became the responsibility of local government. In all, 70% of long-term care beds were transferred to the communes. The counties were to provide elderly citizens only with primary health and other medically essential care. Economic penalties put pressure on communes to receive elderly patients within 7 days after they were discharged from the hospital. This had immediate results, leaving medical wards with redundant capacity. Today, however, there are ethical concerns that patients may be discharged too quickly by the hospital and that home care has not yet developed enough necessary nursing skills for this new frail group (Socialstyrelsen, 1995b).

A third change was the government's 1992 waiting-list initiative. Though the national government was concerned about queues for certain treatments, it could not enforce its views directly. Therefore, a "voluntary" agreement was worked out with the Federation of County Councils, sweetened by a state grant. A patient was guaranteed surgery within 3 months, or else the county had to pay for treatment elsewhere. This initiative made possible a reduction of 20% in waiting lists in the first 2 years; however, it is not clear that the counties will be able to carry this cost in the future.

A final example is from the area of rehabilitation, in which a new policy aimed to jointly optimize separate health service and social insurance budgets by speeding up clinical examinations and rehabilitation. The general Sickness Benefit Insurance and other national plans had paid up to five times more in benefits during waiting time than for the total cost of medical services. Grants from the insurance funds were made to buy extra rehabilitation services or finance investments by the counties that would remove bottlenecks. Following a Dagmar-type negotiated agreement, a trial program was enlarged to full scale in 1992.

One sector, pharmaceuticals, remains to be included in the integrated budget. Whereas prescriptions to outpatients are paid by the state, inpatient prescriptions are covered by the counties. There is a strong connection between drugs and other treatment options, and it is argued that if all costs were covered out of the county budget, the choice between alternative treatments would be more optimal. A commission is at present studying the question and is likely to suggest that the counties take the full responsibility for all costs, including drugs prescribed to outpatients (except for patient copayments).[8]

All these arrangements typically followed the traditional pattern of *administrative corporatism,* in contrast to some market-inspired initiatives. The latter deviated more clearly from these procedures by trying to establish new norms.

A Future for Planned Markets?

The planned-market changes took place within the county delivery systems themselves. Most striking are the attempts to break up organizational hierarchies and replace them by more networklike structures linked together by formal contracts. In these new arrangements, county or district planning agencies negotiated and monitored service delivery contracts. Given the counties' independence in organizational issues, there are strategically meaningful differences in these arrangements (Saltman & von Otter, 1995).

In 1991, Stockholm County Council was one of the first to embark on a full-scale planned-market experiment. The main feature of this new model, which is still in operation, was the creation of an internal market for hospital services in place of planned and sustained global budgeting. A county medical service committee retains overall responsibility but has withdrawn from all operational responsibility for provider units. Nine local area boards are responsible for purchasing health and medical care for the population in their area and receive a population-based global budget from the committee for this purpose. Prices for hospital treatments are determined by a standard price list, by special agreements, or by a simplified DRG system (Saltman & von Otter, 1992).

Differentiated copayment rates have been introduced to encourage patients to use the health centers as their point of entry into the system. To counter planning rigidity with patient choice, no absolute gatekeeper function has been established, and patients can visit hospitals and other specialists without referrals.

Other county models are slightly different. For example, the central concept of the "Dalamodel," adapted for a rural region, is to distribute prospectively set hospital budgets to local primary health care boards. By creating a service-by-contract relationship between the primary care board and the different delivery units, the expectation was that incentives would emerge for the primary care centers to reduce their rate of hospital referrals and to monitor the necessity for specialist services to patients. Production-based payment systems add pressure on hospital clinics to reduce their operating costs. The responsibility for "health for all" objectives, which are strongly emphasized in the model, rests with district boards. The crucial point is that primary health centers will be encouraged to produce more services themselves by increasing the range of diagnostic and treatment procedures performed at the health centers.

An open referral system makes strict limitation of visits impossible, and the local area boards must pay hospitals for "self-referred" patients who receive treatment outside of contracts. The enforcement of patients' rights to choose physician as well as site is seen not only as an instrument of personal satisfaction, but as a kind of personal validation of the planning process that puts pressure on the delivery system. Patient empowerment by the right of exit and lateral reentry at some other point of the system has become a distinguishing characteristic of recent Swedish health policy, setting it apart from British or American "internal markets."

These changes could be considered as a new "market corporatism" replacing the old "administrative corporatism." Moreover, the family doctor reform—and the way it was introduced by the non-Socialist government elected in 1991—was clearly in violation of the old traditions. A *husläkare* (family doctor) for everyone had been a profile issue of the Liberal Party for 20 years. On the model of continental European examples, citizens of all age groups were allowed a free choice of physician without geographic restrictions. Any properly trained physician was free to set up practice, solo or in a group, and to collect a list of 1,000 to 3,000 people. A patient was allowed to reenlist with another doctor or seek a specialist whenever he or she wanted. The restrictions on opening private practices by specialists were also lifted. The family doctor was—and still is—paid for a basic assignment, according to a mixed system of capitated budget and patient copayments. Capitation from the county covers 70% to 80% of family doctors' remuneration and is differentiated according to patients' ages. From the start, there was considerable concern—for example, on the part of the Federation of County Councils (which has been shown to be well founded)—that the proposal would negate important instruments of health planning and cost control. Significant parts of the scheme have been repealed to reestablish planning control since the fall of the coalition government in 1992.

Outcomes and Problems

These "market-based" reforms were attempts to enhance dynamic efficiency rather than straightforward cost-cutting measures. The most important factor in the ultimate success or failure of these reforms was how well the market features were designed to guide patients to less costly levels of treatment and in the process to force hospital specialists to become more productive and more responsive to health policy priorities (Svalander & Åhgren, 1995).

The outcome of all these changes has been mixed. (For an assessment of evaluation reports, see Anell, 1995.) The new institutional incentives introduced at the different organizational levels have led to positive effects on productivity, and waiting lists have been radically reduced. The National Board of Health has recently judged the reforms to be moderately successful, and it favors a phase of stabilization rather than allowing the reforms to move farther ahead (Socialstyrelsen, 1995a).

- Patient choice and competition have proved efficient in animating the public health care apparatus. Competitive bidding has had stunning effects in lowering prices and making clinics more responsive to patient- (or purchaser-) induced demands.

- Contracting has defined a new relationship between purchasers and providers. The most important implication is the change in roles and context of the discussions between the different agents. Hierarchical relationships, which had prevailed between managers and clinics, have been transformed into more equal relationships.

- The obvious contradictions between the *husläkare* program and other health policy targets have unfortunately become apparent, and this reform has already been remodeled to better match the old guidelines for an integrated delivery system. Counties may now again control the right to private practice, and patients' choice of provider has been somewhat restricted.

- Changes in the structure of the delivery system could, contrary to some expectations, not be left to market forces alone. Major structural decisions, such as which hospitals will remain open, have to be decided by a political process. Market outcomes would be too slow, could lead to adverse political consequences, and might have economically inefficient outcomes.

Doctrinaire beliefs in market processes, paradoxically, led to some unnecessary problems when contracting with the private sector. The ground rules of free trade—that competition and financing should be neutral between all providers—were enforced, to the detriment of the long view of building high-trust, cost-effective relationships between purchasers and providers. Contrary to recommendations based on transactions-cost theory, counties were compelled to base decisions on product price and quality alone, rather than on more "sophisticated" criteria such as the trustworthiness of the bidding firms and other long-term perspectives. A consequence has been several "flops" when hospitals and technical services have been brought into the market. For example, a major project to sell one hospital in Stockholm failed because "serious" contractors were not given the long-term commitments they needed to establish themselves in Sweden. Another private hospital had to be bailed out by the county, and several small private clinics have gone bankrupt.

Following a period of extensive experimentation with a range of market experiments with private as well as public providers, the counties are again trying to tighten budget controls. The main payment mechanism for provider institutions, especially hospitals, is being shifted back from production-based budgets to fixed budgets, sometimes with negotiated contracts for volume of service. Although DRG-based and similar systems clearly had very positive effects on productivity by raising volumes, they weakened overall cost control. Either they have now been abolished or a ceiling on reimbursements has been defined. Some new mechanisms, such as target pricing, have taken center stage. It is the firmness of determination to achieve budget discipline rather than specific techniques that seems most important. "Push" is more important than "pull" in changing firmly established bureaucratic structures.

Though a few years ago it was true that nearly all counties were in the process of developing a contract-based purchaser/provider framework, this trend has now come to a halt. This reflects a set of circumstances, including negative feedback from previous experiments and new (Social Democrat) political majorities. Most important is the continuing necessity to give precedence to financial retrenchment over almost all other priorities, such as productivity, convenience, or even service quality. Experience showed the skeptics to be right on almost all counts about the costly effects of unleashing market opportunities, which involved free entry for specialists, lack of gatekeepers, and opportunistic tendencies in contracting. Two conclusions from this important period in Swedish health care history may be made:

1. Economic accountability cannot be relaxed even a little without serious effects on cost control.
2. Market mechanisms can be usefully inserted into a public system, but only if the possibility of market failure predicaments are treated with due respect.

Conclusion

Sweden has a decent record in health care cost control. Its policy is based on a rational financial and delivery structure with limited opportunities to evade budget control and other ceilings on expenditures. Incentives that might drive provision upward have been used very selectively, and it is quite helpful that almost all health care personnel are salaried.

Most important for the success of cost control policies is the active compliance of the medical profession. This chapter has tried to explain how this has been achieved within a policy framework that is described as "administrative corporatism." The "game" played by Swedish professionals—to use the jargon of "game theory"—is quite different from that in many other countries because of Sweden's unique arrangement of institutions, career systems, and professional organizations. The system, despite its public character and concerted planning, is not as monolithic as might be expected. One reason is the sharp division of responsibilities between politicians, managers, and medical professionals. Another is decentralization of the responsibility for running the system to the 26 counties. A third is the relationship between different agents, often regulated by negotiations rather than command.

The regulated and cooperative orientation of the Swedish health care system makes the physicians identify more with the role of a public servant than do their colleagues in many other countries. Many doctors are also quite uneasy about mixing this role with one that is entrepreneurial and oriented to competition. Experiments with planned-market models have had some interesting but mixed consequences.

Though maximum competition is likely to do more harm than good in a system of health services such as the Swedish, the challenge of competition—or rather its weaker form, "contestability"—has already made a big difference within existing public structures. A contestable market does not require the actual presence of a competitor; rather, the possibility of alternatives has a stimulating effect on a system that for too long took a steady flow of patients and resources for granted. Even though the public providers have had their contracts renewed without serious challenge, a new drive is visible. Patient empowerment through choice has contributed to this new responsiveness on the part of providers.

One can conclude, as well, that the policymakers have accepted having to pay a price in lowered dynamic efficiencies to achieve the policy priorities of quality, equity, and cost control. In implementing difficult health policy decisions, it is not enough to rely on the self-healing wonders of the market. One needs to fully appreciate the extent to which the pursuit of personal decisions are intertwined with noneconomic goals and preferences, deeply embedded in social interactions. The shadows of the future and the past are important in shaping cooperative—or evasive—attitudes.

Notes

1. Over the last 30 years, the number of people above 85 years tripled, and by the year 2000 it will have increased by another 30%.

2. Although total expenditure on health is 14.1% of GDP for the United States and 7.5% for Sweden, the public share represents 83% of total expenditures in Sweden and only 44% in the United States (OECD, 1993).

3. The administrative costs of public systems, as in Britain and Sweden, are estimated at between half and a third of those in the United States (see Rehnberg, 1993, for a review of data).

4. An ideal incentive system would be one in which subordinates found it to their interest to share all information and make all efforts to achieve the organization's goals.

5. Some large national registers are kept (for cancer patients and in orthopedic surgery) that provide unique possibilities—even in an international perspective—for outcomes research.

6. In the United States, this argument was raised by Freidson (1988) in support of HMOs.

7. Perhaps they are even less so for lack of experience and a well established system of business ethics.

8. The latter have already been increased, and a ceiling on patient copayments for all kinds of health expenditures of approximately $250 per year has been established (Andersson et al., 1995).

References

Abel-Smith, B. (1992). Cost containment and new priorities in the European Community. *Milbank Quarterly, 70,* 393-418.

Andersson, D., Gunnarsson, B., & Ljungkvist, M. (1995). *A study of the management of cost and utilization of pharmaceuticals in Sweden.* Stockholm: Apoteksbolaget.

Anell, A. (1995). Implementing planned markets in health systems: The case of Sweden. In R. Saltman & C. von Otter (Eds.), *Implementing planned markets: Balancing social and economic responsibility*. Philadelphia: Open University Press.

Bergman, S., & Dahlbäck, U. (1995). *Att beställa häls- och sjukvård: Erfarenheter från landsting med beställarstyrning*. Stockholm: Landstingsförbundet.

Dahlgren, G. (1994). *Framtidens sjukvårdsmarknader: Vinnare och förlorare*. Stockholm: Natur & Kultur.

Erichsen, V. (1992). *State traditions and medical professionalisation: Scandinavian experiences*. Bergen: Norwegian Research Centre in Organisation and Management.

Freidson, E. (1988). *Profession of medicine: A study of the sociology of applied knowledge*. Chicago: University of Chicago Press.

Gertham, U., & Jonsson, B. (1991). Hur hoga är hals- och sjukvårdsutgifterna: En internationell jamförelse. In Landstingsförbundet (Ed.), *Vagvaall-Appendix*. Stockholm: Landstingsförbundet.

Goldberg, M., Marmor, T., & White, J. (1995). The relation between universal health insurance and cost control. *New England Journal of Medicine, 332*, 742-744.

Gustafsson, R. (1994). *Köp och sälj, var god och svälj: Vårdens nya ekonomistyrningssystem i ett arbetsorganisatsoriskt perspektiv*. Stockholm: Arbetsmiljöfonden.

Habermas, J. (1976). *The legitimation crisis*. Boston: Beacon.

Landstingsförbundet. (1995, April). *Landstingens ekonomi*. Stockholm: Author.

Miller, G. (1992). *Managerial dilemmas: The political economy of hierarchy*. Cambridge, UK: Cambridge University Press.

North, D. (1981). *Structure and change in economic history*. New York: Norton.

North, D. (1990). *Institutions, institutional change, and economic performance*. Cambridge, UK: Cambridge University Press.

Organization for Economic Cooperation and Development. (1993). *Health data file 1993*. Paris: Author.

Parsons, T., & Smelser, N. (1956). *Economy and society*. New York: Free Press.

Rehnberg, C. (1993). Administrationskostnader inom häls- och sjukvården. In Statens Offentliga Utredningar (Ed.), *Häls- och sjukvården i framtiden: Rapport från expertgruppen till HSU 2000* (No. 1993:38). Stockholm: Socialdepartementet.

Saltman, R., & von Otter, C. (1992). *Planned markets and public competition: Strategic reform in northern European health systems*. Philadelphia: Open University Press.

Saltman, R., & von Otter, C. (Eds.). (1995). *Implementing planned markets: Balancing social and economic responsibility*. Philadelphia: Open University Press.

Sarv, H., & Carlsson, J. (1994). *Dalamodellen, en analys av effekterna för personalens trygghet, inflytande och utvecklingsmöjligheter* (No. 19/94). Stockholm: Trygghetsfonden.

Socialstyrelsen. (1995a). *Den planerede marknaden i häls- och sjukvården*. Stockholm: Author.

Socialstyrelsen. (1995b). *Utskriven från akutsjukvården, Ädel-utredn*. Stockholm: Author.

Statens Offentliga Utredningar. (1993). *Häls- och sjukvården i framtiden: Rapport från expertgruppen till HSU 2000* (No. 1993:38). Stockholm: Socialdepartementet.

Statens Offentliga Utredningar. (1995). *Vårdens svåra val, Slutbetänkande av Prioriteringsutredningen* (No. 1995:5). Stockholm: Socialdepartementet.

Svalander, P., & Åhgren, B. (1995). *Vad skall man kalla det som händer i Mora? Och andra frågor om styrmodeller. Rapport till HSU 2000*. Stockholm: Landstingsförbundet.

Thompson, G., Frances, J., Levacic, R., & Mitchell, J. (1993). *Markets, hierarchies, and networks: The coordination of social life*. Newbury Park, CA: Sage.

Vetenskap & Praxis. (1995). *Vad tycker invånarna om sjukvårdssystemet.* Stockholm: SBU.

Westerling, R., et al. (1994). *Åtgärdsbara dödsorsaker: En indikator på häls- och sjukvårdens resultat och kvalitet.* Stockholm: SPRI.

Williamson, O. (1985). *The economic institutions of capitalism: Firms, markets, relational contracting.* New York: Free Press.

PART V

The British Experience

CHAPTER 13

Britain's Health Care Experiment

PATRICIA DAY
RUDOLF KLEIN

B ritain's National Health Service (NHS) is at once the envy of the world and its butt. It is the envy of the world because it provides, with remarkable parsimony, a comprehensive service to the entire population. The service is tax financed and free at the point of delivery, with remarkably low administrative costs. Whereas U.S. expenditure on health care is now touching 12% of its national income, Britain's spending has only just topped half that figure. It is the butt of the world because the NHS provides care that, if usually high in quality, is delivered in an often dreary environment to patients trained to defer to the discipline of the queue and service routines. Since its creation in 1948, the British health system has always been undercapitalized and dominated by providers, who have defined the needs of patients rather than responding to the demands of consumers. Not surprisingly, therefore, the NHS has provided illustrations for countless American sermons on health care during its

EDITORS' NOTE: This chapter was originally published as "The British Health Care Experiment," by Patricia Day and Rudolf Klein, Fall 1991, *Health Affairs, 10*(3), pp. 39-59. Copyright 1991 by *Health Affairs.* Reprinted with permission. The research on which this chapter draws was funded by the Economic and Social Research Council, Grant No. G00 23 2419.

40-year history. It is extolled by those who hold up its achievements as demonstrating the virtues of the national health care model. It is excoriated by those who use its failings to chill American spines about the dangers of socialized medicine.

In the future, however, both of these sermons may need revision. On April 1, 1991, the changes in Britain's NHS first announced by Prime Minister Margaret Thatcher's government at the beginning of 1989 came into full effect. They represent an attempt to demonstrate that it is possible to combine the advantages of the national health service model (financial parsimony and social equity) and those of a market system (responsiveness to consumer demands): to show that the acknowledged weaknesses of the NHS, such as provider paternalism and waiting lists, are not necessarily inherent in its design. It is a remarkably ambitious strategy, even though the government has largely stumbled into adopting it rather than marching purposefully toward some ideological vision. It is also a high-risk strategy. Its outcome is uncertain. Any benefits may take the best part of a decade to work their way through—and will be diffused. The costs of implementation, however, are immediate and largely fall on a concentrated, well-organized constituency: doctors, nurses, and others working in the NHS. Moreover, NHS providers have the power to bring about some of their prophecies of doom by resisting or distorting the implementation of change.

In a service that has a record of periodic confrontation between the government and the health care professions—roughly one such crisis every 3 years since 1948—never before has the debate been so ferocious as in the past 2 years. The medical and the nursing professions, the trade unions representing health care workers, and the Labour Opposition fought the administration's legislation and its implementation step by step. Kenneth Clarke, the secretary of state responsible for the reforms, became the most pilloried politician in the country. The British Medical Association (BMA) plastered the country's advertising billboards with its attacks on him. Nor has the battle ended. Health policy reform will be one of the main issues in Britain's next general election. Yet despite all the professional passion and political furor, the service will remain free at the point of delivery to all who seek it. The NHS will still be tax financed and will provide universal coverage.

What has begun to change already, however, is the management structure and style of the NHS, a process that has accelerated since April 1, 1991. This reform attempt rests on the belief that it is possible to achieve the best of all possible worlds by improving management, removing perverse incentives, and dealing with the organizational rigidities that have afflicted the NHS—which has often been held up as an example of the more general British problems of institutional and economic sclerosis (Klein, 1989). These changes, in turn, present a challenge to the existing managerial and professional order in the NHS. In this chapter, we explain the pressures that drove the government to adopt this ambitious, controversial, and risky strategy of reform. We then describe the program of change and analyze why it has had such a dramatic effect on the politics of health care, though not, as yet, on its delivery. We then discuss the extent to which the policy objectives are likely to be achieved. In doing this, we distinguish sharply between policies for hospital services and those for primary health care.[1]

Pressure for Change

Since its birth in 1948, the NHS has always been perceived as being underfunded, a perception encouraged by those working in it. All governments, Labour as well as Conservative, have sooner or later incurred the charge of starving the NHS of resources. In this respect, the 1980s were no different. What distinguished the decade was that the perception of an NHS tottering on the edge of collapse became so intense and pervasive that it pushed the government into its review of the NHS and the subsequent program of reform. The political price of successful cost containment had become too high. This rising sense of crisis can perhaps best be explained by the interaction between three sets of factors. First, there were the actual budgetary constraints on the NHS, reflecting as much the troubled state of the British economy for much of the decade as the government's ideological commitment to keeping down public expenditure. Second, public expectations were rising, in the shape of greater demands for health care responsive to individual wants rather than professionally defined needs. Last, the government's attempts to satisfy rising demands within constrained budgets led to greater pressure on NHS providers to increase productivity. In turn, the aggrieved providers reacted by denouncing the government's meanness and fanning public discontent, thus establishing a cycle of demoralization.

Budgetary Constraints

The 1980s were a decade of financial austerity for the NHS. Continuing a trend set by the previous Labour government in the late 1970s,

TABLE 13.1 Growth in Public Expenditure on the British National Health Service, England Only, Selected Years, 1980-1991[a]

	1980-81	1982-83	1984-85	1986-87	1988-89	1989-90	1990-91[b]
Hospital Services							
Total spending[c]	£6,999	£8,251	£9,208	£10,421	£12,758	£13,765	£15,099
Cash increase		7.3%	5.7%	7.4%	10.9%	7.9%	9.7%
Inflation rate		6.5%	5.8%	6.9%	10.5%	8.0%	7.4%
Purchasing power		0.8%	–0.1%	0.5%	0.3%	–0.1%	2.1%
Primary Health Care							
Total spending[c]	£2,173	£2,894	£3,421	£3,877	£4,871	£5,240	£5,957
Cash increase		15.6%	10.0%	7.6%	13.3%	7.6%	13.7%
Inflation rate		11.6%	6.9%	5.0%	9.6%	6.5%	5.9%
Purchasing power		3.6%	2.9%	2.5%	3.4%	1.0%	7.3%
NHS Current Total							
Total spending[c]	£9,402	£11,478	£13,050	£14,808	£18,181	£19,657	£21,570
Cash increase		9.4%	7.2%	7.5%	11.2%	8.1%	10.7%
Inflation rate		7.4%	6.0%	6.3%	10.0%	7.3%	6.9%
Purchasing power		1.9%	1.2%	1.2%	1.1%	0.3%	3.6%

SOURCE: National Association of Health Authorities and Trusts (1990, p. 22).
a. Current spending only, excluding capital expenditures.
b. Projected.
c. Millions of pounds.

following a series of economic crises, the Conservatives kept health care spending on a tight rein. Public expenditure on hospital services, which accounts for 70% of the total NHS budget, rose by little more than 7% in real terms over the decade (see Table 13.1). There is much debate about how such figures should be calculated. However, there is no doubt that the rate of growth in public spending on the NHS was lower in the 1980s than in the 1970s. The reduced growth rate came as a shock to the system. It challenged the assumption of NHS providers that they could count on an annual increment in the NHS budget—historically set at 2% per year in real terms—to meet the cost of rising demands on the service and their own higher salaries.

No one disputed that demands were on the increase. Britain's population, like that of the United States, is aging; technological innovation is extending the scope for medical intervention; and unexpected tragedies, such as acquired immunodeficiency syndrome (AIDS), create new calls for extra spending. The issue that emerged during the 1980s was whether such demands required an annual increment of 2% in the budget of the NHS, as previously assumed, or whether growth in services could be financed in other ways. The view taken by the Thatcher government was that service expansion could be financed by increasing the efficiency with which existing resources were used within the NHS. To this end, it introduced a series of changes in the NHS managerial structure. It responded to criticisms about inadequate funding by pointing to improving productivity, switching the debate from inputs to outputs. Indeed, there is no doubt that throughout the 1980s the NHS did improve efficiency, productivity, and outputs. Lengths of stay were cut; costs per acute case fell. The number of patients treated in hospitals rose by more than 20% over the decade, a far higher figure than would have been expected from either spending trends or demographic changes.

Increased Demand for Care

The rise in the provision of services in the 1980s went hand in hand with a mounting perception of inadequacy. The gap between what was available and what was required appeared to be widening. Most obviously, the NHS's notorious waiting lists obstinately refused to decline, despite a series of special government initiatives designed to reduce them. By the end of the decade, almost 1 million people were in the queue—mainly for elective surgery—instead of the usual 700,000 or so. In reality, waiting lists are a poor indicator of resource inadequacy or of anything else (Yates, 1987). They are highly manipulable by providers and a good prop in the theater of discontent. They are inflated by the names of people who have moved, have died, or no longer require treatment. No one has yet found a positive correlation between local resource levels and the length of the local queue. Yet despite all this, they command the newspaper headlines, and their persistence helps to explain the growing dissatisfaction with the NHS (Blendon & Donelan, 1989).[2]

More convincing, if still ambiguous, evidence of frustrated demand is provided by the expansion of the private health care sector.[3] The number of people covered by private insurance rose from 3.5 million at the start of the decade to almost 6 million at the end, roughly 10% of the total population. But such statistics should be interpreted with caution. The private insurance industry is, in a sense, parasitic on the NHS. It can offer what are, by American standards, remarkably cheap policies because it offers coverage for acute rather than chronic conditions (the growth in Britain during the 1980s of the private, long-stay sector is a different story, for it has been fueled not by private insurance but by Social Security finance; Day & Klein, 1987). Medical practitioners in the private sector are NHS consultants who supplement their hospital salaries with private practice, a factor that causes friction and conflicts of interest but that also constrains the sector's growth. Overwhelmingly, if not exclusively, the private acute sector deals with quality-of-life procedures, such as arthroplasties or hernia repairs, while leaving the NHS to cope with life-threatening or chronic conditions. So almost 20% of the former procedures are carried out in the private sector. But even the privately insured population use NHS facilities for over half of their hospital stays.

It is, in short, precisely what should be expected if one assumes that the NHS, given resource constraints, gives priority to life-threatening conditions over intervention designed to enhance the quality of life. In this respect, the 1980s conformed to the pattern set in the earlier decades of the NHS's existence. What appears to have changed is the attitude of a growing section of the population that is less tolerant of queuing. In its near half-century of existence, the NHS has been living off a legacy of deference: a mixture of gratitude and respect for doctors and nurses that legitimized the paternalism of the NHS. By the end of the 1980s, this legacy was wearing thin.

Pressure on Providers

This transformation, though potentially threatening to the medical profession, was in turn accelerated by the attitude of the profession itself. The measures taken by the government in the 1980s to increase NHS productivity were increasingly persuading the medical profession to exploit public discontent. Following the 1983 Griffiths Report (Griffiths, 1983), the managerial structure of the NHS was greatly strengthened. Central government set a series of productivity targets for health authorities. The balance between managerial and professional authority began to shift toward the former. As managerial pressure on the medical profession increased, so did the latter's discontent.

The NHS has always been based on an implicit, unspoken concordat between state and profession. The former set the budgets within which doctors operated. The latter, however, had complete autonomy to decide whom to treat and how, within the limits of those budgets; British doctors traditionally enjoyed far greater freedom from scrutiny than their American counterparts. The new managerial activism threatened this concordat. The medical profession reacted by questioning the budgetary constraints within which it had to work and denouncing the inadequacy of the NHS.

Medical indignation was translated, in turn, into public dissatisfaction with the NHS. The culminating point came late in 1987, when the presidents of the Royal Colleges, representing the prestigious specialists, issued a public statement warning that the NHS was facing ruin. This statement, it is said, so infuriated Thatcher that she announced her review of the NHS to the surprise of even her own ministers and civil servants—a review that, against all precedent, excluded the medical profession. So began the process that was to end in the introduction of the program of change.

A New Set of Incentives

The dilemma in which Thatcher and her advisers found themselves when they started their review of the NHS had one obvious solution: to devise a new method for funding health care in Britain in line with its own ideological commitment to rolling back the frontiers of the state. Urged on by many of its own supporters, the Thatcher government investigated the possibility of moving toward an insurance-based system on the German or French models. But, predictably enough, it rejected this option (Klein, 1985). Moving to an insurance-based system, as the experience of other countries demonstrated, did not absolve governments from responsibility for overall spending levels (a seemingly international obsession). Moreover, such systems did not appear to be as successful as Britain's in terms of change; rising public and professional discontent expressed itself in demands for a better NHS (by which was meant a more generously funded one) rather than for a different health care system.

One option, clearly, was simply to soldier on: to continue with the policies designed to improve productivity by strengthening the management of the NHS. To a large extent, this was precisely what happened. Most of the reforms heralded by the 1989 review document *Working for Patients* (Secretary of State for Health, 1989) were built on the foundations laid earlier in the decade. But there was one crucial new element: the revolutionary notion (in the British context) of splitting responsibility for buying health care from that of actually providing services. Hitherto, these had been combined. District health authorities (DHAs) had been funded for running the services within their own boundaries. If those living in a district sought their health care in neighboring health authorities or in prestigious London teaching hospitals, the resulting transfers of money did not reflect real costs. In short, the system of NHS finance did not provide any incentives to increase productivity because greater activity simply added to costs without bringing in any corresponding revenue. Hence, underused operating theaters and hospitals' deliberately restricting the output of their surgeons caught the public eye.

Since April 1991, the system is radically different. The roles of purchaser and provider are separated. DHAs will be funded according to the size and demographic composition of their populations, not according to the services for which they are responsible. Their function will be to buy the best services they can from a variety of providers. The key principle is that money follows patients. Patients can be treated in the district's own hospitals, in other NHS hospitals, in the private sector, or in NHS hospital trusts, a new category created by the 1989 review that allows hospitals to turn themselves, under certain conditions, into self-governing trusts. This status gives hospitals considerable freedom to determine their own policies and salary scales, as well as to raise capital, provided they attract enough patients to generate sufficient income.

The introduction of this new notion, whose full implications are only gradually becoming apparent, dealt with one of the major criticisms of the earlier managerial reforms, which was advanced by Alain Enthoven in his much-discussed reflections on the NHS published in the mid-1980s (Enthoven, 1985; see also Enthoven, 1991). Enthoven's notion of an NHS "internal market," to allow DHAs to buy and sell services, looks remarkably like the solution adopted by the government 4 years later.

Though there is no doubt that Enthoven was extremely influential in helping to shape the vocabulary of debate and extending the range of possible options, there were indigenous influences as well. Those involved in Thatcher's review often draw attention to the government's reforms of the school system, which preceded those in the NHS by some 2 years, as a model (Lee, 1990). These reforms gave schools the right to opt for self-governing status and largely limited the roles of the local education authorities to providing funds for individual schools. Money followed pupils. However, the education changes went much further in one respect. In the case of schools, the dynamic of change was to be parental choice and competition between schools for pupils—one step short of education vouchers, but following much the same logic.

So although much of the rhetoric of *Working for Patients* was about making the NHS "more responsive to the needs of the patient," the reality in the case of hospital services stopped well short of allowing consumer demand to drive the service. Managers will continue to define the needs of patients, explicitly so in the case of the DHAs, which are charged with determining the needs of their populations when drawing up their purchasing plans. Managers also will have greater responsibilities (and powers) for calling the medical profession to account for their use of public resources. Medical audit is to become compulsory. Future consultant contracts will specify in far greater detail what is expected from the jobholder. Distinction awards to consultants, which may double their salaries and greatly enhance their pension entitlements, will in the future no longer be based on clinical excellence alone. Managers will have a voice in making the awards, taking into account the contribution of candidates to the work of the NHS.

This challenge to the autonomy of the medical profession, as much as its manner of production, helps to explain the violent reaction to *Working for Patients*. Not only had the profession been excluded from Thatcher's review—the prime minister chose those she consulted precisely because they were not representative of the profession—but the results of the review appeared to present a direct threat to it. It was no wonder, then, that the medical profession fought the implementation of government's proposals, prophesying that they would create chaos and confusion.

Reforming the Primary Health Care System

In explanations of Britain's ability to deliver a frugal, comprehensive, universal, and reasonably high-quality service, it is customary to stress the system of central financial control. But an important contributory factor in making this achievement possible is Britain's system of primary health care. Every member of the population is registered with a general practitioner (GP) and, on average, makes about four visits a year. The GP is the gatekeeper to the expensive hospital sector and the patient's agent in the choice of route into the complexities of specialist care. In all, there are some 27,000 GPs in England (compared to 45,000 hospital doctors) with an average list size of just over 1,900 patients. The GP is the "family doctor" who, certainly in theory and quite often in practice, provides continuity of care, treats minor and chronic illness, and takes up where high-technology hospital intervention leaves off. Primary health care is a remarkably cheap service. Total expenditure on primary health care represents less than a third of the total NHS budget (Table 13.1). And of this, only 30% is paid directly to GPs and their staffs. A further 46% is spent on pharmaceuticals prescribed by GPs (three quarters of prescriptions are free; there is a flat rate charge for the rest), and the remainder pays for the dental and ophthalmic services.

Nevertheless, the Thatcher government's interest in reforming primary health care predates its program of change in the expensive hospital sector. It published its first set of proposals for change in 1986—that is, well before political and professional agitation persuaded the prime minister to set up her review of the NHS as a whole (Secretary of State for Social Services, 1986). A number of concerns drove the engine of change. First, the Department of Health wanted to harness the activities of general practice more effectively to its own policy objectives, which in the 1980s were increasingly preoccupied with prevention. Second, the British Treasury was putting increasing pressure on the department to stop up one of the few holes in the NHS budget: primary health care spending, which, particularly on prescribing, is demand driven and thus difficult to control. This, of course, is why, as Table 13.1 shows, expenditures have been rising at a much faster rate than in the hospital sector. Third, within the profession itself, and especially in the Royal College of General Practitioners, powerful voices were arguing for action to improve the quality of general practice, with particular anxiety about the inadequacy of many practices in inner cities.

Last, as in the case of hospital consultants, there was a feeling that GPs should be made accountable for their use of public resources. British GPs are independent contractors with the state. They achieved this status in 1911 and have defended it fiercely ever since, with the result that they gained virtual immunity from scrutiny of their activities. However, by the 1980s, ministers (and others) were getting increasingly restive about the variations in GP practices and the implications for expensive hospital services and NHS budgets. At times, there were 20-to-1 variations in the hospital referrals made by GPs, without any obvious explanations.

These concerns largely shaped the government's first set of proposals. These were designed to provide incentives to improve quality and to introduce a tighter system of accountability, thereby giving a larger and more active role to managers. The proposals also introduced a new policy theme, reflecting the Thatcher government's bias toward consumerism and the market principle. Although the system of remuneration introduced in 1948 maintained the principle of capitation payment first introduced in 1911, at the birth of national health insurance, this principle was subsequently eroded by a variety of salary elements—for example, allowances to encourage GPs to settle in underdoctored parts of the country. By the mid-1980s, therefore, only 46% of GP income was derived from capitation. The Thatcher government decided that this trend should be reversed. With list sizes falling, the danger was no longer that GPs would accumulate excessive numbers of patients but that they would be indifferent or unresponsive to consumer demands. Hence, they should derive a higher proportion of their income, say 60%, from capitation fees to give them an incentive to compete for patients.

There followed a stately pavane of consultation with the BMA and others. Though persisting with its strategy, the government made some concessions. Yielding to the profession's objections to merit awards for GPs deemed to be practicing high-quality medicine, the government put forward another battery of incentives: payments dependent on the achievement of specific targets for immunization and vaccination rates. However, the stately pavane turned into a frenzied dance with the publication of the government's 1989 review. If the prospects of achieving an agreement between government and profession had always been uncertain, now they were extinguished. The knives were out.

The profession viewed two new proposals for change that emerged from the review as particularly threatening. First, the review brought in the notion of "indicative drug budgets" for individual GP practices—that is, a budget ceiling for prescribing costs. Although ministers stressed that reasonable overshoots would be allowed—that the budgets were indicative, and no more—the medical profession, not without reason, saw this as a victory for the Treasury and a move toward capping their prescribing budgets. Second, the review introduced the idea of GP practice budgets: practices with more than 11,000 patients (subsequently reduced to 9,000) could opt for a budget, out of which they would buy a range of diagnostic and hospital services for their patients (in effect, becoming miniature health maintenance organizations). This move was denounced by the profession, echoed by the Labour Opposition, as being designed to encourage GPs to pinch pennies rather than to pursue the best interests of their patients. This denunciation appeared to assume either that GPs had previously been indifferent to financial considerations (singularly unconvincing, given their toughness in pay negotiations) or that they were overly susceptible to corruption (an unflattering conclusion).

There followed further negotiations between the Department of Health and the medical profession. A package acceptable to the profession's leadership was worked out; however, it was promptly repudiated by the representatives of rank-and-file GPs. Finally, Secretary of State for Health Kenneth Clarke—who throughout enraged the profession with his combative manner and his lack of deference to them—imposed a new contract on the profession, for the first time in the history of the NHS. As it turned out, in its billboard advertising campaign, the profession had simply advertised its own impotence: its failure to block, or even significantly dent, government policies. When it came to the point, Britain's GPs had no stomach for a fight; the threat of withdrawing from the NHS was an empty one, given their dependence on income from the state.

The new contract symbolized the changed status of GPs: accountable, at last, for what they did and with explicit obligations to carry out certain contractual tasks (General Medical Services Committee, 1985). Under the previous contract, GPs had defined their own obligations. If family health services authorities, the managerial bodies responsible for primary health care, choose to do so, they can henceforth monitor the implementation of the GP contract as never before, as they can monitor referral and prescription patterns.

Implementation: The Short-Term Impact

The new-style NHS is very much the product of the Thatcher era. Nevertheless, there is no reason to expect any change of policy, as distinct from style, in the post-Thatcher years while a Conservative government remains in power. With the legislation pushed through successfully and the new machinery put into place, the government's tone has become more conciliatory—a process that was apparent even before the change of cast. But John Major's government is firmly committed to the reforms. If there remains much uncertainty about the impact of the changes, it is because the new NHS is, in a very real sense, an experiment whose outcome cannot be predicted with confidence.

Hospital Services

Consider first the case of the hospital services. The timetable of change allowed little more than 2 years between the announcement of the program of reforms and getting new machinery running. Little preparatory work had been done, and at times the civil servants at the Department of Health appeared to be inventing the machinery on the hoof. Yet it is difficult to exaggerate the complexity and demanding nature of the managerial task involved. The notion of splitting the purchaser and provider roles not only meant developing a new grammar and language of management. It also meant creating a database capable of generating the information needed to operate the new system. Traditionally, the NHS has been information-poor, if awash with statistics. But if doctors were to be held more accountable, it was necessary to know more precisely what they did. If the money was to follow patients, it was essential to know how much services cost. Thus, a massive investment was needed to develop the NHS's primitive information system, an investment that produced large dividends for management consultancy firms and others with relevant experience, often imported from the United States.

Given the exacting, expensive, and exhausting managerial transformation involved, it is not surprising that the government was widely criticized for its hurried root-and-branch approach to reform. Those hostile to the principles shaping the changes denounced the government for imposing an untried set of ideas on the country without testing them first. Even among those sympathetic to the reform package, many argued it would have been wiser to start with some demonstrations to eliminate bugs and to show doubters that the system could be made to work (Smith, 1989).

It is not quite clear whether such a step-by-step strategy would have been feasible. Social experiments seldom settle political arguments, as U.S. experience shows all too clearly. Furthermore, demonstration projects tend by definition to be atypical. But, in any case, the argument for a more cautious strategy has been largely made redundant by events. True, the new system was in place nationally as of April 1, 1991, but it is already clear that change is being implemented incrementally—that both purchasers and providers are exploring their new roles tentatively and interpreting them variously and that there is, in effect, a series of experiments, reflecting local circumstances and understanding of what should be done.

The point can best be illustrated by looking in more detail at how the principle of separating the roles of purchasers and providers is being interpreted in practice. This principle represents the key element in the new NHS. Moreover, it has also encouraged the myth that Britain has adopted the U.S. model of competition in the health care market. In the outcome, there is not going to be much competition or much of a market. British purchasers (i.e., the DHAs) are mostly going to stick to the hospitals in their own or neighboring districts that have traditionally produced services for their populations. Most of the purchaser/provider service agreements are block contracts designed to ensure continuity in the provision of health care.[4] To quote one of Britain's most sophisticated management teams:

An examination of purchaser/provider relationships in industry and commerce suggests that the most successful companies are those which work closely with supplier partners. . . . A partnership framework for developing service agreements is particularly suited to the Oxfordshire District. This is because, if the DHA is to maintain convenient access for local residents to good quality services, an Oxfordshire provider will often be the only reasonable choice. The rationale for developing explicit service agreements within such a framework is therefore to enhance accountability, *not to encourage competition*. (Oxfordshire Health Authority, 1990, emphasis added)

The story, and the strategies, may be rather different in districts with a large export and import business and where there is an imbalance between their income (calculated on the basis of the size and composition of their populations) and the facilities within their boundaries. In such cases, competing for customers and contracts may be a condition of financial survival. However, such authorities are a minority and largely concentrated in London. In this, as in so many other respects, the situation in London—with its concentration of teaching hospitals that draw in customers from a wide catchment area—tends to be atypical of the rest of the country. It does, however, attract a disproportionate share of the comment about the NHS because of the propinquity of the media. Too often, the NHS is viewed through the distorting mirror of London, which turns even minor hiccups into headline-catching crises.

If the move toward competition is going to be, at most, incremental and marginal, much the same is true of the transformation of NHS hospitals into self-governing trusts. Such trusts, be it remembered, still remain NHS property, with more freedom to run themselves and to raise their own capital for development. They are also revocable (NHS Management Executive, 1990b). Equally, this status is optional: No hospital has been compelled to change its status, although the government has employed both cajolery and bribery to make sure that this model is up and running. Nevertheless, few proposals in the government's reform package have encountered more opposition. Self-governing status has frequently been denounced as privatization by another name. The freedom of trusts to negotiate their own terms of service for their employees, instead of being bound by national agreements, has been seen as a threat by professional as well as trade union bodies. Right to the end, the process of setting up trusts was accompanied by demonstrations and opposition, often orchestrated by the Labour Party. Surprisingly, for those who thought that such trusts could turn out to be worker cooperatives dominated by consultants, the medical profession has been split. As often as not, consultants have voted against opting to set up trusts when managers have tried to set them up.[5] Only 56 of the 1,700 hospitals in England achieved self-governing status in the first wave, although that number will probably triple in April 1992, when the second wave is due. There is therefore every opportunity for testing out the model before it becomes generalized.

Rather than a sudden plunge into a competitive health care system, the NHS's "internal market" for hospital care will be a special kind of market, with managers trading with each other and with the consumer conspicuous by his or her absence. Moreover, the trading may have more to do with the reliability, accessibility, and timeliness of services provided than with the price. Managers will be seeking, not the cheapest form of intervention for individual patients, but the service package that appears to offer best value and the services required by their population.

Thus, it is not competition that is going to distinguish the new-style NHS. Rather, it is the move from the notion of trust to one of contract. For its first 40 years, the NHS left explicit treatment decisions to clinicians. Now, however, contracts will spell out what was previously left implicit. The crux of the purchaser/provider relationship is precisely that, for the first time ever, the nature of the services to be provided in the NHS will have to be defined in the contracts or service agreements made. In the context of the NHS culture, this move from the implicit to the explicit, from trust to contract, is truly revolutionary and has perhaps the farthest-reaching long-term implications.

General Practitioners

What goes for hospital providers also applies to GPs. The first impact of changes in the NHS may, paradoxically and perversely, blunt the incentives to compete and limit consumer choice. Most immediately, and perhaps most importantly, the change has been a financial bonanza for many (perhaps most) GPs who were already vaccinating, immunizing, and screening most of their patients before the contract introduced bonus payments for meeting specific targets. Similarly, GPs who practice in inner cities—and thus qualify for the special "deprivation payments" introduced by the new contract—get extra compensation for the difficulties involved in reaching these targets when dealing with a mobile population. Add to this the surge in spending on subsidies to GPs for employing practice staff, 70% of whose salaries are met out of the public purse up to a limit of two per practitioner, and it is clear that they have emerged from their battle with the government a great deal richer, if not happier.

This conclusion needs to be qualified in one respect. Financially, the new deal is an exercise in redistribution of income among GPs, sweetened by what the government hopes will be a once-and-for-all injection of extra funds. The new system of pay is designed to steer money toward those GPs who practice the best medicine, largely defined in terms of their preventive activities and their capacity to organize their practices to achieve the various targets. Conversely, GPs who practice old-style reactive medicine and, often because they practice solo, lack adequate information systems will lose out, although the government conceded a system of transitional payments to ease the pain. It is too early to draw up a balance sheet of gainers and losers; first indications, however, are that only a small minority of GPs will suffer a loss of income. There will also be some opportunities for entrepreneurial GPs to add to their incomes by engaging in fee-for-service activities made possible by the new contract, notably minor surgery and health promotion clinics. But here the profession has a collective incentive to discourage excessive exuberance. The income of GPs is determined by an independent tribunal, which sets the average net remuneration for the coming year.[6] Multiplied by the number of GPs, this then determines the profession's collective income. If this is exceeded as a result of hyperactivity by some physicians, the excess will be deducted from the following year's settlement. This inhibition does not apply to GPs who boost their incomes by increasing the number of patients on their lists because one GP's gain is another's loss.

Overall, however, it is clear that most GPs will have no pressing reason to engage in competition for patients. Similarly, it is likely that the most contentious component in the government's package—the introduction of budget holding for GPs—will also dampen competition. Specifically, budget holding permits GPs to shop around, on behalf of their patients, for the kind of diagnostic and elective procedures that are the core of the waiting-list issue. At the same time, it gives them an incentive to deal with patients' problems themselves instead of passing them onto the hospital service. Budget-holding GPs thus will be forced to examine the financial implications of their clinical decisions. This caused the BMA, as well as the Labour Party, to pronounce anathema on the whole concept. The judgment of GPs, it was argued, would become corrupted. Instead of thinking only about the patient, they would be worrying about their bottom line. They would exclude expensive patients from their lists.

If developments since 1989 have not stilled the objections of principle to budget holding, they have demonstrated the feasibility of what at first seemed a rather crackpot notion. A surprising number of GPs have voted with their feet against the BMA line; the BMA has been forced to moderate its root-and-branch excommunication for fear of splitting its membership. Some 300 practices became budget holders in April 1991— roughly 10% of those eligible—and this number is likely to double in April 1992. In part, this reflects the generous handouts for the pioneers, particularly for the installation of information systems. In part, however, it reflects a realization among GPs that budget holding gives them power.

Instead of being dependent on the good will of hospital consultants, the situation may be reversed: Consultants may actually come to see them as valuable customers and woo them accordingly. In addition, budget holding has come to be seen as the cure for the occupational disease of British GPs: boredom. Instead of being preoccupied with dealing with chronic complaints, they face a new, acute challenge. This helps to explain, perhaps, the enthusiasm and skill that has been brought to developing the information systems required to make budget holding work. But the converse of this enthusiasm is that budget holding gives GPs an incentive to build up larger practices and even to form buyer cooperatives with other local practices, limiting competition and choice.

Whether intended or not, budget holding is therefore an experiment; only the experience of the first 300 practices, over time, can yield any kind of evaluation. But two tentative conclusions can already be drawn. The first is that the sheer crudity of the process of determining the level of budgets provides safeguards against predicted dangers. The budgets have mostly been negotiated on the basis of the previous activities of the practices concerned; hence the very considerable variations in the allocations, on a per capita basis, between them. This is precisely the same strategy as that adopted in the case of determining funding for prescribing. But the fact that the budgets are settled by negotiation rather than by formula does offer protection against abuse. If GPs engage in adverse selection, for example, they will be penalized accordingly in the determination of their budgets. Account can also be taken of patients with special needs. Also, it has become clear that GPs will have only weak financial incentives to skimp on patient care. Any "profits" must be plowed back into practice improvements; they cannot be taken out in cash. So although underspending may improve the practice's long-term financial prospects by funding investment, it gives no immediate yield and could, if too blatant, lead to a downward revision of the budget.

The other shift in powers made transparent by the process implementing the reforms is that from the medical profession to the managers of primary health care. The managers are the midwives of innovation. They determine GP budgets, prescribing ceilings, and the allocation of funding for the practice staff. Similarly, managers will monitor the way in which the new system works, particularly if budgetary limits are overshot. At every stage, therefore, managers will have an opportunity to mold general practice and to call GPs to account for their use of public resources. The emphasis in all of this is on persuasion and dialogue; the rhetoric is very much about the enabling role of management, rather than about its powers. But here again there must be uncertainty about how the new system will develop over time, and in particular about the danger that the new regulatory machinery will be captured by the medical profession.

Future Indefinite

What will Britain's health care system look like by the end of the 1990s? No confident answer can be given to that question, given that the NHS operates in a turbulent and uncertain economic and political environment. If Britain's economy prospers, so will the NHS budget. Conversely, if the economy remains sluggish, health care will continue to be on short commons. In this respect, the Conservative changes have done nothing to diminish the service's financial vulnerability to political decisions taken in the light of the government's overall policies of economic management. Similarly, if the Labour Party were to be returned to office at the next general election, due by mid-1992, change would go into reverse gear. Labour has committed itself to both increasing expenditure on the NHS and dismantling most of the Conservative reforms, although its willingness and ability to carry out these pledges would of course depend on its economic inheritance and the timing of the election (Labour Party, 1990). If this were later rather than sooner, a Labour government might well plead the problems of disruption and confine itself to some resonant symbolic changes. Abolition of hospital trusts, which inspire much emotion but are marginal to the principle of the internal market, is one such gesture. Whether Labour would also honor its commitment to end GP budget holding might, however, depend on how this worked out in practice and whether a constituency had been created for its survival. However, the purchaser/provider split looks set to survive any change of government.

Assuming, however, that Major's government wins the next general election, what then? Even if April 1, 1991, has not marked an immediate transformation of the NHS as experienced by its consumers, what will happen as the changes work their way through the system? Regarding costs, it is clear that spending on administration in the NHS—hitherto an extraordinarily parsimonious system—has risen and will continue to do so. Apart from the investment in information technology, probably justified in terms of improving services for patients, there will be the extra costs of billing under the contract system. Using American technology will, in this respect, lead to an American-style cost problem, if stopping far short of it. More intangibly, the move toward demanding greater accountability from the medical profession could backfire if it leads to sullen resentment. Although the NHS may have relied excessively in the past on the relationship of trust between doctors and managers, this still remains one of its greatest assets. It has ensured a degree of medical commitment to the NHS that goes far beyond anything that could be guaranteed by the letter of a contract; most hospital consultants, for example, put in more hours than required by their contracts (Wilkins, 1990). Much will therefore depend on whether ministers and managers succeed in their efforts to smooth down the ragged tempers of the medical profession and to restore good will.

The move toward explicit contracts is, nevertheless, responsible for some of the most immediate benefits that are emerging. It has forced into the open issues that have remained undiscussed for 40 years. Thus, there has been an upsurge of interest in how to specify quality and how to ensure its delivery. Similarly, there has been a newfound zeal for devising standards for patient treatment. This, indeed, is a transformation, even if it will take some time before the effects trickle down to the patients. Again, the emphasis on prevention and health promotion in GP contracts marks a radical shift in public policy, although some of the enthusiasm for regular checkups and screening may be a touch promiscuous. It is not quite clear that it will have the hoped-for effect on health outcomes. In all of these (and other) respects, the NHS has become more self-critical and self-aware. Nothing will ever be quite the same, therefore, even if the program of reform is put into reverse or on hold.

So far, then, the balance sheet seems to come out in favor of the reforms, despite the burdens imposed on managers struggling to implement an extraordinarily complex task against a ferocious timetable. But there remains the question of whether the new-style NHS—whatever improvements it may bring—will actually meet the aspirations of its creators: whether, to return to the argument we began with, it will combine the advantages of the national health service model (financial parsimony and social equity) with those of a market system (responsiveness to consumer demands). Here the verdict must be an open one. For what is most significant about the new-style NHS—and the point most frequently neglected in discussions about it—is that it actually incorporates two different models. Whereas the hospital model is management and provider led, the primary health care model is much more consumer led. Even if competition is going to be mainly conspicuous by its absence in both models except at the margins, the nature of the markets will be very different. In the hospital model, purchasers are proxy consumers, whereas in the primary health care model, GPs are proxy consumers.

The two models are incompatible in at least one crucial respect. The responsibility of purchasing authorities is to determine the health care needs of their populations and to buy services accordingly. This is very much in the paternalistic tradition of the NHS; equity has always been defined in terms of experts identifying needs and allocating resources accordingly. In this sense, the hospital model represents the apotheosis of the health expert. In practice, of course, things will be much less tidy; health authorities will also have to provide quick fixes in response to political or consumer pressures. But, quite clearly, the model is at odds with the demand-led primary health care model. For if responsibility for buying services is to be diffused among GPs, not in accordance with some ideal population-based strategy but in response to the needs (and pressures) of patients as interpreted by individual practitioners, then population-based health care planning is in tatters. To the extent that the achievement of equity does indeed depend on sticking to a needs-based model, then clearly it cannot be combined with a market based on a plurality of buyers. Conversely, to the extent that responsiveness to consumer demands depends on a plurality of buyers, it cannot be combined with equity based on giving a purchasing-power monopoly to expertise. So which model will win out?

Clearly, the big battalions are on the side of the monopoly purchaser, hospital model. Hospital consultants have been remarkably slow to realize the way that GP budgets could tilt the balance of power toward primary health care. But together with the equally threatened hospital managers, they form a potentially powerful coalition. They might therefore be expected to seek to abort the GP budget-holding experiment by a mixture of outright opposition and preemptive change, by demonstrating their willingness to adapt their practices to GP demands. Such strategy could well succeed, particularly if the first wave of GP budget holders produces a crop of financial fiascos or much-publicized inequities in the treatment of patients—a perfectly conceivable outcome, given that some failures are inevitable in any experiment. Moreover, GPs who are unwilling or unable to become budget holders might well applaud the collapse of the experiment—as would the BMA—for they are in the position of small shopkeepers threatened by the rise of the supermarket.

Another consideration is pulling in the opposite direction—one at the heart of the debate that prompted the Thatcher government's plunge into reform in the first place. This is the question of which model is most likely to ensure financial control. Here, on the face of it, the hospital model is a clear winner. Once a purchaser has decided what services to buy, within the constraints of the existing budget, expenditure is eminently controllable. In contrast, the primary health care model—as yet untested, in any case—diffuses spending decisions among GPs with no experience of budgetary control or tradition of public accountability. So, in terms of financial control, there would appear to be no contest. However, the balance of argument changes when we turn to political considerations. Here the strength of the hospital model turns out to be its weakness, whereas the converse is true of the primary health care model. In the past, resource allocation decisions in the NHS have been largely implicit—part of the concordat between state and profession, which has left the individual doctor to ration at the point of delivery. The new system, however, forces purchasers to be more explicit about what services will be provided for their populations. The purchasing authorities will have to give visibility to decisions about what to buy and, more important, what not to buy. Although the concentration of financial power and decision making reinforces control, it also increases the risk of political embarrassment. Without intending to do so, the government may have created a system that will add to the pressures for more public expenditure on the NHS. Significantly, the public spending plans for fiscal year 1991-92 envisage a larger rise, in real terms, in the NHS budget than at any time in the 1980s. Conversely, although the primary health care model is weaker on financial control, it diffuses the decision-making process. It makes the consequences of resource constraints much less visible and, in this respect, would mark a return to the traditional British approach of making rationing largely invisible by leaving it to individual physicians and disguising it as clinical decisions.

So, in effect, two quite different futures for the NHS are on offer, apart from the possibility of muddling through with an unresolved conflict at the heart of health care policy. One would represent a reversion to tradition, modified at the edges; the other would mean a more radical break with the past. The present mix, however, is likely to prove unstable. The way in which future governments jump will depend on a variety of factors: the outcome of the present experiments, political ideology and expediency, economic prospects, and the attitude of the medical profession. Only one prediction seems reasonably safe: that Britain's health care system will continue to change before it reaches a stable state. In the meantime, it will continue to send out confused and conflicting messages to those who want to use it as a text for sermons.

Notes

1. Throughout, we refer to "hospital services" where, strictly speaking, we should be referring to hospital and community services: that is, to the outreach programs, such as

community nursing, which conventionally are grouped under the hospital heading, particularly in public expenditure statistics.

2. Note that British public opinion is not independent of the medical profession's attitudes but largely shaped by them.

3. *Laing's Review of Private Health Care 1989/90;* this is the most comprehensive, up-to-date source of information about private health care.

4. NHS Management Executive (1990a) provides some illuminating specimen contracts.

5. The splits have been gleefully reported by the *British Medical Journal;* see, for example, the reports in the issues of May 5 and June 16, 1990 (pages 1158 and 1539, respectively).

6. This is the Review Body on Doctors' and Dentists' Remuneration. Although its recommendations are not invariably accepted by governments, over time it effectively determines medical pay.

References

Blendon, R., & Donelan, K. (1989). British public opinion on National Health Service reform. *Health Affairs, 8*(4), 52-63.

Day, P., & Klein, R. (1987, March). Residential care for the elderly: A billion-pound experiment in policy making. *Public Money,* pp. 19-24.

Enthoven, A. (1985). *Reflections on the management of the National Health Service.* London: Nuffield Provincial Hospitals Trust.

Enthoven, A. (1991). Internal market reform of the British Health Service. *Health Affairs, 10,* 660-670.

General Medical Services Committee. (1989). *NHS regulations.* London: British Medical Association.

Griffiths, R. (1983). *NHS management inquiry: Report.* London: Department of Health and Social Security.

Klein, R. (1985, Spring). Why Britain's Conservatives support a socialist health care system. *Health Affairs, 4,* 41-59.

Klein, R. (1989). *The politics of the NHS* (2nd ed.). London: Longman.

Labour Party. (1990). *A fresh start to health.* London: Author.

Laing's Review of Private Health Care 1989-90. (1990). London: Laing & Buisson.

Lee, T. (1990). *Carving out the cash for schools* (Bath Social Policy Paper No. 17). Bath, UK: Centre for the Analysis of Social Policy.

National Association of Health Authorities and Trusts. (1990). *Health care economic review, 1990.* Birmingham, UK: Author.

National Health Service Management Executive. (1990a). *Contracts for health services: Operating contracts.* London: HMSO.

National Health Service Management Executive. (1990b). *NHS trusts: A working guide.* London: HMSO.

Oxfordshire Health Authority. (1990). *The Oxfordshire approach to developing service agreements.* Oxford, UK: Author.

Secretary of State for Health. (1989). *Working for patients.* London: HMSO, Command No. 555.

Secretary of State for Social Services. (1986). *Primary health care: An agenda for discussion.* London: HMSO, Command No. 9771.

Smith, R. (1989). Word from the Source: An Interview with Alain Enthoven. *British Medical Journal, 298,* 1166-1168.

Wilkins, G. (1990). Survey of the work and responsibilities of consultants in the NHS: 1989. In G. Wilkins (Chair), *Review Body on Doctors' and Dentists' Remuneration, 20th Report.* London: HMSO, Command No. 937.

Yates, J. (1987). *Why are we waiting?* Oxford, UK: Oxford University Press.

•

CHAPTER 14

The Reforms of the British National Health Service

JOHN APPLEBY

The British National Health Service (NHS), nearly 7 years after major structural and economic reform, and hovering on its 50th birthday, is having a turbulent middle age. The complex and interacting pressures of politics, changes in medical technology and demography, the public's expanding expectations, the uncertainty within the NHS about future direction (despite, or perhaps because of, the recent change in government), and low morale among health care professionals suggest a service that is in some difficulty. Moreover, inequalities in health status persist across income and socioeconomic groups.

And yet the NHS remains the most popular of state institutions (easily beating the monarchy—especially of late). An affection for the commitment of nurses—"angels"—and a somewhat awestruck appreciation of the medical magic of clinicians are no doubt significant factors contributing to such popularity, however. Every year, the NHS appears to treat more patients, supply more drugs, and make further inroads into waiting times for treatment. And, *pace* Bunker, Frazier, and Mosteller's (1994) quantification of the contribution of health care to health, trends in the main causes of death continue to fall. Public financing—although perhaps low by international standards—has at least been maintained: The NHS share of national public spending has held fairly steady at around 15% of the total, and currently, the NHS consumes over £40,000 million out of total public spending of £274,000 million. The NHS is also a major employer in all areas of Britain; in many towns it is in the top five, with its employees providing a signif:cant financial input to local economies.

Such contradictions are not necessarily new to the NHS. For many, the NHS has always been seen as an embodiment or upholder of "good things"—fairness, care, the right to a healthy life—and motivated by things other than money. On the other hand, it has also suffered from a degree of criticism about its waiting lists, the shabbiness of its hospital waiting areas, and its paternalism. Moreover, given the chance to rectify the widespread feeling that the NHS was underfunded, over the last decade and a half the public invariably voted into office administrations committed to cutting taxes.

Structural and organizational reform has also been an almost constant item on the agenda of the NHS since its inception. New tiers of management have come and gone, hospitals have been reorganized, and new forms of management have been introduced. However, although the changes introduced in 1991, in particular the creation of an internal market, can be viewed as just the latest reorganizational fad, their origins and the depth and breadth of the change they embody suggest that unlike previous reorganizations they have set the NHS on a significantly new course. Moreover, health care reform in Britain has been paralleled and to some extent mirrored in many other countries. Although approached from different starting points and arising from different policy concerns, health care reform around the world appears to be creating a new conventional wisdom about how countries address fundamental issues common to all health care services such as scarcity, choice and prioritization, value for money, and the role of incentives. At the risk of overgeneralization, international trends in health care reform over the last 5 to 10 years have explored the potential of managed or regulated markets: For centralized or integrated systems such as Britain's, this has meant the creation of limited and tightly regulated supply-side competition within an overarching framework of state control. For other countries, such as the Netherlands, the competitive pressure has been introduced on the demand side.

This chapter examines the rise and progress of market-based reforms in Britain. It outlines the origins of the reforms of the NHS, reviews evidence of their impact on the service, and, on the basis of current and emerging trends—in particular, the election of a new government—tentatively speculates about the next 5 years.

The Origins of Reform

The NHS—almost alone among the big state organizations—escaped the 1980s Thatcherite zeal for rolling back the frontiers of the state through privatization. This was perhaps a tribute to its perceived uniqueness in the public's mind. While many rushed to buy shares in privatized industries and firms such as gas, telecommunications, electricity, British Airways, and water, it would have taken a politician terminally out of touch with public feeling to try and devise a share issue for the NHS. Nonetheless, the NHS was not immune from a governmental desire to introduce market-based disciplines and incentives to encourage efficiency.

However, the NHS, unlike other health care systems around the world, was not suffering from problems such as soaring costs (in the opinion of many, quite the opposite) or, to any significant degree, problems of coverage or access. And save for annual rows about (admittedly only a handful) of delayed operations due (in part) to shortages of funds, neither was there any vociferous public clamor for a shake-up of the NHS. Although there was no doubt that there was room for improvement, the NHS was certainly not bust and in need of fixing. In the absence of some terminal disease requiring radical surgery, what were the origins of the reforms of the NHS? Perhaps the best way to understand the changes is in terms of the prevailing government orthodoxy at the time: the importance of a strong economy, the belief that there was no inherent reason for the superiority of public over private production, and the assumed ubiquity of organizational inefficiency in the public sector. Within this philosophical context, Butler (1994) identified four formative foundations of the 1991 reforms of the NHS:

1. The growth of *managerialism* in the public sector and the NHS in particular
2. The encouragement to public sector bodies to *generate income* to boost public funding
3. The policy of *contracting out* or market-testing services provided by the public sector (particularly local government and, within the NHS, support services such as laundry, catering, and cleaning)
4. The growth of *internal markets*

Together with the (perennial) minifinancial crisis in the NHS in 1987, such developments during the 1980s provide a credible explanation for the underlying forces that led to Margaret Thatcher's somewhat eyebrow-raising surprise announcement on the BBC TV news program *Panorama* of a review of the NHS. To Butler's list of policies leading up to the reforms of the NHS could perhaps also be added Margaret Thatcher's particular (and rather un-Tory) aversion to the Establishment, in this case in the guise of the medical profession, whose representative bodies, the British Medical Association and the Royal Colleges, had produced a report in the late 1980s castigating the government for its underfunding of the NHS. The quote "If they want change I'll give them change, but not the change they expect" may be apocryphal but nonetheless rings true.

The eventual outcome of the governmental review was the white paper *Working for Patients* (Department of Health, 1989), which, at its core, advocated the need for an internal market in the NHS—based on ideas expressed by Alain Enthoven (1985). The white paper also proposed a number of other changes in the organizational structure of the NHS and, as a direct consequence of the creation of the internal market, changes in the way financial resources were to be allocated throughout the service. Table 14.1 summarizes all the key changes of *Working for Patients*.

On April 1, 1991 (dubbed "Year Zero" by the unlikely revolutionaries within the Department of Health), the reforms of *Working for Patients* were implemented in England and Wales, to be followed a year later in Scotland and Northern Ireland.

The aims of the reforms, as stated by the government in *Working for Patients,* were to install

> a funding system in which successful hospitals can flourish . . . [to] encourage local initiative and greater competition. All this in turn will ensure a better deal for the public, improving the choice and quality of the services offered and the efficiency with which these services are delivered. (Department of Health, 1989, p. 22)

Thus, the internal market was expected to improve patient choice, service quality, and provider efficiency. Although emphasis on these goals was criticized for ignoring another important aim of the NHS—namely, equity—the then Prime Minister, Margaret Thatcher (1989) stated in her introduction to the white paper that "the National Health Service will continue to be available to all, regardless of income, and to be financed mainly out of taxation." Here was a restatement of the notions of equity of delivery (equality of access based on need rather than ability to pay) and equity of financing (due to the mildly progressive nature of the U.K. tax system, the rich pay a higher proportion of their income to fund the NHS than the poor).

TABLE 14.1 *Working for Patients:* Key Changes

Introduction of weighted capitation to distribute money voted by Parliament for the NHS to regions and on to districts.

NHS trusts charged for the use and acquisition of capital, including interest and depreciation.

GP practice budgets ("fundholding") for large practices that wished to purchase a (selected) range of health care for their patients.

In place of the traditional demand-led drug expenditure, indicative prescribing amounts for GPs to control drug costs.

Audit of the NHS accounts to be carried out by the independent Audit Commission.

The separation of the provision and purchase of health care; the so-called "internal market."

Extension of hospital clinical budgeting.

Creation of NHS trust units with greater freedoms to set pay levels, borrow for capital projects, etc.

Changes in the composition of health authority and family practitioner committee membership; boards created along private sector lines.

Devolved management, together with stronger lines of accountability from top to bottom in the NHS.

Consultants' management service to be taken into account in their meritorious service and distinction awards. NHS managers to have more say in these awards.

Consultants' contracts to be more detailed. Trusts to hold and negotiate their consultants' contracts.

Medical audit to be extended throughout the NHS.

One hundred additional consultants to be appointed over 3 years.

Tax relief on private medical insurance for elderly people.

Nevertheless, the key aim of the reforms was to promote efficiency through the use of a form of competitive "quasi market." Inasmuch as there exists a trade-off between efficiency and equity, the reality, if not the rhetoric, of government policy appeared to be that the efficiency goal takes precedence over equity.

Where Are We Now?

Since the passing of the NHS and Community Care Act of 1990 and its implementation in 1991, the reforms have developed an impetus and evolutionary path of their own. This was inevitable given the rather sketchy nature of the reforms in the first place (more outline than

TABLE 14.2 Developments Since *Working for Patients*

Mergers of health authorities ("purchasers") from around 190 in 1991 to around 100 in 1995.

Inquiry into London's health services recommends reduction in hospital bed numbers and investment in primary care. Other urban areas attempt similar reductions.

GP fundholding scheme extended to encompass "total fundholding," practices allowed to buy all types of care.

Some GP fundholding practices form "multifunds," loose purchasing alliances involving up to 80 GPs.

Regional health authorities in England abolished; new (and fewer) regional offices start in 1995. Staffing at regional and national levels cut by around a quarter.

12% real increase in the NHS budget between 1991 and 1993.

The Waiting Times Initiative continues to reduce waiting times through targeted additional funding and heavy political pressure on NHS managers.

"Hospital League Tables" detailing the performance of named hospitals published in June 1994.

Department of Health fund "evidence-based health care" initiatives such as the NHS Centre for Reviews and Dissemination and the Cochrane Centre at Oxford.

The white paper *The Health of the Nation* (Department of Health, 1992a), published in 1992, sets health outcome targets for the NHS to achieve over the next 10 to 20 years.

The Patient's Charter (Department of Health, 1992b), published in 1992, sets standards for service quality and patient satisfaction.

Private financing of NHS capital schemes strongly encouraged by the Department of Health and the Treasury.

Health authorities encouraged to "market-test" clinical services through open tender.

---

blueprint). But there was also an inherent fuzziness to the changes; one of the benefits of setting up a market is that excessive and detailed central planning and prescription is (to an extent) made unnecessary. It was therefore up to the NHS itself to explore and develop the new opportunities created by the market framework. This it did, and as experience has been accumulated, so the reforms changed and new emphases developed (see Table 14.2 for just some examples of developments in the NHS since 1991).

So, from the early outlines of reform, how has the NHS moved on? In 1991, 57 (out of around 600) NHS hospitals became self-governing trusts, cutting their managerial (and guaranteed budget) ties with their local health authorities and setting off as new businesses (although still accountable to the Secretary of State for Health) in search of income. By 1997, all hospital and community units applied and had become trusts, shedding their "directly managed" status. The fear that there would be trusts that failed financially has not been realized, although a number have struggled and have been given financial assistance. (The notion of freedom of exit from the market is not one that politicians welcome as much as the freedom of entry.)

The GP fundholding scheme also expanded. By 1997, around 40% of all GPs were part of fundholding practices, covering about the same proportion of the population and in command of around £3,200 million of the £42,000-million NHS budget. Changes in the scope of the fundholding scheme since its inception meant that GPs could take on the entire health care budget for patients on their lists. Around 30 pilot projects were established to assess the viability of this form of health care purchasing. Further changes since 1991—designed to encourage more practices to apply for fundholding status—created a "community services" category in fundholding, allowing practices to buy a restricted set of community services (and not secondary care).

Fundholding, initially seen as something of an afterthought, was increasingly promoted as the "cutting edge" of the reforms, with GPs applying more pressure on providers through market mechanisms than health authorities. The independent contractor status of GPs and hence their rather tenuous lines of accountability perhaps contributed to their more aggressive stance with providers. Although only a handful of practices withdrew from fundholding, a significant minority were resistant to the concept of fundholding. Indeed, many fundholders were not entirely happy with the scheme but felt they had to take part for fear of losing out in some way.

Health authority purchasers merged with family health service authorities (FHSAs—the organizations that channel payments to GPs and general dental practitioners) to become health commissions. Mergers between purchasers have slowed down, and there are now around 100 commissions across the United Kingdom—about half the number in 1990—serving populations of around 600,000 on average.

The relationship between the two sets of public sector purchasers—fundholders and health authorities/commissions—did not always develop smoothly. Problems with GPs' accountability, clashes between commissions' responsibility for the health care needs of their entire population (including fundholder patients), and differences in size and purchasing leverage all contributed to a degree of friction between these two purchasing units. The fact that it is GPs who refer patients to hospital (and not commissions) also meant that commissions' purchasing arrangements have sometimes been upset by changes in fundholder referral patterns. Many commissions realized that cooperation on the purchasing side was vital if coherent purchasing strategies were to be pursued (and, indeed, if Department of Health policies were to be implemented). Learning to work with GPs, to involve them in the purchasing decisions and contracting process, was an undoubted benefit of the reforms, although not an objective stated anywhere in the original white paper outlining the reforms.

Such cooperation has been one development in the contracting process. Purchasers also explored the possibilities of market testing and tendering of clinical services rather than negotiating contract variations with existing providers (Appleby, 1995). Such market testing was encouraged by the Department of Health and the Treasury—the latter being especially keen to see virtually all publicly provided services put through the market-testing process (H.M. Treasury, 1991).

Alongside these developments in contracting came a greater awareness of the need to regulate and to an extent manage the evolving market in health care. One of the roles for the new regional offices (which replaced the regional health authorities) was the implementation of market regulation guidance issued in 1995 (NHS Executive, 1995). This guidance essentially covered some of the issues dealt with by the existing Monopolies and Mergers Commission (which pursues similar goals to the U.S. Department of Justice in its antitrust work). The regulatory guidance aimed to curb the exercise of monopolistic and collusive behavior and to review and approve provider and purchaser merger plans. Unlike the independent offices of regulation that have been created as public utilities have been privatized (e.g., OFWAT for the water supply industry, OFGAS for the gas industry), regional offices' (OFSICK?) market management powers were not based on price regulation but relied on rules of accountability and formal review of purchasers' and providers' management decisions.

Organizationally, the NHS reached some sort of equilibrium by 1995. Figure 14.1 shows how the organizational map has changed between 1991 and 1995.

Structurally, then, the reforms fell into place, although new developments continued to emerge as the key actors in the game—fundholders, commissions, providers—learned more about the new economic framework in which they had to operate. The crucial question, however, is the effect the reforms have had on the key goals the NHS pursues, such as efficiency, effectiveness, equity, comprehensiveness, and quality. Unfortunately, evaluative research to date has not been able to provide a definitive answer to this question. Government-funded research has been directed at answering the equivalent of cost-minimization questions (What is the cheapest way of implementing the reforms?) and not at cost-benefit questions (Is it *worth* implementing the reforms?). With no official evaluation or monitoring, it has been left to other organizations to carry out assessments. As a consequence, such evaluation as has been carried out has been rather fragmented and uncoordinated. Nevertheless, some

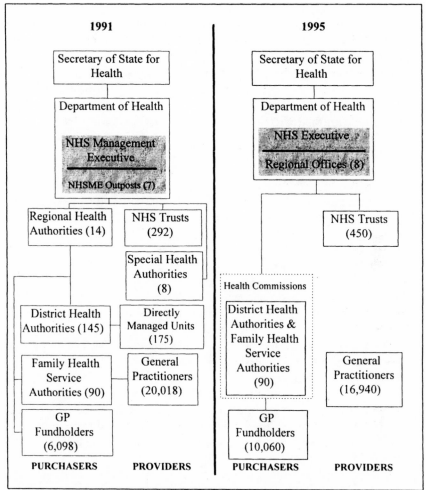

Figure 14.1. Organizational Map of the NHS: 1991 and 1995

indications of the reforms' impact can be gleaned, although there are significant problems in carrying out evaluations and interpreting results.

Theory and Practice: Evaluating the Reforms

As LeGrand and many others have noted (Appleby, Smith, Ranade, Little, & Robinson, 1994; LeGrand, 1994), evaluating the impact of the reforms on the NHS (and in particular how the NHS's key aims and objectives have been affected) is deeply problematic. The assessment difficulties are not unique to the NHS, but given the importance, scale, and the untested nature of the 1991 reforms, they are particularly acute. The complicating factors are familiar to nearly all social research and include parallel policy and other organizational and environmental changes that either obscure or totally obliterate the links between the policy under consideration (the reforms of the NHS) and its outcomes. In addition, there are problems of definition and measurement. If, as seems likely, we are interested to know the impact of the reforms on equity (of delivery and finance of health care), what definition of *equity* should we adopt? Moreover, how is efficiency to be defined, and how is it to be measured?

To facilitate evaluation, economists often assume conditions of *ceteris paribus*—other things being equal. But since 1991, the NHS has been subject to a host of developments within the context of the initial reforms framework laid down by *Working for Patients* and in addition has been influenced by other policies and, importantly, some of the largest annual increases in its budget for over 20 years. To illuminate the researcher's nightmare, Table 14.2 lists just a few of the developments in the NHS since the implementation of *Working for Patients*.

Again, as LeGrand and others have pointed out, if we take two of the most commonly cited measures of "success" of the reforms—waiting times and the numbers of patients treated by the NHS—it would be surprising indeed if real increases in NHS spending had *not* had some positive effect on these measures. But additional funding and policies such as the Waiting Times Initiative (which presumably had some impact on waiting times) were not part of the package of reforms brought in by *Working for Patients*.

Another evaluative problem is the choice of performance or outcome measure(s). The NHS, like most public service organizations, tends not to focus on one bottom-line performance measure (such as profit or return on capital). Instead, it strives to improve its performance on a number of (often conflicting) fronts, such as efficiency (usually crudely defined in terms of unit costs of treatment), equity (defined as equal access for those in equal need), and quality (with no agreed-on definition!). Other goals of the NHS include acceptability (of services and treatments to patients), appropriateness (of treatments), comprehensiveness (of the range of services available), and effectiveness (clinically).

Evaluation on all these fronts is a tall order. However, there are five issues—two general (efficiency and equity) and three specific (waiting times/lists, transaction/management costs, and patient activity)—on which it is perhaps worth concentrating. These are looked at in turn below.

Efficiency

Although the internal market's main aim was to promote the efficiency with which services were provided, primarily through supply-side competition, its structure lacked the classic market incentives. Though trusts competed for their business and hence income, there were no equivalent (and automatic) incentives for district health authority purchasers to pursue efficient purchasing policies. For this reason, the Department of Health required health authority purchasers (although not GP fundholder purchasers) to meet annually set efficiency targets (usually of around 2% to 3%). Monitoring of these efficiency targets was and is carried out via the Efficiency Index. The index is a fairly crude (and much criticized—see Appleby & Little, 1993) measure of technical or productive efficiency that is calculated as the ratio of annual changes in activity to changes in real funding. Figure 14.2 shows how a similar index, the Cost Weighted Activity Index, has changed between 1981 and 1992.

The figure suggests that productive or technical efficiency increased more than its trend in the first year of the reforms but settled back to the trend line in the second year. Clearly, to form any conclusive interpretation on just two observations would be presumptuous. Even when figures for the last 2 years become available, there are some serious doubts about the validity of this measure of efficiency.

First, around 20% of the services and treatments carried out by the NHS are not included in the index. Second, no allowance is made for expenditure that does not increase activity but that does contribute to, say, improvements in quality (and arguably, improvements in efficiency). Third, activity in the first few years of the reforms was artificially inflated as trusts came to grips with more accurate counts of the patients who passed through their doors. (Trusts' income depended on this.) Fourth, there has been and remains considerable scope for collusion between purchasers and their providers to inflate the Efficiency Index in that both sides tend to view it not only as a spurious and bureaucratic measure of efficiency but also as one that contains perverse incentives (e.g., increasing the volume of treatment regardless of the appropriateness of doing so). Finally, even if none of these problems existed, changes in the value of the index could not be unambiguously attributed to the introduction of the reforms.

Perhaps the safe if somewhat lame conclusion to draw from this evidence is that it is still too early to draw any conclusions. Nevertheless, this immediately raises the question as to when it will be appropriate to draw conclusions about the impact of the internal market on efficiency and, subsequently, what level of efficiency gain we should consider adequate to pronounce the reforms a success.

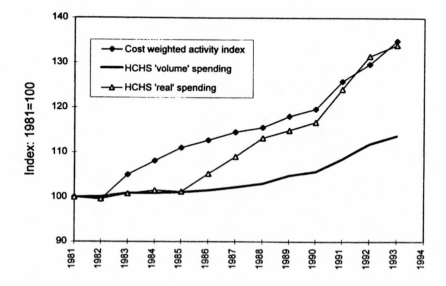

Figure 14.2. Cost Weighted Activity Index: Changes in Technical Efficiency: English NHS

Equity

There are two dimensions to the issue of equity: finance and delivery. The Aristotelian concepts of *vertical* and *horizontal* equity are usually applied to questions of health care financing and delivery respectively. Treating unequals (in terms of income) *un*equally when it comes to paying for health care (in particular, where the rich pay proportionately more for care than the poor) is generally accepted as an equitable situation. (There are, of course, arguments about *how* much more the rich should pay relative to the poor.) In the United Kingdom, paying for health care means paying taxes. Given that the funding source for the NHS remains as it was before the reforms (i.e., largely from general taxation), changes in the tax system need to be examined to ascertain changes in the equity of financing of the NHS. A particular trend in the United Kingdom's tax system over the last 10 to 15 years has been the switch away from direct taxation to indirect forms such as VAT. In general, therefore, there has been a move away from progressive taxes and toward more regressive forms of revenue raising. Moreover, direct taxes such as income tax have become less progressive as the higher tax bands have been abolished. Although the

United Kingdom's tax structure is mildly progressive, it has become less so over the last decade. Quantifying the impact of these changes on the equity of NHS financing is difficult, but the conclusion must be that qualitatively equity of financing has suffered.

Despite being perhaps the most important criterion informing the creation of the NHS, equity of delivery (where equals—in terms of need—are treated equally) has always been problematic for the service. Many studies carried out over the last 20 years have produced contradictory conclusions. For example, LeGrand (1978) concluded that higher social groups received more than their fair share of health care resources, and this conclusion was supported by Hurst (1985); Collins and Klein (1980, 1985) disputed these results, however. Since 1991, there have been no definitive studies of the equity of delivery of services by the NHS.

Whitehead (1994) attempted to synthesize what evidence there was in this area. However, much of it is anecdotal or subject to criticism on grounds of poor research methodology. Whitehead's tentative conclusions were that in many respects the equity goal of the NHS had been downgraded relative to other aims. In some particular instances (e.g., the fundholding scheme), there was evidence to suggest that equity had been unambiguously damaged. The fact that GP fundholders have been able to secure faster treatment than nonfundholders as a result of holding budgets and being more prepared to argue with providers has not been disputed by ministers. In fact, such outcomes have been held up as examples of the success of the reforms, and it has been argued that such improvements for fundholder patients have eventually percolated through to nonfundholder patients. The evidence for this is thin, however. Moreover, the fact that some patients, suffering exactly the same problems, receive more prompt treatment simply because they have the good fortune to belong to fundholding practices is an inequitable position. This is not redeemed by the possibility that there may be some "trickle down" of improved access to other patients some time in the future.

Waiting Times/Lists

The NHS is perhaps universally known and often criticized for the existence of waiting lists, and many studies have shown that these are one of the primary reasons for people to use private health care and to buy private medical insurance coverage (see Higgins, 1988). Of course, all health care systems have waiting lists. Indeed all products have waiting lists (I am currently on a waiting list for a bigger, newer car—it's just that I cannot afford one at the moment). NHS waiting lists are just more overt than those of other health care systems. The importance of waiting lists (and, more importantly, times) in the public's perception of the NHS and the government's competence in general has not been lost on health ministers. Examination of the trends in waiting lists and times since 1988 suggests that far fewer people are now waiting very long times for admission to hospital after the reforms (see Figure 14.3).

Should this be taken as an unambiguous success story for the NHS? The answer, for a number of reasons, is probably not. First, NHS waiting lists are not simple queues operating on a first-come, first-served basis. Urgent cases are admitted more promptly than nonurgent cases (with clinicians deciding on the clinical urgency of each case). The reductions in the very long wait cases have therefore been among those cases that were deemed nonurgent (a very large proportion being plastic surgery patients). Even if this had not occurred at the expense of other, more urgent cases (and there is some evidence to suggest that it has), it raises the question as to whether treating the long waiters was the best use of scarce resources.

But as with many of the performance indicators used to measure the impact of the reforms, waiting lists and times have been subject to policies unrelated to those contained in *Working for Patients*. In particular, over the last 10 years or so the Department of Health has targeted additional funds at specific waiting list "black spots" and has applied considerable political pressure (through, e.g., the Patient's Charter standards) to NHS managers to deal with waiting-list problems.

Patient Activity

An often quoted statistic used by ministers as illustrative of the positive effect that the reforms have had on the NHS is the number of extra patients treated each year since 1991. Just taking figures for England, between 1990 and 1994, there has indeed been an increase in patients treated of around 1.3 million, an increase of nearly 15%. Delving a bit deeper and examining long-run trends reveals a more complicated picture, however. As Figure 14.4 shows, the bulk of the recent increases in hospital activity have arisen from the increase in day case work, with ordinary inpatient numbers leveling off from 1988 and day cases increasing more sharply from that year. It thus seems very unlikely that this apparent switch to day case treatment or the increase in numbers overall can be attributed to the reforms of the NHS.

Furthermore, as has been noted in relation to the Efficiency Index, there is no doubt that in the first few years of the reforms activity was artificially

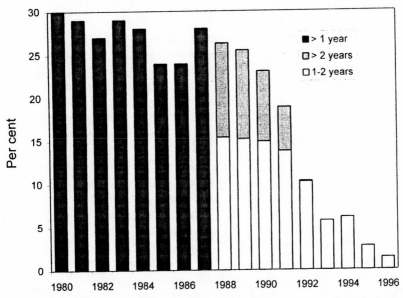

Figure 14.3. Percentage of Ordinary Cases Waiting Over 1 and 2 Years for Admission

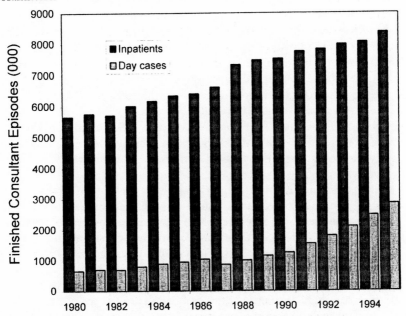

Figure 14.4. Hospital Activity: Inpatients and Day Cases, England

inflated as trusts learned to count their patients with more accuracy. Also, crude counts of volumes of treatment reveal nothing about either the nature of the treatment delivered or its necessity (nor, of course, anything about its impact on patients' health status). As with the other indicators of performance, we are left in a rather inconclusive position with regard to the reforms' effects.

Transaction/Management Costs

A common complaint leveled at the NHS reforms is that they have led to a vast increase in administrative costs. Traditionally, the NHS has been viewed as a rather cheap system to manage—the integrated nature of the system and the rather low (by international standards) staff pay being the primary reasons for this. The introduction of a system (the internal market) that required a new set of bureaucratic procedures (e.g., contracting) and the freedom for trusts to set their own pay levels would suggest that administration (and transaction) costs would inevitably rise. Has this been the case?

There are no officially collated figures for transaction costs in the internal market and indeed no official definition of what constitutes such costs. On the one hand, there are the salaries and wages of managers and administrators and fractions of salaries of medical staff who devote some of their time to management and market duties. On the other hand, there are the unrecorded opportunity costs associated with contracting, dealing with the extra accounting duties required by the market (pricing, calculating capital charges, etc.), and managing the service in general.

In terms of the readily measurable, as a proportion of total spending on the NHS in England between 1990-91 and 1992-93, managerial costs have increased from 9.8% to 10.3%; establishment costs (printing, postage, telephones, etc.) have stayed constant; and consultancy and audit costs have risen from 0% to 0.7%.

Even this crude analysis suggests that there has been an increase in the sort of costs associated with completing transactions in the internal market. Whether these costs are justified in terms of the benefits obtained from the introduction of the market is another question, and one that brings us full circle to the difficulties of establishing the impact of the reforms on the NHS in the first place.

In conclusion, although ideally an evaluation of the effect of the 1991 reforms should focus on the outputs of the NHS in terms of the health of the U.K. population, in practice this is very difficult, not least because of the difficulties in drawing valid and robust connections between the work or process of the NHS and population health measures such as infant mortality and life expectancy. Few if any independent commentators on the NHS would (or could) unequivocally pronounce the reforms either a complete failure or a roaring success. What evidence does exist suggests that aspects of the reforms have brought benefits but that these have often been achieved at some cost to other objectives and goals. Moreover, given the rather equivocal nature of the outcomes of the reforms so far in comparison with the energy, resources, and time spent by managers, clinicians, and others on the reforms' implementation, one is forced to ask whether it has been time and money well spent.

One thing the reforms have not had, however, is time to prove themselves: The general election of May 1, 1997, saw the Labour Party return to power after 18 years in opposition. The future of the reforms and the direction of the NHS over the next 5 to 10 years will be dependent on the policies of the new government.

A New Direction?

One of the key drivers of future change for the NHS and health care in general in the United Kingdom is politics. The Labour Party currently have a working majority in Parliament that exceeds the total number of seats won by the Conservatives and have an apparent mandate from the people for radical change. Labour had entered the election with a policy statement on health and health care (*Renewing the NHS*; Labour Party, 1995). Since the election, it has firmed up this statement and produced a white paper on the future direction of the NHS.

In *Renewing the NHS,* the Labour Party set out its priorities for health and health care. It stated that a future Labour government would tackle inequalities in health care, improve the services of GPs, extend patient choice, promote care of proven effectiveness, and support the needs of the growing numbers of elderly (the words "motherhood and apple pie" immediately spring to mind). But, as the old joke goes, reaching these destinations would be a lot easier if the Labour Party could have chosen to start from somewhere else.

Renewing the NHS proposed a combination of renaming (contracts become "comprehensive health care agreements"), real if slow change (GP fundholding to be abolished—but over 5 years), and a reemphasis of objectives that have taken a back seat over the past 5 or 10 years (an avowed "attack on inequalities in health").

Along with the creation of a new ministerial post for public health designed to coordinate interdepartmental action to tackle health inequalities, *Renewing the NHS* also proposed to revamp community health councils, extending their powers and renaming them as "local health advocates." However, it was the internal market and the separation of purchasers of health care and providers that presented the most overt challenge to Labour's traditional values. Was there an alternative to the internal market that did not return the NHS to pre-1991 days?

Labour's criticisms of the internal market hinged around its perceived unpopularity with the public, unnecessary restrictions on GP referral freedoms, and a U.S.-style mountain of paperwork and added bureaucracy. Interestingly, a 1986 report from the former NHS Management Board (now the NHS Executive) produced very similar arguments against the internal market idea. But in response to their own criticisms, Labour now treads carefully.

The publication of the white paper, *The New NHS* (Department of Health, 1997) has drawn on previous policy statements such as *Renewing the NHS*. However, it does so in a different context. Labour are in power (not opposition); they have a majority (albeit unexpected in its sheer size), which suggests a significant political mandate for change; and they have stuck to their preelection pledge to carry through the previous administration's somewhat parsimonious public spending plans until 1999. Table 14.3 summarizes the new white paper's key proposals.

Along with the changes noted in Table 14.3, the government have committed themselves to increasing NHS funding by more than the rate of general inflation for the rest of their term in office (although no particular figure has been mentioned). Funding sources are to remain the same—that is, largely general taxation, supplemented where feasible by miscellaneous sources such as patient charges for prescriptions and dental services. The Private Finance Initiative (PFI), whereby private groups fund, design, build, run, and lease back hospitals to the NHS, will continue.

Although the new white paper proposes to abolish the internal market in the NHS, its attempt to find a "third way"—by retaining the separation between purchasers and providers of health care, insisting on very long term agreements (aka "contracts"), and emphasizing cooperation over competition—requires some faith.

One problem is the extent to which cooperation has the power to enforce change when change is required. The white paper's answer is to give health authorities a planning/regulatory role backed up by national and local performance targets for waiting times, readmission rates, and

TABLE 14.3 *The New NHS:* Key Proposals

Creation of an NHS information "superhighway": The "NHSnet" will connect GP surgeries, pharmacies

Creation of "Health Action Zones": Worst areas of poor health targeted, bringing together the NHS with other agencies to tackle health problems

Revamped Patient's Charter: Annual surveys of users and caregivers

Abolition of the internal market: split between purchasers (renamed as "commissioners") and providers to remain; new "commissioning" organizations (e.g., primary care groups) to be established, centered on general practitioners with support from and accountability to health authorities

Abolition of general practitioner fundholding scheme: primary care groups to take their place

National performance framework: to set performance targets on health improvement, efficiency, effectiveness, etc.

Creation of the National Institute for Clinical Excellence (NICE): to provide guidance on clinical and cost-effective health care

Creation of Commission for Health Improvement (CHI): to oversee and enforce, if necessary, improvements in clinical quality

Unification of local health budgets: Hospital and community health services, GP prescribing, and general practice infrastructure to become one, cash-limited budget

Revamped Health of the Nation *strategy document:* fewer and lower targets for the NHS to achieve

Public Health Green Paper: with emphasis on dealing with health inequalities

---

financial incentives for the new GP-led commissioning groups. But when push comes to shove, how does a health authority—divorced from the day-to-day management and control of health care providers and dealing with commissioning groups dominated by GPs (who are independent contractors, not NHS employees)—actually pursue a course of action that is in the best interests of patients but not of providers (which, confusingly, can include GPs)? The power of commissioners to enforce change is further undermined by the proposed involvement of hospital trusts in helping to plan their local Health Improvement Programme. Although the competitive incentive implicit in the internal market has been somewhat muted, at least there existed a clear and powerful lever of control for purchasers to pull, even if only as a last resort after cooperative negotiation had failed.

However, if there has been one important lesson from the last 7 years, it is the gap that can open up between the intentions of a white paper and the reality of its implementation. The reality of the internal market never lived up to the expectations of competition; cooperation—of sorts—was always an important practicality in order to get health care delivered.

Moreover, it was hard to predict at the time of *Working for Patients* just how important and influential the GP fundholding scheme would be in changing not only services but the locus of power within the NHS. Although *The New NHS* will abolish fundholding (seen as a source of unnecessary bureaucracy, inequity, and queue jumping), the importance of the role of GPs within the NHS is recognized in the proposals to integrate general practice into the mainstream of NHS planning and decision making through GP commissioning groups and primary care groups.

Overall, given its starting point, it is hard to see exactly what direction Labour's health policy could have taken other than that proposed in *Renewing the NHS* and now, with some greater depth added, in *The New NHS*. Ultimately, the main aim and justification for the NHS is the effective and appropriate care of the population. Achieving that goal requires more than a reemphasis of priorities, however. Some tough decisions will have to be taken on the way that will not always please some of the more powerful stakeholders in the NHS. Whether the essentially managerial levers, targets, and performance incentive systems that Labour proposes will prove powerful enough to keep the NHS changing and adapting to meet the health needs of the population remains to be seen.

References

Appleby, J. (1995). *Testing the market: A national survey of clinical services tendering by purchasers* (Research Paper 18). Birmingham, UK: National Association of Health Authorities and Trusts.

Appleby, J., & Little, V. (1993). Health and efficiency. *Health Service Journal, 103*(5351), 20-22.

Appleby, J., Smith, P., Ranade, W., Little, V., & Robinson, R. (1994). Monitoring managed competition. In R. Robinson & J. LeGrand (Eds.), *Evaluating the NHS reforms*. London: King's Fund Institute.

Bunker, J. P., Frazier, H. S., & Mosteller, F. (1994). Improving health: Measuring effects of health care. *Millbank Quarterly, 72*, 225-258.

Butler, J. (1994). Origins and early development. In R. Robinson & J. LeGrand (Eds.), *Evaluating the NHS reforms*. London: King's Fund Institute.

Collins, E., & Klein, R. (1980). Equity in the NHS: Self-reported morbidity, access and primary care. *British Medical Journal, 304*, 1307-1308.

Collins, E., & Klein, R. (1985). *Self-reported morbidity, socioeconomic factors and GP consultations* (Bath Social Policy Papers No. 5). Bath, UK: University of Bath, Centre for the Analysis of Social Policy.

Department of Health. (1989). *Working for patients*. London: HMSO, Command No. 555.

Department of Health. (1992a). *The health of the nation*. London: HMSO, Command No. 1986.

Department of Health. (1992b). *The patient's charter.* London: HMSO.

Department of Health. (1997). *The new NHS*. London: HMSO.

Enthoven, A. C. (1985). *Reflections on the management of the NHS* (Occasional Paper No. 5). London: Nuffield Provincial Hospitals Trust.

H.M. Treasury. (1991). *Competing for quality*. London: HMSO, Command No. 1730.

Higgins, J. (1988). *The business of medicine: Private health care in Britain*. London: Macmillan.

Hurst, J. (1985). *Financing health care in the United States, Canada and Britain*. London: Nuffield/Leverhulme Fellowship Report, King's Fund.

Labour Party. (1995). *Renewing the NHS*. London: Author.

LeGrand, J. (1978). The distribution of public expenditure: The case of health care. *Economica, 45,* 125-142.

LeGrand, J. (1994). Evaluating the NHS reforms. In R. Robinson & J. LeGrand (Eds.), *Evaluating the NHS reforms*. London: King's Fund Institute.

National Health Service Executive. (1995). *The operation of the internal NHS market: Local freedoms, national responsibilities*. Leeds, UK: Author.

Thatcher, M. (1989). Introduction. In Department of Health, *Working for patients*. London: HMSO, Command No. 555.

Whitehead, M. (1994). Is it fair? Evaluating the equity implications of the NHS reforms. In R. Robinson & J. LeGrand (Eds.), *Evaluating the NHS reforms*. London: King's Fund Institute.

CHAPTER 15

Policy Lessons From the British Health Care System

Donald W. Light

The basic decisions that the British made in using the paradigm of managed competition to transform the National Health Service (NHS) offer valuable lessons for American policymakers (Light & May, 1993; Light, 1997a). For even if the NHS does not deliver the style or quality of health care that Americans prefer, its *design* ideas (as distinct from their execution) merit attention. Moreover, the 1991 reforms, which converted a governmental welfare service into a system of interlocking contracts, became the fullest example of managed competition in the world. Every health authority, responsible for the health care of every resident, was transformed from a governmental administrative office into

AUTHOR'S NOTE: This study was made possible by Paul Ginsberg and the invitation of the Physicians Payment Review Commission to draw policy lessons from the British experiences in transforming the world's largest single health care system into a set of interlocking managed markets. The essay is partially based on the Jan Brod Lecture delivered at Green College, Oxford University, on May 18, 1995. I am also indebted to Albert Wessen for his extraordinary editing skills. Two outstanding GPs provided detailed reviews, Andrew Farmer (a Harkness Fellow) and Peter Orton. An authority in public health, Alison Hill, and two senior members of the NHS also reviewed the manuscript. I am grateful to them all for their many helpful suggestions.

a purchaser. Every physician, hospital, and clinical team was transformed from a line-item budget recipient into a seller seeking contracts. This British experience deserves the attention of Americans as they ponder their policy options.

This chapter will discuss *adaptable policy lessons* that Americans might draw from the British NHS. Extracting such lessons is a highly selective process, and for brevity's sake, much of the local detail, politics, and history that are unique to Great Britain will be passed over. The lessons here are the attempt of one analyst to extrapolate from his study of and work with the NHS. Others might draw other lessons. To some degree, the lessons are distinct and could be adopted separately by other systems, though they make up a rather integrated whole in the British context. Some are in tension with others because all health care systems contain within them conflicting visions and models of what a system should be (Light, 1994a).

Eight Basic Policy Lessons About Universal Health Care

Before turning to the lessons of the British experiences with managed competition, one must attend to the prior lessons learned when the British confronted the limitations and inequities of voluntary health insurance schemes and decided to create an equitable, universal health care system with a strong primary care base. These decisions are important both in their own right and because they frame the experience with managed competition. For several features of the British design seem particularly suitable for meeting the health care needs of an aging population in the 21st century (Fox, 1993). The first five concern the basic parameters of national health insurance and efforts to make health care both equitable and efficient. The last three focus on shaping a strong primary care system.

Lesson 1: The Value of Universal, Equitable Funding

During the 19th and early 20th centuries, the British had their own mixture of voluntary health insurance through friendly societies, commercial insurance, cash payments, and public health services for the poor (for a brief overview, see Hollingsworth, 1986, pp. 6-64). To overcome the most egregious problems of destitution from illness, Parliament passed a modest national health insurance plan in 1911 that paid for sick low-income workers (but not their dependents) to receive free general practice medicine as well as cash benefits to replace lost wages. The money was collected through general taxes. Thus, early on, the principle of universal funding was established for the poor and working classes. Over time, this principle came to be applied to everyone.

The costs of this system, however, were high (Royal Commission, 1926), and it allowed the inequitable distributions of doctors and hospitals to grow. Moreover, financing became increasingly inequitable. The middle class "received no concessions at all in the finance of its medical requirements and it was forced, by indirect means, to subsidize the medical coverage of the rest of the population" (Eckstein, 1958, p. 9). The middle classes also found that private voluntary health insurers charged more or provided less coverage for their sicknesses—the "inverse coverage law" (Light, 1992). These basic problems trouble the American health care system today as well.

The British solution was universal funding through the tax system. Medical care was to be free for all at the point of service. It achieved, in the words of Charles Webster (1993), the NHS's most eminent historian, "the maximum redistributive effect and potentially the greatest gains for the poorest and most needy sections of the community. . . . Funding the NHS from general taxation was simple, unbureaucratic, and egalitarian" (pp. 15-16).

When the Thatcher administration considered financing health care through insurance premiums rather than taxes, they decided against insurance because it would require a second, costly piece of bureaucratic machinery to collect the money alongside tax collection and was likely to be more complex and less equitable (Fowler, 1991; May, 1993). As Sir Roy Griffiths, the most distinguished business executive concerned with British health policy, said, "Once you start getting into insured schemes, the amount of paperwork is disastrous" (quoted in May, 1993, p. 27).

Lesson 2: The Importance of Strict Budget Limits

From the British point of view, the problem of health care "hijacking" other social programs and personal income will continue in the absence of a health care budget. American policy bodies such as the Physician Payment Review Commission (PPRC) can deliberate on target formulas or think about the criteria for setting a budgetary goal, but such exercises are ultimately futile in a nation that has no actual global health care budget.

Funding health care from general revenues, as the British have done, is the toughest approach to cost containment because health care must fight directly every year for its share against the military, education, welfare programs, social security, economic development, transportation, and other major programs. Faced with these competing demands, the British Treasury held health care expenditures to less than 4% of GDP through the 1950s and 1960s. Expenditures did not exceed 4.5% until the mid-1970s and did not reach 6% until the 1980s (Webster, 1993).

In the eyes of many British citizens and some policymakers, pitting health care against other social budgets has been too stringent, and the quality of health services has suffered as a result. Rationing takes place primarily by limiting supply—beds, clinics, specialists, equipment—and then having patients' doctors make clinical decisions within that context (Aaron & Schwartz, 1984). The infamous waiting lists of the NHS for elective surgery and other procedures and tests are in part a result of what most perceive as underfunding. The NHS does emergency care and a very broad range of community and primary care well but uses waiting lists for elective specialty care as a budgetary escape valve.

Lesson 3: The Value of Free Care at the Point of Service

Many American business leaders and policymakers believe that health care costs rise because patients do not pay for them with their own money. As the PPRC (1994) put it, the central argument for cost sharing is "to make consumers more sensitive to the price of services and, it is hoped, alter their behavior to avoid using unnecessary health care" (p. 165). This conviction seems uniquely American.

The British principle has long been that services should be "free at the point of delivery." There is a good reason why. If a nation's goal is a universally accessible service, direct charges or copayments represent a conflicting set of principles about how to make health care affordable and accessible. As the NHS's chief historian put it, "The entire population was promised a comprehensive health service, free of direct charges and almost entirely financed by general taxation" (Webster, 1993, p. 15). From this point of view, copayments are "a tax on the sick." Yet small direct charges (British English for copayments) for prescriptions and dental and eye services began in 1951 and slowly increased. Then, during the 1980s, the Thatcher government increased direct charges for dental and optical services and brought them increasingly to the point where they were hardly part of NHS services (Webster, 1993). Nonetheless, for the most part, the NHS remains free at the point of service.

Lesson 4: The Need for Equal Access and Distribution of Services

The complement of the principle of universal, equitable funding from general taxes is equal access to needed services. As people in other countries have realized, however, the British found that universal health insurance and various compensatory programs were not enough to provide equal access or distribution after decades of inequitable social, economic, and medical distribution. The policy lesson from Britain is that providing equal access and distribution of services is a long and complex process.

A major goal of the NHS was to equalize access and distribution, which by 1946-48 seemed quite uneven. A Medical Practices Committee was established to identify underserved primary care areas and to authorize new practices in them. Areas already well served were "closed" so that over time equal distribution was ensured. Local practice committees addressed more specific barriers to access by having the power to assign people turned away by one GP to another. These practices continue today.

Reducing inequalities is a slow process under tight budgets because there is not much money for reallocation or new building. The policy implication of the British experience is that politically one can equalize only by upgrading inferior parts of the system and underserved areas; thus, equalizing takes a lot of money. Although in 1962 the government launched a 15-year program to modernize hospitals and reduce some inequalities in the process, by 1975 the British economist Alan Maynard (1975) concluded that "the geographical distribution of the hospital bed stock is very unequal" (p. 206), ranging from 13 to 7.7 beds per 1,000 population in different regions. The poorer regions, which treated more sick patients, had the fewest beds. Maynard attributed this chiefly to prewar inequalities and tight budget constraints.

Closely related to hospital bed inequalities have been historic patterns of funding that have favored more affluent regions. By 1976, the richest region was receiving 36% more than the poorest, and variations by smaller areas (districts) were even greater (Allen, 1984). To address this more fundamental layer of inequality, a Resource Allocation Working Party developed a formula based on population adjusted for age, sex, and standardized mortality. Such large reallocations as the formula implied, however, are very dislocating for both the regions that lose and those that gain. One needs several years to retrain, retool, close down, and build up, especially if for political reasons no region is to suffer significant cuts. This slowed the equalization process, and inflation reduced the value of what monies could be found for developing the poorer areas. Nevertheless, the regional range in funding per capita steadily decreased up to the Thatcher reforms, from a 36% gap to one under 18%, and district-level equalizations were even greater. The British experience shows that it takes more than having national health insurance, or even controlling the entire health care budget, to correct these and ensure equal access for every sick patient.

Lesson 5: The Need for Streamlined Organization and Better Management

All health care systems, it seems, think they have too many bureaucrats and are inefficient, even if by international standards they have small overheads and provide a lot of clinical medicine for their money. Such is the case with the NHS, which has been struggling with "an administrative structure that in England and Wales alone involved some 600 administrative bodies [and] was subversive to integrated planning" (Webster, 1993, p. 17). By the 1960s, all agreed that the NHS needed to be greatly simplified and unified around services managed at the district level.

Discussions, distractions, and discontinuities dragged on until the 1974 reorganization, which provided "a slight extension in unification at the cost of greatly increased bureaucracy" (Webster, 1993, p. 18). The reorganization also included attempts to make services more responsive to patients by establishing community health councils.

Continued dissatisfaction with the performance of the NHS led Margaret Thatcher, soon after her election, to turn to a team of four businessmen, headed by Roy Griffiths, for advice on how to make the NHS more efficient. Griffiths, a successful and prominent executive, set an example by conducting his review in record time, using a small staff, and issuing a very brief report in 1983 that minced no words. He argued that the buck-passing vagueness of "consensus management" by teams of doctors, nurses, and managers needed to be replaced by strong general managers who would be accountable for performance. The now famous Griffiths Report initiated sweeping changes, instituting strong general management in each unit and district and transferring executive responsibility for the NHS from the Department of Health to a national Management Board.[1] Yet implementation was slow as doctors resisted ceding their power, and habits of consensus management continued.

There followed a series of efforts to improve cost-effectiveness in the operations of the NHS. First, management budgeting was introduced to make service providers aware of the costs they incurred and to make them assume accountability for their allocation and expenditure (Packwood, Keen, & Buxton, 1991). Unfortunately, the scheme was not linked to the overall budgeting and planning process, and information systems did not provide good enough cost data on clinical activities to enable clinicians to review their activities. Moreover, it was seen as a top-down, budget-dominated strategy. Clinicians distrusted both the information and the process. After 2 years, the experiment in management budgeting was ended.

"Resource management" represented the next effort to streamline organization and strengthen management. It was a major, high-profile experiment that placed clinicians at the center of the process. The NHS also developed performance indicators for all managerial areas. Data, costing, and coding again dominated much of the project's efforts. Participants found that creating true clinical management teams across service units involved sorting out different perceptions, values, and ways of thinking in order to build trust and share sensitive information. To some, it seemed like consensus management reincarnated. The outcome of the resource management program is unclear, however, because, before the process was completed, the Ministry of Health changed the structure, rules, and funding. The evaluators ended up wondering if rhetoric and process had not become ends in themselves. Thus, strengthening management and streamlining organizations became more complex, elusive, and expensive than its designers had imagined.

From the point of view of those involved, resource management had been tried at only a few sites in a partial way and thus had not been given time to prove itself. However, the government felt it had played its hand out trying to squeeze more services out of a flat budget through "efficiency savings" and better management. Moreover, as Alan Maynard (1993) observed, "These processes may have achieved some efficiency gains but, in doing so, they made the implicit and ubiquitous processes of rationing more explicit" (p. 29).

Meanwhile, ministers took a new tack. They built "efficiency savings" into the actual budgets of hospitals, eliminating any real increases and forcing hospitals to find such savings themselves. One mandatory source was competitive bidding by NHS staff and outside corporations for catering, cleaning, laundry, and other routine services. This appears to have saved money in some cases, but in others it simply shifted both employees and funds to newly formed companies. In 1988, an Efficiency

Unit was established to review the civil service as a whole. It advocated a system of "quasi-autonomous, self-regulating agencies responsible for fulfilling contracts and meeting performance targets set by ministers" (May, 1993, p. 25).

This quite different blueprint for how to maximize efficiency foreshadowed the NHS reform proposals. Faced with widespread charges of underfunding and charges that patients were dying for lack of care, Mrs. Thatcher announced a surprise review in 1988 that concluded that inducing competition would greatly increase efficiency. With the issuance of the white paper *Working for Patients* in 1989 (Secretary of State for Health, 1989), on transforming the NHS into a system of managed markets, the "internal market" era was born. With competition as the new watchword, a great deal of time and money went into making hospitals ready for self-governance, learning how to contract with purchasers of care, and developing their own kind of resource management. On the other hand, fewer resources went into general management, again (as twice before) without good evaluation. No independent observer would characterize the conversion to an "internal market" as streamlining organization or saving money. Rather, it represented a return to the top-down, management-led orientation of management budgeting on a sweeping scale.

The government handled the sudden policy shift by declaring resource management a success and incorporating it into the "self-governing trust" concept of hospitals as independent commercial agents in competing markets that would reward efficiency. That concept had informed a number of schemes developed earlier in the 1980s for hospitals to generate extra income: shopping arcades in unfilled hospital corridors; health clubs in unused basements; car parks on unused land; advertising space sold on blank walls; and mail-order services (Butler, 1994; Sheaff, 1991). Although such innovations did not produce much additional income, they signaled a new ethos. Competitive tendering (contracting) for domestic services, food services, and the like implied that the core responsibility of society to provide needed services had been reduced to merely seeing that they were available. The mandate that hospitals should generate income put into question the implied commitment to fund universal health care from general revenues.

Competitive contracting and attaining efficiency through competitive markets differ most profoundly from the concept of strong general management up the chain from districts to regions to the Management Executive of the NHS. Even within the "stronger management" school were two orientations: Those who advocated strong general and central

management differed from those committed to strong clinical directorates. These differences would cause problems for years. The advocates of
clinical directorates have such natural advantages in determining what
should be done, how money should be spent, and how to increase
cost-effectiveness that they cannot be ignored. Ironically, however, this
leads one back toward team management. In short, though the British
keenly appreciate the need for greater efficiency and a more streamlined
management structure, they have found the road to attaining these goals
to be long and difficult.

Lesson 6: The Need for Strong General Practice

In the opinion of health services researchers in Great Britain and
abroad, nothing is so vital to equity and cost restraint as establishing a
strong group of general practitioners (GPs) who serve as personal doctors
and who coordinate all care (Starfield, 1992). British general practitioners
are trained more broadly than most American primary care physicians and
treat everyone in the family from newborns to aging grandparents. Thus,
pediatrics, internal medicine, gynecology, and geriatrics are only referral
subspecialties to which more complex cases are referred. All Britishers
choose their GP and usually stay with him or her for years. This long-term
relationship is critical to making health education, prevention, and comprehensive clinical management a reality. As Andrew Farmer (1993) put
it, "GPs are responsible for more than 90 percent of patient contacts but
cost only 10 percent of the NHS budget. . . . General practice costs the
equivalent of [$150] per person (including the cost of drugs) each year"
(p. 58).

Evidence about how the British primary care system works was provided by a representative survey of British elderly in 1990. It found that
83% reported seeing their GP within the previous year, and 34% within
the previous month (Jones, Lester, & West, 1994, pp. 138-142). Increasingly, they also saw a practice nurse. They and their caregivers also used
district nurses, mental health nurses, and health visitors. About 10% of
those surveyed received a home visit both during and after practice hours.
Satisfaction rates ranged from 95% to 99%.

This kind of strong primary care base facilitates more prevention,
cheaper yet better care, earlier intervention, fewer referrals, and higher
patient satisfaction (Franks, Clancy, & Nutting, 1992; Grumbach & Fry,
1993). It also provides an anchor for the rest of the system. After an operation or hospitalization, the patient goes back to his or her GP for follow-
up care and continuing clinical management of remaining problems.

British style general practice goes well beyond using primary care physicians as "gatekeepers" in managed-care systems. The term *gatekeeper* connotes a stranger whose main job is to keep most people out, a far cry from the broader role of GPs as clinically expert counselors, advocates, and managers of services for their patients' health over a long time. GPs work in small groups located in the community where their patients live. By contrast, American primary care gatekeepers work in large regional managed-care corporations and increasingly do not know the communities, lives, or personalities of their ever-changing panels of patients.

The British have seen no reason to fragment or dilute the GP role in an era of increasing subspecialization. On the contrary, they have concluded that it is better for the specialist—rheumatologist, cardiologist, oncologist, or psychiatrist—to refer the patient back to the GP and to work with him or her than to take over the care of the patient. Patients often have multiple problems and need the broad yet professional perspective of a GP to orchestrate all aspects of care for them and for others in the household. At present, the GP role is itself evolving toward that of the GP consultant to primary care nurses or nurse practitioners.

Lesson 7: Relatively Equal Pay for All Doctors

Britain's medical elite, largely based on social class and collegial ties, formed before the advent of modern medicine. During the 19th century, general practice acquired a firm organizational, financial, and social locus through friendly societies that treated the working class. Thus, when specialization arose around the better hospitals, specialists were paid much more than GPs, not only because of their specialties' prestige but also because of the hospitals to which they belonged, the higher degrees they had often obtained, the clubs and societies to which they belonged, and the social status of their private patients. These mutually reinforcing factors also contributed to high concentrations of specialists and voluntary hospitals in metropolitan and fashionable areas.

Thus, when the NHS was established, it came as no surprise that consultants won high, uniform salaries. They also won control over a generous merit pay system, life tenure, clinical autonomy, and the right to continue seeing private patients. As a group, consultants also gained effective control over the regional hospital boards. Teaching hospitals, in which leading consultants were concentrated, received special status and treatment.

A uniform salary scale for specialists has several advantages. The principle of making life earnings as equal as possible means that physicians can choose their specialty without reference to financial considerations. Equal earnings tend to end invidious comparisons among physicians. They give those specialties that deal with the most needy patients, such as geriatricians and psychiatrists, parity with procedure-oriented specialties.[2]

The British faced the gap between earnings of GPs and specialists 30 years ago. Until 1966, the financial status of GPs relative to specialists had steadily declined. The share of general medical services dropped from 10.1% of the NHS budget in 1949 to 7.5% in 1966. Good students avoided general practice, and its quality seemed to be deteriorating. GPs became increasingly upset—many emigrated—and in 1965, GPs threatened to resign en masse if the government did not improve their conditions of work. The result was the Family Doctor Charter of 1966. Among other changes, it raised the career earnings of GPs to about the same level as those of specialists.[3] Their pay scale was increased according to seniority, at 7, 12, and 21 years. This, together with other improvements discussed below, has made a significant difference in the quality of students applying for general practice and the quality of services.

Lesson 8: The Uses of Low-Risk, Mixed-Incentive GP Contracts

A hazard of capitation is the "perverse" incentive it offers doctors to maximize revenues and minimize work by attracting enrollees and then providing them with minimal care. The Family Doctor Charter reduced capitation payments to about 50% of the contract and provided GPs direct grants for most of their overhead and operating costs.[4] The new contract also provided incentives for practicing in groups and for hiring both office and clinical staff. Separate fees were also paid for immunizations, an idea that was expanded in the revised contract of 1990. Clear rules were issued prohibiting undertreatment and defining when home visits must be made. As well, unhappy patients could lodge their complaints with a GP service committee, which reviewed each complaint. The general point is that the British have balanced incentives in primary care so that the contrasting incentives of lump sums, fees, and capitation largely neutralize each other. The implicit principle is that most operating expenses should be provided so that capitation covers mostly the doctor's own time; in addition, lump-sum or "chunky" fees provide incentives for meeting specific health goals.

Investment in Prevention

The 1990 GP contract involved a considerably increased investment in prevention. GPs received new payments for screening patients for heart disease, cervical cancer, and childhood disorders. Bonus or target payments were granted for such practice measures as immunizing a target percentage of children. For example, for each 2,000 enrollees, GP practices receive the full targeted chunky fee of about $3,700 if they complete the childhood immunization schedule on 90% of their children, $1,250 if they complete immunizations on 70% to 89%, and nothing extra if they complete immunizations on fewer than 70%. There are similar fee structures for other specific targets of prevention and for maintaining complete health records on patients.

Extra Pay for GPs in Disadvantaged Areas

GPs also receive extra pay in proportion to the number of their patients who live in deprived and/or rural areas (Farmer, 1993, pp. 60-61). Because poor patients are more often sick, have more chronic conditions, and are often more difficult to treat because of their limiting circumstances, the British developed a scale to rank areas in terms of degree of deprivation. Developed in the early 1980s by a general practitioner, Professor Brian Jarman, the scale combines demographic measures of deprivation with measures that make clinical care more difficult and expensive (Jarman, 1983). The Jarman scale is based on reports by GPs concerning factors that increase the difficulty of practice in a community. These include the proportion of older or very young people, the proportion unemployed or in poor housing, and the proportion of ethnic minorities, single-parent households, elderly living alone, and so forth. Service factors for the area are various measures of insufficient resources. Such measures were weighted and aggregated for small geographic practice areas in Britain, and each area was given an Underprivileged Area Score. Then patients enrolled in a GP's list were assigned the score for their area.

The Jarman scale became widely accepted by patients, politicians, and providers. It is used principally to increase the funds allocated to a practice, based on the number of patients from residential areas with different levels of deprivation; a provider group gets more money in proportion to the number of patients it treats from underprivileged areas.[5] This is an important way to reduce class differences in health care, the opposite of what one finds in the United States and other countries, where more money goes to providers in *affluent* areas.

Providers in affluent areas do not get less pay. Affluent people are generally no more healthy than average people; it is deprivation that correlates with health problems. In sum, despite being poorer and having much less money for health care, the British pay GPs considerably more for treating socially and economically underprivileged citizens.

The "Internal Market" Reforms and Their Effects

Nowhere in the world has the American paradigm of managed competition been so fully implemented for an entire health care system as in the United Kingdom, where the NHS meets the basic criteria for managed competition (Enthoven, 1988) better than in the United States, where none of the criteria is in place. Moreover, the British applied the model to the entire system as completely as one is likely to find when any model is adopted by a nation. Therefore, the lessons of these reforms, both positive and negative, are invaluable for policymakers elsewhere who want to bring competition more fully into health care.

The NHS meets nearly all of the stipulations for avoiding the many forms of market failure noted in Enthoven's most fully developed and balanced versions of managed competition (Enthoven, 1988). For example, the NHS already had a single, comprehensive benefits plan and universal health insurance in place. The usual systems for certifying providers, for reviewing quality, and for accountability were also in place, though in need of strengthening. There was a mature system of national and regional offices to manage the market, which needed only to be retooled and upgraded; the Management Executive could manage the overall market, and the health authorities could serve as unified purchasers, somewhat like the health alliances proposed by the Clintons.

The Thatcher administration and conservative think tanks developed ideas about managed competition for health care in the context of a universally funded and accessible foundation of primary care doctors with referral services, operating within the parameters of free care and tight budgetary constraints. Given the natural tendencies of markets to differentiate by cost, complexity, and price, this framework is vital because, as Enthoven (1988) advocated, it contains those tendencies within an equitable and universal system.

By changing every health authority from an administrative office into a "health alliance" or comprehensive market manager and every hospital, specialist, and community or home health service into a seller, the reforms of 1991 leapfrogged American manifestations of the Enthoven model, where unmanaged conditions prevailed and still do. Rarely, if ever, has an organization with a million employees and a $50-billion budget been redesigned so rapidly into something so profoundly different from what it was.

To compensate for the higher costs of treating people who are poor, old, at high risk, or living in rural areas, providers are paid more for them. To minimize skimping and underservice, the NHS version of managed competition includes significantly increased professional and consumer checks: medical audit of treatment effectiveness, a Patient's Charter of rights, an expanded complaints system, and comparative assessment of performance. Its emphasis on "fundholding"—local, community-based, and small-scale practices of what might be called primary managed care—creates the possibility of communication, accountability, and coordination with other community-based services and public health efforts.

In the following pages, we shall present five positive lessons on basic design and then turn to five sobering lessons on implementation that raise questions about whether managed competition is the right policy for Britain. The concluding section draws three lessons from recent tendencies of the NHS to shrink back from the hazards and costs of managed competition and move toward community-based purchasing (Light & May, 1993).

Five Lessons on the Design
of Managed Competition

Lesson 1: The Possibility of a Budget-Limited
Internal Market

Theoretically, competition should not work within a budget limit, and the architect of managed competition, Alain Enthoven, has repeatedly emphasized that his concept should not be subject to budget limits. But British leaders did not dare (and the Treasury would not allow them) to drop the key feature that has held NHS expenditures in check. Why not create markets of competitive contracts among doctors and hospitals within the budget limits of the NHS as a whole? The resulting design was called "the internal market." Because firms outside the NHS hold contracts too, a more accurate term might be "supply-side competition."

Lesson 2: Funds Based on Needs; Services Based on Effectiveness

This was ultimately the most profound feature of British-style managed competition, one that is now transforming the reformed health care system itself. Although HMOs and Enthoven's model of managed competition are implicitly based on the health needs of enrollees, intense annual competition between buyers distorts this goal in a number of ways. On the one hand, increasing market-induced demand is emphasized, lest a given managed-care system lose money. On the other hand, the considerable needs of patients with high risks or chronic disorders are costly and to be avoided in a market where buyers are seeking to attract the healthiest customers (and perhaps discourage the neediest).

The British approach of "supply-side managed competition" allocated to district health authorities a population-based budget roughly adjusted by risk.[6] At the level of primary care practices, the variations in budgets caused by years of differences by social class, politics, and area are greater and more inequitable. In response, the NHS is moving toward equalizing these primary care budgets so that the variations reflect needs rather than clinical practice styles and historic biases in funding. Ironically, it was a Conservative government that reduced inequities in the name of establishing a fair market (Appleby, Smith, Ranade, Little, & Robinson, 1994).

British supply-side managed competition means that each district has a single purchasing authority with the long-term responsibility to maximize the health and well-being of its population. In the context of American policy debates, it would be called *single-payer managed competition,* a combination not usually considered.

Within the first 2 years of the reforms, the British started using the term *commissioning* to signify that district purchasing authorities should do more than purchase existing services "off the shelf." Rather, "commissioning" focuses on how best to spend allotted funds so as to meet a population's needs in new, more cost-effective ways. Commissioning also aims to reduce future needs by addressing their causes. Sometimes those causes involve behaviors such as smoking or drinking. Sometimes they are ecological or community based, such as poor housing, dangerous neighborhoods, or pollution. They require providing such "nonmedical" services as teaching better skills to young mothers or providing adult caregivers of the disabled or infirm.

For a health care system built up around hospitals, major academic centers, and the elaboration of subspecialized medicine, the implications of a needs-based health care budget based on a stable population are more radical than those of managed competition. The center of *medical* care becomes the periphery of *health* care; traditional medical care becomes a "service of last resort" after one does as much as possible to prevent or diminish problems.[7]

Once it is established that services are needed, the goal is to use effective ones. The United Kingdom is going through a long, research-based process to measure effectiveness by results or outcomes; the British call this "evidence-based medicine." The point is that needs-adjusted limited budgeting for a stable population aligns priorities and incentives in fundamentally new ways. It may also highlight the extent of underservice and thus make the low level of British funding intolerable.

Lesson 3: Competition Should Take Place at the "Wholesale" Level

The American model of managed competition focuses on the "retail" consumer—patients—choosing among health plans by price and reputation. However, a good argument can be made that the complex, esoteric, and contingent nature of health care calls for professional agents to compare alternate services and buy the best services in volume for groups of consumer/patients.

The British version of managed competition uses this "wholesale" approach of having professional agents for patients negotiate bulk contracts with provider groups. The buyers are the district health authorities, though larger GP practices have also been given funds to buy some specialty and community services for their much smaller, local patient panels. This approach may be justified by evidence indicating that British patients are a long way from being the informed, smart buyers posited by the American model (Light, 1995). One is struck by the results of surveys showing how few Britishers even know what the reforms are about or have any idea about their impact on their care (Jones et al., 1994; Mahon, Wilkin, & Whitehouse, 1994). Nor do patients have much interest in going beyond their local area for better care.[8] After the reforms, only one patient in 20 asked his or her physician about other hospitals to which he or she might go. Two thirds did not know to which specialist their GP had referred them before receiving an appointment letter with their name on it. Most patients are focused on their own doctor(s) and nearby hospital(s) and put their faith in them. Even if this were not so, there are serious questions about how much time patients would be willing to devote to the kind of systematic review of competing services expected of full-time professionals.

Lesson 4: GP Fundholding as *Clinically* Managed Primary Care "HMOs"

Besides restructuring health authorities into purchasers responsible for the health needs of a population, the NHS reforms set up a program by which qualified GP groups could receive and manage the budget for a specific list of low- and medium-risk specialty and hospital services, prescriptions, home health care, community services, dietetic and chiropody services, and services for people with outpatient mental health problems and learning disabilities (Glennerster, Matsaganis, Owens, & Hancock, 1994, p. 76; Ham, 1994, p. 20).

Essentially, GP fundholding created "mini-HMOs" run by GPs. It has one of the few truly new innovations in health services design since World War II (Fry, Light, Rodnick, & Orton, 1995). It addressed a number of frustrations and wishes of GPs, who said they wanted (a) to hold funds in order to coordinate services and improve quality of care for their patients, (b) to select the specialists and hospitals with which they worked on behalf of their patients, (c) to develop a better on-site constellation of services, and (d) to have the budget to develop their own comprehensive primary care service (Glennerster et al., 1994, pp. 83-86).

GP fundholding practices and their more recent variants have distinct advantages over American-style full-service HMOs. They are small, local, and personal. They are run by the GPs themselves, so they are *clinically* managed care that is directly accountable to patients. They allow GPs to make their patient services more comprehensive.

One implication of GP fundholding is that competitive contracts do not have to cover all services or all risks, as American policy makers mistakenly believe they must (Fry et al., 1995, Chapter 8). The all-services, all-risk approach to managed competition in the United States is forcing doctors and patients into large managed-care corporations because nothing smaller can deliver the full range of services and absorb all the financial risks. This approach thus greatly reduces choice to a few large plans per area. By contrast, GP fundholding gives GP groups the funds for a wide range of relatively low-risk services, and their risk is limited to $7,500 per patient per year. After that, costs are absorbed from a reserve fund held by the area commissioning authority.

The concept of a primary care mini-HMO is ideally suited to meeting the major challenges of 1990s: providing a base for prevention and extending health promotion upstream; coordinating the growing portion of short-stay and ambulatory specialty procedures, reflecting the shift from institutions to households; developing shared care and improved management of chronic health problems; coordinating health care with other local services; and meeting threats to health such as unemployment, poverty, and HIV and other infectious diseases.

From an American point of view, four principles underlie GP fundholding (Fry et al., 1995). One is to give GPs the fiscal ability to offer their patients comprehensive primary care services. This gives patients and the system a foundation of clinically managed care rather than "MBA-managed care" and much more choice in small cities, large towns, and even semirural areas.

The second principle is to pass on enough risk to motivate GPs but not so much that they can make or lose large sums. In the NHS, a poorly run practice cannot actually lose real money, even if it goes over budget (which few do). GP fundholders do not physically hold the money; it is held in their account at the district level. If a practice "loses money" so that its account shows a negative balance, the area authority must replenish it. Before that happens, however, financial and management teams go out and review all aspects of the practice in order to turn it around.

The third principle is that profits must be plowed back into the practice. If GP fundholders try to pocket the profits personally, it is a criminal offense.

The fourth implicit principle is continuity of care, for health care is locally integrated by one's personal physician.

GP fundholding profoundly changed the organization and power structure of medicine, giving GPs the power of the purse over some specialty and hospital services. GPs got specialists to work more closely with them and be more responsive to the needs of both their patients and themselves (Farmer, 1993, pp. 62-63; Glennerster, Matsaganis, & Owens, 1994). They are also more invested now in developing good ways to care for the disabled and people with chronic problems so that they can reduce hospital admissions and specialty consultations.

Despite these design advantages, GP fundholding created serious hazards. It eliminated the purchaser/provider split that is the foundation of managed competition and may have compromised the commitment of GPs to their patients. Conflicts of interest were inherent. The organization of specialty services easily became fragmented as different fundholders made uncoordinated purchasing decisions. Fundholding decisions were uncontrolled, and no quality checks were put in place, though the situation is likely to change soon. Decentralized services and administration were inherently more costly, even if they had other clinical and political advantages. A number of the GPs felt swamped with managerial work, and overall stress was high. GPs varied greatly in their managerial competence. Inevitably, some practices were not well run, though few went into receivership. More serious, GP fundholding created a two-class system in which some patients were "sponsored" by real funds, whereas patients in nonfundholding practices were not. GPs need practice managers (which they are getting), and specialists need more stability in their budgets and professional lives than has thus far been provided.

Lesson 5: The Value of Local, Nonprofit, Community-Based Services

The limited-risk primary care contracts and the emphasis on using NHS resources when possible kept managed competition largely local and nonprofit. Although the NHS reforms were clearly intended to create a level playing field for private, for-profit providers and hospitals, for-profit medicine did not win much of the main business in acute care.[9] In 1991-1992, Appleby, Smith, Ranade, Little, and Robinson (1994, pp. 51-52) found that only 0.5% of purchasers' contracting partners were from the private sector. In 1992-1993, the private contractors accounted for only 0.04% of providers' contracts.

NHS facilities—now "self-governing trusts"—have natural advantages in competitive markets, and they learned quickly how to use them. Their capital debt is small, and they are usually more fully staffed and equipped than are private institutions. It has been NHS staff members who have done most of the private work anyway. For these reasons, as well as old ties, values, and customs, the local NHS trusts won the lion's share of the business. Vertically integrated managed-care systems could form, as in the United States, but they would have to be sufficiently more efficient to pay for the system's overhead and management costs. It is unlikely that even the best American managed-care systems could match the cost-effectiveness of current NHS arrangements. Four years of competitive contracting have not generated much movement in that direction. In the future, the reforms are likely to become even more community based because these facilities are seen as the key to cost-effective programs.

Six Negative Lessons From the British Experience With Managed Competition

Managed competition has been costly and disruptive. Many of the improvements attributed to it are continuations of earlier trends, and most innovations (such as GP fundholding) have significant drawbacks. The following lessons are drawn here from studies, observations, and interviews over the past several years.

Lesson 1: Undesired Political Consequences of Competition

The British experience with managed competition is sobering for any country that is serious about holding costs down. For since managed competition began, the British had to find more and more funds to pay for more managers, more consultants, more data, more marketing, more consumer pressures, more consumer complaints, more funds for under-budgeted areas, and more demands for high quality.

The government's own awareness of the dangers dawned soon after the reforms began. As Butler (1994) observed, before the fall of 1990 the proposals were a blueprint for a highly commercial and competitive market in health care. Early enthusiasm was also evident

> in the jubilant reception accorded the white paper [*Working for Patients* (Secretary of State for Health, 1989)] from the right wing of the Conservative party, in the hawkish early documentation produced by the NHS Management Executive on how the market would work, and in statements of ministerial intention to allow the market to produce its benign effects with minimal interferences from the Government. (Butler, 1994, p. 22)

Soon, however, ideology met up with reality, and the government realized that competition unleashed very powerful forces that historically have been used to promote economic *growth,* not restraint. The government also realized, from the poor business plans of the first self-governing trust hospitals and from the inability of health authorities to purchase, that the reform to which it was committed could quickly become a disaster. In response, the government took a number of actions to minimize the very competition it was boldly promising.

By December 1990, the Secretary of State for Health admitted that the government had been carried away in its application of business thinking to health care. A "sea-change" took place behind the scenes, one evident in language changes by 1991. "Buyers" became "purchasers" and then "commissioners." "Sellers" became "providers," acknowledging their distinct and central role in medicine. Most important, "marketing" became "needs assessment." Ever since, the government has found itself in the awkward position of setting up the structure for a highly competitive market, yet caging its forces and denying to an anxious public and suspicious press that any such thing has taken place.

The policy of managed competition has been a command performance by a powerfully centralized government. One might call it *dictated competition*, perhaps a contradiction in economic theory but not in politics. Ironically, however, politically dictated competition meant that actual competition was minimized. The Department of Health and the Management Executive issued orders, directives, executive letters, and advisories by the hundreds that specified the terms on which competition would take place.[10] First, the government required a practice year of "shadow purchasing," during which the provider units and their administrative offices were required to provide the same services from the same sources with nearly the same budgets but were to make up "shadow" contracts. Next, the government required that the first year of real contracts must go largely to the same providers, for nearly the same services, so that there would be a "steady state" and a "smooth take-off" for the internal market. There followed hundreds of pages of terms, guidelines, and prohibitions from the Management Executive and the Department of Health.

The chairs of all health authority boards were and are appointed by the Secretary of State for Health. This eliminated the famous civil service professionalism of Great Britain, replacing it with survival of the politically loyal.[11]

Finally, the government quickly reined in the ability of trust hospitals to borrow money. They had to earn 6% return on assets in use, to break even each year, to stay within their external financing limit, to set prices equal to average costs, to have no cross-subsidization between services, to make no capital investment that could not be demonstrated to be fully recovered from contract income, to not dispose of their surpluses, and to obtain most of their income from contracts with NHS authorities and fundholders. Trusts cannot go bankrupt. Bartlett and LeGrand (1994) concluded that "the independence and autonomy available to trusts is highly circumscribed, and the incentives to improve performance, which might be expected to be associated with an ability to retain financial surpluses earned through improved management performance, are eliminated" (p. 56).

How much competition and change, then, have occurred? The empirical studies that exist find much less change than declared by senior officers or perceived by those in the market (Whitehead, 1994). GP fundholders universally thought they were changing referral patterns and waiting lists much more than the evidence indicated. In one of the few well-designed studies comparing fundholders with comparable GP practices not holding funds, Angela Coulter's team (Coulter & Bradlow, 1993) showed that fundholders did not scrimp on referrals to save money and were not less restricted in referring outside the district and to the private sector than were nonfundholders. Nor were waiting lists and waiting times shortened; in fact, they rose slightly, but with a shifting of waiting time from fundholding patients to nonfundholding patients. A related study found that fundholding practices spent less on drugs, largely because of a one-time switch to generics.

GP fundholding succeeded in getting consultants to be more responsive to both patients and providers, to write up clinical notes promptly, to review treatment plans with GPs, and to see patients at or near the referring GP's practice site.[12] A major change was that differences in the quality and promptness of services for patients emerged between fundholding and nonfundholding practices (Whitehead, 1994). A parallel study of hospitalized patients found few changes and "no marked improvement from 1990 to 1992" (Jones et al., 1994, p. 150).

Consultants probably experienced the most change—largely for the worse, they would say. The reforms crumbled their fortified walls unlike any previous changes in the system; for their operating budgets became destabilized and were at the mercy of district health authorities, hospital managers, and GP fundholders. In the future, their salaries and pensions may become subject to local and multiple negotiation as well.

British specialty services were a major example of embedded inefficiency (Light, 1991b). Something had to be done to make them more responsive to clients, more efficiently coordinated with primary care teams, and more accountable. But the cross-cutting arrangements went so far that they threatened the minimal stability needed to run a good clinical service for patients. Moreover, low morale, battles with lay managers, disruptions in service, and the costs of new arrangements meant that "savings" may have cost more than they saved. However, there were no systematic evaluations of the reforms on major medical and specialty services.

On the purchasers' side, systematic evidence showed that past funding patterns were altered only at the margins and often at variance with declared priorities. "In other words, there is a sharp contrast between priority talk and priority decisions" (Klein & Redmayne, 1993, p. 17). On the whole, Klein (1993) found that policy was "driven by concern about the details of the contracts, instead of determining the nature of contractual arrangements" (p. 6). Time pressures and lack of good data made this almost inevitable.

Purchasers' first priorities were to maintain acute medical services, to set up the machinery for purchasing, and to respond to a flood of demands for different priorities from Whitehall, from different sectors of clinical care, from consumers, and from managers—all within about the same budget as the year before. Yet each authority had a unique configuration of services and institutions, local issues, and power structures. Reallocation of existing funds came hard. When some authorities got explicit about rationing and presented proposals to GPs or the public, protests against exclusions as "the thin end of a very undesirable wedge" forced them to abandon the effort (Redmayne, Klein, & Day, 1992). Purchasers, Klein (1993) concluded, "are caught between two millstones. On one hand, there are the top-down constraints and priorities and, on the other, the bottom-up pressures" (p. 76). Purchasers muddle through competing demands and constraints in an incremental way. Klein argued that in fact the diffuse process of incrementalism reflects the nature of organizational knowledge more accurately than does the rational model.

Given the political nature of markets in medicine, the British found that they had to impose safeguards and damage controls, which resulted in little economic competition taking place. Without failure and exit, there cannot be much competition, and in most national health care systems trying to contain costs, there is not much entry of new competitors either. Moreover, a national system with a history of tight budgets and taut supply or choice means that little can change. The question for other countries drawn to the theory of managed competition is whether they dare let health care markets "run" freely. Are they ready to watch as competitors drop unprofitable services, expand profitable ones to oversupply, and drive less well-managed hospitals into bankruptcy? For if they are not, then they will end up with all of the extra costs of competition and few of its potential savings.

Competition, even within budgets, unleashes and rewards entrepreneurial forces that constantly expand the system. Even when hospital beds are closed and nurses are replaced by nurse's aides, other parts of the system expand. The inevitable result is a pressure to increases revenues— that is, costs. The expansionary pressures are clear, even though in theory competition is supposed to focus only on increasing efficiency *within* budgetary constraints.

Lesson 2: The Need for Good Market Information and Effective Purchasers

At the outset, the government neglected the obvious fact that effective competition depends on there being good market information and strong purchasers. Surveys in 1991 and 1992 of NHS managers found high agreement that the "information required was limited, non-existent, inaccurate, or late. . . . Progress on needs-assessment was also fitful" (Appleby et al., 1994, pp. 34-35). Eighty percent of the purchasers surveyed said they had difficulty obtaining comparable cost data in 1991, a figure that dropped to only 70% in 1992. Sixty-five percent said they also lacked data on patient flows. Over 70% of provider/sellers surveyed also said that obtaining cost data was a problem. As a result, health authorities had no choice but to purchase largely by means of block contracts with hospitals and units in their vicinity, hardly what advocates had in mind as competition. By 1992-1993, 88% of all contracts were still block contracts, and only 10% were based on costs per procedure (Appleby et al., 1994, pp. 40, 42-43).

Exacerbating this basic problem was a widely perceived migration of talent from buyers to sellers. Talented managers from health authorities (the purchasers-to-be) and even from the Management Executive rushed to be chief executives of the new trust hospitals because the money and action were there.

GP fundholders appeared to be an important exception, and they quickly gained a reputation for being astute purchasers. Because they knew their patients and their problems, they could induce change at the margins (Glennerster et al., 1994, p. 100). But their reputation as good purchasers exceeded the degree of change that actually has taken place (Coulter & Bradlow, 1993; Roland & Coulter, 1992).

The British did perceive the need for good information about quality of care and made "medical audit" part of the reforms. But an independent assessment concluded that because it was done by clinicians of their own work, medical audit was largely "an extension of the profession's current self-management arrangements" (Kerrison, Packwood, & Buxton, 1994, p. 157). Audit funds went specifically to senior doctors, not to purchasers or even managers. They defined what aspects of medicine were to be audited (mainly technical aspects) and by what measures. Purchasing was not tied to the results of audit, and clinicians did not emphasize resource use as an important focus of medical audit.

Lesson 3: Providers Can Become Entrepreneurs and Potential Monopolists

At the same time that the reforms began with little market information and weak purchasers, their design rewarded providers who changed from thinking of themselves as public servants to thinking of themselves as entrepreneurs and exploiting their monopolistic advantages. Overall, few sellers compete with one another in the NHS; yet one needs choice and therefore slack in a market if competition is to make producers more efficient. In the case of the NHS, careful planning and tight budgeting over the previous decades had kept duplication to a minimum, so that introducing competition tended to strengthen the hand of provider/sellers rather than buyers. In short, competition in taut, highly imperfect markets can backfire and turn carefully budgeted providers into active monopolists. The dangers of monopolistic action by provider/sellers are abetted by several factors: the weakness of buyers, as discussed above; the disinclination of patients to travel very far, so that de facto markets are small; and the existence of restrictive collegial behaviors that are regarded by economists as anticompetitive (Light, 1994b, p. 363). Moreover, the "product" being bought and sold is often difficult to define because medical services are ordered only as diagnosis and treatment unfold and are contingent on information and responses to previous efforts (Light, 1993). Property rights are fuzzy. It is not even clear who is buying and who is selling, for the seller/providers often decide what is to be done (bought) and serve as the buyer's (patient's) agent. Independent information on what is being bought (however that gets defined) is difficult and costly to gather. The seller/providers control much of the information needed to decide what to buy and can easily manipulate this information if given the incentives to do so. Patients, moreover, often want it this way. All of these problems became evident within the first year, and several still plague the British reforms.

So far, entrepreneurial exploitation by British doctors has been minimal, in part because the government has severely restricted such behavior and in part because the cultural shift to a commercial ethos takes many years, as it has in the United States since the end of World War II (Light, 1997; Starr, 1982). But the dangers of commercialism may well increase. GPs have now been given a high economic stake in a wide array of services, and although they may not pocket profits, there are ways of plowing them back into the practice so that doctors benefit. Consultants (chiefs of services) have had to become small businesspeople and increasingly to market their services. Trust hospitals have only begun to exercise their powers to alter staff mix, compensation, and contracts. The potential for underservice, "wallet biopsy," distrust between patients and providers and among providers, exploitation of patients and markets, and increased inequality is ominous. The commercialization of medicine in the United States since the late 1960s has produced all these effects while greatly increasing costs. To what extent will the NHS reforms also spur entrepreneurial expansion while increasing transaction costs?

Competition aims to turn physicians and others into entrepreneurs, driven by incentives to maximize their self-interests on the grounds that perfect markets improve services and efficiency for everyone. There is considerable ambivalence about this in Britain. Even the market managers at the Management Executive want doctors to retain their dedication to patients and their service ethos. They are disturbed by suggestions or evidence that doctors assume a commercial ethos, even as they promote it (personal interviews).

Lesson 4: Competition Created New Inefficiencies and Costs

Even though it was supposed to save money overall, competition in health care created new inefficiencies and costs that were often not discussed in advance. Very large costs went into constructing the basic market itself—defining what the "products" were, determining costs, setting prices, gathering market information, contracting, monitoring— because the bureaucratically organized NHS had little need for itemized costs or prices. There has also been a wide and diverse effort to obtain data on every aspect of productivity, quality, and cost-effectiveness. The cost of collecting all these data was estimated early on to subtract about 10% of the budget from clinical services (Light, 1990c). Large sums were invested in computer systems and data systems that often did not work, did not provide the necessary information for purchasing, or were not compatible with each other. At the annual meeting of the Federation of NHS Trusts in 1995, it was determined that the majority of trust hospitals still lacked the information necessary to assess their cost-effectiveness and thus to make competition a viable enterprise.

The fact that in a competitive market there are winners and losers leads to further potential problems (Light, 1991b). Winning institutions may find themselves swamped with more business than they can handle. Quality and efficiency may decline as a result. Meanwhile, losers become still more inefficient as their unused capacity rises. Because it is extremely difficult to shut down a health care facility, the increased inefficiencies of losers may be dragged along in the system for some time as part of everyone's costs. In short, winning and losing may not produce efficiencies if markets clear slowly and if the costs of losing institutions have to be carried.

Contributing to the costs of competition was the granting of new freedoms and power to qualified hospitals as "self-governing trusts." This gave those deeply entrenched institutions more powers and more incentives to persist and grow at a time when the nation needs to dehospitalize and reallocate the large sums locked up in hospital-based services.

Some of the dislocations resulting from the reforms are good in the sense that they show the market is working. Increased use of local secondary care has left major tertiary care centers in financial crisis. Perhaps the most notable cases resulted from the decisions by purchasers around London to buy specialty services nearby rather than send patients to the very expensive, major academic hospitals in London. This certainly highlighted the inefficiencies, waste, and oversupply of academic medical centers, but the size and scope of dislocations were so great that the government essentially administered the situation in an old-style state planning mode, closing or consolidating facilities by administrative fiat.

The generous allocations to GP fundholders depleted the budgets of district health authorities so that some could not pay for nonemergency care. This, in turn, created a two-tier market between the "sponsored" patients of fundholders and the unsponsored patients of GPs who do not hold funds. Whitehead (1994) nicely summarized the evidence that the patients of fundholders received preferential treatment. It also created budget refugees, known as "extracontractual referrals," because some patients see consultants not under contract with their home authority or GP. These inequities, however, have been counterbalanced by the unprecedented reductions in inequities between regions, between districts, between hospitals, and between GP practices obtained by recalibrating budgets on a needs-adjusted capitation basis.

During the first 3 years of competitive markets, managerial costs in the NHS approximately doubled, from 5% to 11% of total expenditures. The number of managers in the system approximately tripled, in large part to handle the complex and relentless requirements of contracting.[13] Managerial salaries rose two to three times faster than doctors' or nurses' salaries. Compensation for the senior executive of trust hospitals approximately doubled between 1990 and 1995.

Managers have become increasingly professionalized and a countervailing power to the medical profession. They claim improved efficiency and productivity, though the data are lacking to support this, and U.S. data indicate that the managerial revolution there primarily benefited managers (Woolhandler & Himmelstein, 1994).

Lesson 5: Ideological Conviction Precluded Evaluation

The conclusion that using competition to solve the problems of health care involved more ideological conviction than reality testing is a judgment that is widely held in the United Kingdom (May, 1993; Webster, 1993). By international standards, British health care had one of the lowest administrative overheads and smallest per capita budgets in the Western world. If "efficiency" is measured by services per million dollars, then the NHS was among the most efficient. Although Mrs. Thatcher declared that crises due to underfunding were caused by inefficiencies that managed competition would rectify, there is considerable evidence that underfunding itself was (and is) a major source of inefficiency. Beds and services routinely had to be closed down because a given hospital or unit ran out of money before the year's end. In fact, underfunding may be one of the major sources of inefficiency in the NHS because units have to carry the dead weight costs of underused capacity (Light, 1990b, 1991a).

Compared to the previous two decades, funding for units of service slowed down during the 1980s (Robinson & Judge, 1987). Yet costly technological advances, rising expectations, and the burdens of an aging population all accelerated the volume of services. The government was repeatedly attacked in the late 1980s for underfunding and letting desperately ill patients wait for treatment and even die while waiting (Butler, 1994). The presidents of three senior Royal Colleges called on the government to "save our health service, once the envy of the world" (Hoffenberg, Todd, & Pinker, 1987, p. 1505). An editorial in the *British Medical Journal* declared the NHS to be in terminal decline (Smith, 1988). Thus, a strong case can be made that many of the problems, and certainly the ones that pushed Mrs. Thatcher into making the market reforms, were largely due to underfunding. Efficiency gains from the managerial reforms and the contracting out of services during the earlier part of the 1980s meant that "there was little more scope within the existing system for greater yields without the addition of further resources" (Webster, 1993, p. 19).

It was easy to blame the problems of the NHS on the public administration of welfare services and to imagine that competition would greatly
enhance value for money, ignoring the fact that private health care systems
have far more costly forms of specialty and academic dominance, much
larger administrative overheads, and many of the same micro- and macro-
inefficiencies. Thus, British conservative policy followed Enthoven's
(1985) influential policy analysis of NHS inefficiencies and attributed
the problems of the NHS to "perverse incentives" and "gridlock."
When people are paid a wage or salary, or institutions receive a budget,
Enthoven argued, they face "perverse incentives" not to improve quality
or efficiency.

One problem with this diagnosis is that it ignored the impressive gains
in efficiency that these salaried providers and public administrators had
actually accomplished. During the 1980s, NHS hospital specialists and
administrators shortened length of stay for medical cases by 29% and for
surgical cases by 13%, while increasing throughput by 47% (National
Association of Health Authorities and Trusts, 1992). They decreased the
average cost of geriatric cases by 24% and of acute inpatient cases by 10%
in constant pounds. For nearly the same amount of constant pounds in
1989 as in 1980, they treated 16% more inpatients and 19% more
emergency cases and did 73% more ambulatory surgery. One would be
hard pressed to find a better record of improved efficiency and continuous
adaptation than under these conditions of "gridlock" and "perverse incentives." The question for the 1990s is whether managed competition can
match this record.

The ideology of competition emphasized more choice and an end to
the infamous "efficiency trap" caused by fixed budgets so that money did
not follow patients. In fact, however, managed competition in health care
limits choice and makes patients follow contract money.

The government also chose ideology over reality by not examining
closely the character of the inefficiencies it wished to reduce. Had it
done so, it would have found that many of the inefficiencies were
embedded in professional standards, clinical habits, the organization
of work, the division of labor, hierarchies of power, and organizational
rules (Light, 1991b). Some of the embedded inefficiencies found in the
NHS at the start of managed competition included wasted bed days,
underused theater (operating room) time, overused theater time, subspe-
cialists being embedded in hospitals, high staff turnover, uncoordinated
staff leaves, bureaucratic elaboration, and the overuse of hospitals (Light,
1990a, 1990c). Such embedded inefficiencies are likely to be carried
forward within the calculations of costs and the structure of contracts as

part of the taken-for-granted nature of work when competitive bidding is established.

The government chose ideology over reality by ignoring the well-known imperfections of health care markets and not discussing carefully how it would address them. It acted ideologically by overpromoting the highly visible features of the reforms, even while losing sight of the overall goal of cost-effective purchasing based on needs. Thus, it accepted applicants for trust status despite their submitting poor business plans and then avoided trouble by quietly reining in what "self-governing" trusts could do (Light, 1991c). It was as if the government was more interested in the semblance of competition than in allowing much competition to take place. Although creating a market within the NHS was supposed to depoliticize cost control, the government was also not willing to bear the political consequences of failures or bankruptcies. Ironically, for reasons explained below, the NHS is more politicized now than it was ever before.

The government also accepted almost any GP group that wanted to be a fundholder and offered generously estimated budgets, even though this load on the budgets of district purchasing authorities jeopardized their ability to pay for hospital care. Thus, the government chose the highly visible fundholding scheme, which was largely unregulated and not needs based, at the cost of gutting its design of comprehensive, supply-side competition as a means of meeting community and individual health needs.

Finally, the government did not commission empirical studies of the services or the markets it was creating because independent evaluation of performance was not thought to be "necessary." Further, it changed the ways in which data were collected or classified, thus making before-and-after comparisons difficult. This antiempirical stance seems to have softened by 1995. Yet as recently as December 1994, the *British Medical Journal* published details about suppressed data, use of the Official Secrets Act to block information about services, and gag clauses in trust contracts prohibiting doctors from saying anything critical about the quality of medicine they observed (Smith, 1994).

In these ways, the British policies advocating competition to bring tough-minded realism to health care were not rooted in reality or in a clear vision of where the NHS should go and a strategic plan for getting there. After summarizing the central elements of the reforms, Butler (1994) asked, "Yet what was it all for? What were the goals or purposes or objectives of the white paper? . . . What was the theory underlying the Government's belief in the capacity of the internal market to enhance the efficient use of resources?" (pp. 9, 20).

The ideology of competition promised to depoliticize cost containment (Enthoven, 1985). Instead, health care services have become more politicized at the same time that market forces have come into play. The choice, then, is politicized health care without economic competition or with it (Klein, 1991). With it, the political stakes get considerably higher because risks get higher and services become destabilized.

When choosing an ideological solution to real problems led to undesirable consequences, the British government's response was to announce success by declaration. This involved three notable policies. One required that no one in a national position speak critically of government actions. This in effect produced a blackout of realistic exchange about the problems. One experienced an almost surreal disjuncture between the blunt, smart, realistic reporting of problems by good British journalists and the vague, elusive, sweet responses from high officials. It was unclear whether those who were managing the market—on whom the success of managed competition completely depended (Enthoven, 1988, 1993)—really did not hear the problems or merely denied them publicly. This "we can do no wrong" posture greatly limited what could be done to repair a decision that is not working.

Another way that feedback on problems was minimized stemmed from the lack of consumer or "retail-level" involvement in markets. Of course, consumerism appeared to be one of the basic platforms of the market reforms; the key document is entitled *Working for Patients* (Secretary of State for Health, 1989). Yet the government had commissioned little research on the role and dynamics of patient preferences, and a good case can be made that working "for" patients meant that consumer choice was irrelevant because the NHS would provide the best possible care for everyone (Mahon et al., 1994). Patients were little involved in choosing a hospital or consultant, yet seemed highly satisfied with the choices made.

Beyond Managed Competition: Three Positive Lessons

Lesson 1: Focus on Commissioning Rather Than on Competition

By the second year of the reforms, many NHS executives and purchasers began to express in interviews their exasperation with competing against one another, especially in markets that the central management was constantly altering. Wasn't the point of needs-based purchasing to *work together* to figure out how best to spend a limited budget to help people with health problems? Didn't this mean that the act of purchasing—or even better, commissioning—was what really mattered (Light, 1994c)?

The conversion of administrative authorities into purchasers with budgets for the health care of a fixed population has transformed thinking from a focus on clinical intervention to an emphasis on prevention, health maintenance, new configurations, and accountability. Purchasing or commissioning promotes accountability, value for money, and a structured process of reflecting on what one is doing that administering services does not do. For instead of service groups getting a new year's budget based on their last year's budget, they must come together to agree on a common needs-based budget and think through (or fight out) more cost-effective ways to reallocate funds and reconfigure their services.

The principal lesson that has emerged from the British experience with systemwide managed competition seems to be that *almost all the benefits of the health care reforms stem from the act of purchasing, and almost all the hazards, inequities, and cost run-ups come from competing.* This conclusion may seem strange, for how can one purchase without competition resulting? Certainly, some competition is inherent in purchasing, but it can be very little, and the policy focus makes a great difference. The paradox of purchasing without (much) competition is solved by setting rules for equity, universality, and cost containment that have the net effect of minimizing supply-side economic competition in a market prone to distortions and market failure.

Cooperative purchasing between parties or enterprises that have a common goal (such as maximizing the health of a people) is similar to the Japanese approach toward economic growth, in which protected entities (like health authorities) have long-term relationships with the best producers they can find and work mutually with them to improve service and product (Best, 1990; Johnson, 1995). This neglected 19th-century theory of economic growth differs markedly from Anglo-American ideas about competition (Fallows, 1993). Competition focuses on the process of buying and selling between units. It assumes that this process will increase wealth for everyone. Cooperative and regulated purchasing focuses on maximizing production (in this case of health) for entire communities and society.[14] Whereas the results of competition are unplanned, with a roller-coaster of profits and losses, cooperative and regulated purchasing is based on long-term planning. Competition assumes there will be more and more money and wealth, so that everyone can keep winning. However, in the zero-sum situation produced by a global health care budget, competition maximizes losers and disruption in a frustrating contest of everyone against everyone else.

Lesson 2: The Value of Needs-Based
Joint Commissioning

The focus on purchasing within limited budgets leads inexorably to "promoting the health of the population, involving it in a wide range of relationships extending beyond the NHS itself" (Functions Analysis Group 7, 1994, p. 1). Purchasing for the health needs of a population fundamentally requires asking, "How can we best spend this money to meet the health needs of our area?" That question, in turn, quickly engenders complex but important debates about what "need" means, how to measure it, and how to decide which needs get priority over others. All this has led the British to reconceptualize purchasing as "commissioning"— that is, the creative rethinking of what kinds of services will best maximize the health of a population or community. Needs-based commissioning, in turn, calls for *joint* commissioning—that is, the joining of budgets so that integrated plans can be carried out.

Joint commissioning initially referred to joining the GP budget for primary care with the health authority budget for specialty and community health care.

> With GPs responsible for referring patients to hospital . . . and health authorities responsible for placing contracts with hospitals, there was an obvious requirement that [they] should work together to decide what services should be purchased and where contracts should be placed. (Ham & Spurgeon, 1992, p. 7)

Joint commissioning centers on the creative process of figuring out how best to spend limited funds to maximize the health of a population. It is now the revolutionary force in the NHS.

As early as the second year, purchasers were advocating it (Ham & Heginbotham, 1991). They found that they could best assess health needs together. Starting in the second year of managed competition and expanding rapidly in the third, top administrators started forming joint commissioning authorities (even though these were illegal because each partner was required to purchase in its own domain). The senior managers developed elaborate informal procedures and accounting mechanisms to obey the spirit of the law while breaching it in reality. Parliament hastily began to write a law to make the inevitable legal. As these and other developments have strengthened purchasing, providers have combined organizationally and politically to match the size and power of the joint authorities. The fragmenting effects of GP fundholding on needs-based purchasing and on addressing the overall needs of a population also require coordination.

Yet joint commissioning is not easy. Overcoming professionalism and its battle-hardened tactics of turf protection entails a complex, long, and sometimes painful effort to reconcile quite different visions of needs, and beliefs about which interventions are most effective. Further, GP fundholders operate at a local, clinical level that somehow has to be put in the context of a district's overall health needs. "The dilemma here is that health authorities and fundholders offer a starkly contrasting approach to purchasing. . . . In simple terms, the choice is between needs-based purchasing for large populations and demand-based purchasing for small populations" (Ham & Spurgeon, 1992, p. 32). Yet all agree that it is the larger goals of preventing illness and death to which all purchasing should be directed.

Joint commissioning also refers to joining the health services budget with that for community care services (which are now part of local or municipal social service budgets). This is very complicated and politically charged, for NHS services are not means tested, but local services are. Is nursing home care a social service, a part of public housing with a nurse or doctor coming in now and then, or is it a part of health care? Similar questions are being raised about many other services for people with chronic conditions. *Joint commissioning* can also refer to joining the budget for public health with those for clinical services. Britain, like many countries, has a master plan for prevention, but it must be expressed in priorities for funding and decisions about the reorganization involved in joint commissioning. Community health and social services, which are much more extensive than in the United States, are part of this integration. Many interesting and original models for integrating medical and social programs are being developed. The obvious need to work with authorities involved in reducing crime and violence, providing safe and adequate housing, generating more jobs, and training the workforce widens that circle still further. In short, the British have discovered that underlying managed competition for cost-effective medical services is the agenda to prevent illness and death, promote health, and mobilize community-based health programs.

Lesson 3: The Need to Emphasize Long-Term Responsibility and Continuity

The lesson for American managed competition is that multiple purchasers competing to maximize profits in fluid markets are unlikely to address the most pressing health needs or serve the most needy well. In fact, if they do, they will lose money and therefore undermine the investor confidence needed for survival. Given that so much cost goes to the care of so few very sick people—about 72% of costs consumed by only 10% of a population—incentives to avoid them or disenroll them are intense.

The British have focused on joint purchasing authorities that have a long-term responsibility for enhancing health and improving services for a resident population. This is the only way that effective programs can be developed and implemented to good effect. Trust and accountability are maximized, in contrast to the high rates of switching and the spot markets that characterize the more "advanced" American system. In the case of health care, almost everyone agrees that improvement should center on the health status and functioning of people in the community.

In many ways, these last three adaptable policy lessons reinforce the goals and vision with which the NHS started, but which were only partly attained after 1948. The eight lessons with which we began all concern a *medical* service. Through the transformation from budgeting services to purchasing for improving the health of populations, the NHS has sharpened its focus on the reasons for its existence. The first eight adaptable policy lessons, together with these last three, will prepare the United Kingdom (or any other nation) to address the tidal wave of chronic conditions—many of which can be prevented, minimized, or postponed—that will extend well into the 21st century.

Notes

1. Composition, operation, and evaluation of the Management Board and the management of the markets could be the subject of another report.

2. A corollary of this principle, practiced in Great Britain, is that medical education should be free; training doctors is as much a public good as training police.

3. The complexities of calibrating career earnings, given different career structures, length, and structure of pensions, requires separate treatment.

4. These grants were based on detailed and complex formulas that reflected the size and location of practice as well as other factors.

5. The scale ranges from –62 to +73, with 0 being set at the national average. Negative scores are assigned to areas with less deprivation than average. Deprivation pay is given per capita according to the proportion of patients living in election wards with a high Underprivileged Area (UPA) score. A practice receives a supplement equal to 40% over its capitation rate for adults aged 18 to 65 for each enrollee from a ward with a UPA score of 30 to 39, 52% extra for each enrollee from a ward with a UPA score of 40 to 49, and 70% extra for those from an area with a score of 50 or more. Assuming that a pound was worth $1.50, the capitation rate in 1994 was $21.90 per year for enrollees aged 0 to 65, $28.95 for enrollees aged 65 to 75, and $55.95 for enrollees over 75. The Jarman deprivation payments added

362 THE BRITISH EXPERIENCE

$10.25 per year per patient from areas with a score of 30-39, $12.44 for scores 40 to 49, and $17.90 for scores over 50 (Lillie Road GP Fundholder, 1994).

6. This leveling of the playing field means that large past inequities between affluent and poorer areas are being rectified. Because implementing this formula all at once would mean that some regions would experience serious budgetary reductions from historical budgets based on utilization and politics, the change is being phased in gradually.

7. This approach reflects the work of Archie Cochrane, a pioneer in social medicine after whom the Cochrane centers around the world were named and whose tenets make up the Cochrane test for an efficient and effective health care system (Light, 1991a).

8. Three quarters of the patients who had waited for more than 1 year for an elective procedure were unwilling to travel more than 10 miles, no farther than 77.5% of those seen within a month said they were willing to travel (Mahon et al., 1994, pp. 118-121).

9. Private for-profit and nonprofit providers have become a major presence in the care of the elderly, the mentally handicapped, and the mentally ill, thanks to a funding door that Mrs. Thatcher opened to the Treasury. As a result, expenditures rose over 100-fold in these areas, not quite what Mrs. Thatcher had in mind when she championed the efficiency of the private sector.

10. See the extraordinary set of brief articles assembled by the editor of the *British Medical Journal* and entitled "The Rise of Statism in the NHS" (Smith, 1994). The Management Executive is formally part of the Department of Health, but it is so powerful that its influence has become at least parallel to, if not greater than, that of the department itself.

11. Thus, even low-level staff personnel in the second and third years explained in confidential interviews that they felt they must either report "doctored" data on the success of the reforms so that their superiors would have their expectations confirmed by "facts" or be criticized for turning in "bad" reports.

12. A study of older patients, who use services most and have the most health problems, found few changes or changed perceptions between 1990 (the year the reforms started) and 1992, except that waiting times *increased* (Jones et al., 1994).

13. The increased number is due partly to supervising nurses being reclassified as "managers"; this is a principal way for them to receive increased remuneration.

14. Ironically, the United Kingdom used this approach to become the strongest industrialized nation in the world and then started to lose its strength when it shifted to laissez-faire, Adam Smith competition (Fallows, 1993; Lazonick, 1991).

References

Aaron, H., & Schwartz, W. (1984). *The painful prescription*. Washington, DC: Brookings Institution.

Allen, D. (1984). Health services in England. In M. Raffel (Ed.), *Comparative health systems* (pp. 197-258). University Park: Pennsylvania State University Press.

Appleby, J., Smith, P., Ranade, W., Little, V., & Robinson, R. (1994). Monitoring managed competition. In R. Robinson & J. LeGrand (Eds.), *Evaluating the NHS reforms* (pp. 24-53). London: King's Fund Institute.

Bartlett, W., & LeGrand, J. (1994). The performance of trusts. In R. Robinson & J. LeGrand (Eds.), *Evaluating the NHS reforms* (pp. 54-73). London: King's Fund Institute.

Best, M. (1990). *The new competition: Institutions of industrial restructuring*. Oxford: Polity.

Butler, J. (1994). Origins and early development. In R. Robinson & J. LeGrand (Eds.), *Evaluating the NHS reforms* (pp. 13-23). London: King's Fund Institute.

Coulter, A., & Bradlow, J. (1993). Effect of NHS reforms on general practitioners' referral patterns. *British Medical Journal, 306,* 433-437.

Eckstein, H. (1958). *The English health services.* Cambridge, MA: Harvard University Press.

Enthoven, A. (1985). *Reflections on the management of the National Health Service: An American looks at incentives to efficiency in health services management in the UK.* London: Nuffield Provicial Hospitals Trust.

Enthoven, A. (1988). *Theory and practice of managed competition in health care finance.* Amsterdam: North-Holland.

Enthoven, A. (1993). The history and principles of managed competition. *Health Affairs, 12*(Suppl.), 24-48.

Fallows, J. (1993). How the world works. *Atlantic Monthly, 172*(6), 61-87.

Farmer, A. (1993). The changing role of general practice in the British National Health Service. In D. Light & A. May (Eds.), *Britain's health system: From welfare state to managed markets* (pp. 57-66). New York: Faulkner & Gray.

Fowler, N. (1991). *Ministers decide.* London: Chapman.

Fox, D. (1993). *Power and illness: The failure and future of American health policy.* Berkeley: University of California Press.

Franks, P., Clancy C., & Nutting, P. (1992). Gatekeeping revisited: Protecting patients from overtreatment. *New England Journal of Medicine, 327,* 424-429.

Fry, J., Light, D. W., Rodnick, J., & Orton, J. (1995). *Reviving primary care: A US-UK comparison.* Oxford, UK: Radcliffe Medical Press.

Functions Analysis Group 7. (1994). *Local strategy and purchasing.* London: National Health Service Management Executive.

Glennerster, H., Matsaganis, M., & Owens, P. (1994). *A foothold on fundholding.* London: King's Fund Institute.

Glennerster, H., Matsaganis, M., Owens, P., & Hancock, S. (1994). GP fundholding: Wild card or winning hand? In R. Robinson & J. LeGrand (Eds.), *Evaluating the NHS reforms* (pp. 74-107). London: King's Fund Institute.

Grumbach, K., & Fry, J. (1993). Managing primary care in the United States and the United Kingdom. *New England Journal of Medicine, 328,* 940-945.

Ham, C. (1994). *Management and competition in the new NHS.* Oxford, UK: Radcliffe Medical Press.

Ham, C., & Heginbotham, C. (1991). *Purchasing together.* London: Kings Fund College.

Ham, C., & Spurgeon, P. (1992). *Effective purchasing* (HSMC Discussion Paper No. 28). Birmingham, UK: Health Services Management Centre.

Hoffenberg, R., Todd, P., & Pinker, G. (1987). Crisis in the National Health Service. *British Medical Journal, 295,* 1505.

Hollingsworth, J. (1986). *A political economy of medicine: Great Britain and the United States.* Baltimore: Johns Hopkins University Press.

Jarman, B. (1983). Identification of underprivileged areas. *British Medical Journal, 286,* 1705-1709.

Johnson, C. (1995). *Japan: Who governs?* New York: Norton.

Jones, D., Lester, C., & West, R. (1994). Monitoring changes in health services for older people. In R. Robinson & J. LeGrand (Eds.), *Evaluating the NHS reforms* (pp. 130-154). London: King's Fund Institute.

Kerrison, S., Packwood, P., & Buxton, M. (1994). Monitoring medical audit. In R. Robinson & J. LeGrand (Eds.), *Evaluating the NHS reforms* (pp. 155-177). London: King's Fund Institute.

Klein, R. (1991). The politics of change. *British Medical Journal, 302,* 1102-1103.

Klein, R. (1993). Rationality and rationing: Diffused or concentrated decision making? In M. Tunbridge (Ed.), *Rationing of health care in medicine* (pp. 73-81). London: Royal College of Physicians.

Klein, R., & Redmayne, S. (1993). *Patterns of priorities: A study of the purchasing and rationing policies of health authorities.* Birmingham, UK: National Association of Health Authorities and Trusts.

Lazonick, W. (1991). *Business organization and the myth of the market economy.* Cambridge, UK: Cambridge University Press.

Light, D. (1990a). Biting hard on the research bit. *Health Service Journal, 100,* 1604-1605.

Light, D. (1990b). Labelling waste as inefficiency. *Health Service Journal, 100,* 1552-1553.

Light, D. (1990c). Learning from their mistakes? *Health Service Journal, 100,* 1470-1472.

Light, D. (1991a). Effectiveness and efficiency under competition: The Cochrane test. *British Medical Journal, 303,* 1253-1254.

Light, D. (1991b). Embedded inefficiencies in health care. *Lancet, 338,* 102-104.

Light, D. (1991c). Observations on the NHS reforms: An American perspective. *British Medical Journal, 303,* 568-570.

Light, D. (1992). The practice and ethics of risk-rated health insurance. *Journal of the American Medical Association, 267,* 2503-2508.

Light, D. (1993). Escaping the traps of postwar Western medicine. *European Journal of Public Health, 3,* 223-231.

Light, D. (1994a). Comparative models of "health care" systems, with application to Germany. In P. Conrad & R. Kern (Eds.), *The sociology of health and illness.* New York: St. Martin's.

Light, D. (1994b). Health care systems and their financing. In J. Walton, G. Owen, & P. Rhodes (Eds.), *The new Oxford medical companion* (pp. 355-364). Oxford, UK: Oxford University Press.

Light, D. (1994c). *Strategic challenges in joint commissioning.* London: North West Thames Regional Health Authority.

Light, D. (1995). Homo Economicus: Escaping the traps of managed competition. *European Journal of Public Health, 5,* 145-154.

Light, D. (1997a). From managed competition to managed cooperation: Theory and lessons from the British experience. *The Milbank Quarterly, 75,* 297-341.

Light, D. (1997b). The restructuring of the American health care system. In T. J. Litman & L. S. Robins (Eds.), *Health politics and policy* (3rd ed., pp. 456-474). New York: John Wiley.

Light, D., & May, A. (1993). *Britain's health system: From welfare state to managed markets.* New York: Faulkner & Gray.

Lillie Road GP Fundholder. (1994). *GP payments: 1994.* Unpublished manuscript.

Mahon, A., Wilkin, D., & Whitehouse, C. (1994). Choice of hospital for elective surgery referral: GPs' and patients' views. In R. Robinson & J. LeGrand (Eds.), *Evaluating the NHS reforms* (pp. 108-129). London: King's Fund Institute.

May, A. (1993). Thatcherism, the new public management, and the NHS. In D. Light & A. May (Eds.), *Britain's health system: From welfare state to managed markets* (Chapter 2). New York: Faulkner & Gray.

Maynard, A. (1975). *Health care in the European Community.* Pittsburgh: University of Pittsburgh Press.

Maynard, A. (1993). Market reforms and the funding of the NHS. In D. Light & A. May (Eds.), *Britain's health system: From welfare state to managed markets* (pp. 29-38). New York: Faulkner & Gray.

National Association of Health Authorities and Trusts. (1992). *Healthcare economic review 1990.* Birmingham, UK: Author.

Packwood, T., Keen, J., & Buxton, M. (1991). *Hospitals in transition: The resource management experiment.* Philadelphia: Open University Press.

Physician Payment Review Commission. (1994). *Annual report to Congress, 1994.* Washington: Author.

Redmayne, S., Klein, R., & Day, P. (1992). *Sharing out resources: Purchasing and priority setting in the NHS.* Birmingham, UK: National Association of Health Authorities and Trusts.

Robinson, R., & Judge, K. (1987). *Public expenditures and the NHS: Trends and prospects.* London: King's Fund Institute.

Roland, M., & Coulter, A. (1992). *Hospital referrals.* Oxford, UK: Oxford University Press.

Royal Commission on National Health Insurance. (1926). *Report.* London: HMSO.

Secretary of State for Health. (1989). *Working for patients.* London: HMSO.

Sheaff, R. (1991). *Marketing for health services.* Milton Keynes, UK: Open University Press.

Smith, R. (1994). The rise of statism in the NHS. *British Medical Journal, 309,* 1640-1645.

Smith, T. (1988). New year message. *British Medical Journal, 296,* 1-2.

Starfield, B. (1992). *Primary care: Concept, evaluation, and policy.* New York: Oxford University Press.

Starr, P. (1982). *The social transformation of American medicine.* New York: Basic Books.

Webster, C. (1993). The National Health Service: The first forty years. In D. Light & A. May (Eds.), *Britain's health system: From welfare state to managed markets* (Chapter 1). New York: Faulkner & Gray.

Whitehead, M. (1994). Is it fair? Evaluating the equity implications of the NHS reforms. In R. Robinson & J. LeGrand (Eds.), *Evaluating the NHS reforms* (pp. 208-242). London: King's Fund Institute.

Woolhandler, S., & Himmelstein, D. (1994, September 19). Giant H.M.O. 'A' or Giant H.M.O. 'B'? *Nation,* pp. 265-266.

PART **VI**

Health Care Reform:
Toward a Synthesis

CHAPTER 16

Structural Differences and Health Care Reform

ALBERT F. WESSEN

B y the early 1970s, the health care systems of most developed nations had attained a state of relative stability and maturity. By *maturity*, we mean that they had developed systems of provision for primary, secondary, and tertiary care that were available to their populations on acceptable terms and with assurances of financial accessibility to all or most inhabitants. In every country, attainment of this state of "maturity" was the result of a long historical process involving both the private and the public sectors, and, usually, the piecemeal attainment of near-universal access to care through successive enactments of social legislation.[1] This was certainly the case in the four countries discussed in this volume.

During the past 20 years, these "mature" health systems have experienced increasing strains resulting from changing demographic and socioeconomic conditions (see Chapter 1 of this volume). In every country, these strains manifested themselves most compellingly with respect to financial matters. The progressive and seemingly endless increases in health care costs led to perceived "crises" in every country. Whether the symptoms of these crises involved actual or projected budget deficits, increased and "onerous" charges to consumers or payers for medical care, or frank inability to provide or pay for needed services, all countries attempted remedial measures to moderate the costs of care. Although

369

most countries were quite successful in slowing the rate of increase, the specter of unsustainable financial burdens continues to hover over modern health care systems.

Table 16.1 provides comparative data on health care costs as a percentage of gross domestic product (GDP) for the period from 1970 to 1992.

In all four countries studied in this book, health care accounted for a larger share of the GDP in 1992 than had been the case in 1970. Except for Sweden, health care's share of the GDP was about half again as great (or more) at the end of the period as had been the case at the beginning. Among the three European countries shown in this table—and for the OECD countries' mean—the growth rate slowed markedly during the 1980s and early 1990s; indeed, Sweden actually reduced its costs as a proportion of the GDP during this period. Canada and the United States are exceptions. The burden of increased costs is more dramatically demonstrated by the explosion of per capita costs during the period. In dollar terms, the per capita increases ranged from about fivefold (in Sweden) to almost ninefold (in Germany and the United States).[2]

At the same time, demands for more and better health care continue. Aging populations, with their burden of chronic illness and disability, require increased services. Continual technological innovations offer the alluring promise of more effective intervention—and the near certainty of increased expense. Rapid and sometimes destabilizing social changes have created new health risks that may entail major long-term burdens on the health care system: Witness, for example, the AIDS epidemic. Distributional problems hinder the attainment of equity in health care in every nation. And better educated and more assertive populations have raised the threshold of what constitutes acceptable health care, demanding more responsive and holistic forms of care and a greater range of alternatives in time of need.

Thus, policy makers have been forced to consider further changes in their health care systems. As would be expected, however, countries differ both in terms of the specific problems on their health policy agendas and on the types of solutions attempted. It is the aim of this chapter to consider some of these variations on the theme of reform and to inquire whether structural differences are associated with these variations.

Factors Affecting the Response to Continued Cost Inflation

Health economists have long agreed that a major determinant of the amount of resources a nation allocates to health services is its overall

TABLE 16.1 Health Care Costs as a Percentage of GDP, 1970-1992

Year	Germany	Canada	Sweden	Britain	U.S.A.	OECD Average
1970	5.9	7.1	7.2	4.5	7.4	5.4
1975	8.2	7.2	7.9	5.5	8.4	7.1
1980	8.4	7.4	9.4	5.8	9.3	7.0
1985	8.7	8.5	8.9	6.0	10.8	7.2
1990	8.3	9.4	8.6	6.2	12.6	7.6
1992	8.7	10.3	7.9	7.1	13.6	8.1
1992 as % of 1970	147.5	145.0	109.7	157.8	183.8	150.0
1980 as % of 1970	142.4	104.2	130.6	128.9	125.7	129.6
1992 as % of 1980	103.6	139.2	88.8	122.4	146.2	115.7

SOURCE: Abstracted and calculated from Schieber, Poullier, and Greenwald (1994, p. 101) and Schieber and Poullier (1991, p. 109).

wealth (Culyer, 1989; Newhouse, 1977; Organization for Economic Cooperation and Development [OECD], 1987). Thus, it is not surprising to note that Great Britain, with the smallest per capita GDP among the nations studied in this book, has also consistently allocated the smallest proportion of its GDP to health services. At the same time, the United States, with its relative affluence, has devoted the largest proportion of its resources in this area (see Table 16.1).

Moreover, although all the nations in our study were affected by the economic difficulties of the past 25 years, the timing and intensity of these problems varied from country to country. Thus Sweden—in 1970 the most wealthy of the nations studied—was plunged into an extremely deep recession during the 1980s, with its cherished low unemployment rate vanishing as its competitive position was increasingly threatened by globalization of the economy and structural rigidities. Its high tax rates were increasingly seen as a barrier to recovery, and its national debt was increasingly worrisome. Germany also experienced a prolonged increase in unemployment and an increasingly difficult competitive position; these problems were substantially aggravated during the 1990s by the unexpectedly high costs of reunification with East Germany. Canada, too, suffered prolonged recession in the 1980s and early 1990s, with persistently high unemployment and an escalating federal government deficit. By contrast, Great Britain led Europe toward recovery from recession and—perhaps—began to profit from the success of the Thatcher government's economic policies. Such an analysis would help to account for the fact that after 1980 Sweden actually was able to reduce the relative proportion of its GDP allocated to the health services and that Germany was successful in attenuating its increase. Canada, on the other hand, experienced continuing health care inflation.

In all the countries studied in this volume, financing of the health care system is largely a governmental responsibility—through national taxation in Britain, a combination of national and provincial taxes in Canada, mostly county taxes in Sweden, and statutorily mandated payroll contributions to sick benefit societies in Germany. What seems to explain differences in the effectiveness of cost containment, however, is not the source of financing but the ability of governments to impose global budgets on the health care system (Abel-Smith, 1992; Reinhardt, 1993). In the British National Health Service (NHS), this is attained through the Exchequer's ability to limit expenditures through the mechanism of the national budget. In Sweden, each of the counties can achieve the same results through its annual appropriations for health services; moreover, each is bound by limitations on its taxing power imposed by the *Riksdag*. In Canada, the federal government has successfully reduced its financial contribution to the provinces for health care while maintaining its requirements that the latter ensure reasonable access to comprehensive health services on uniform terms and conditions. This has left the provincial governments with the problem of how to cope with increasing costs. And in Germany, rates of payroll contributions for health insurance have historically been set by a plethora of autonomous sick benefit societies after negotiations with health care providers.

Since its inception in 1948, the British NHS has been subject to the iron constraints of the Exchequer. Although funding levels have improved as British prosperity has increased, the drag of obsolescent facilities, together with the cost of technological progress and the imperatives of increased demands for service, have kept the NHS in what most experts agree is a chronic state of underfunding. Sweden, too, was able to take concerted action to restrain health care inflation. Limits on the power of the counties to raise taxes spurred them to limit health service expenses through a combination of judicious budget trimming and experiments in health service administration. Although health care inflation has largely been halted, many Swedes feel that the quality and availability of health care may now be adversely affected. But because both Britain and Sweden underwrite almost the whole costs of their systems through advance appropriations, they have been able to restrain health care costs effectively.

Neither Germany nor Canada has found it easy to do this. Both health care systems reimburse physicians for ambulatory care through a fee-for-service system. In Germany, hospital services were historically financed hospital services by negotiated reimbursement for costs of care. Such controls as could be placed on health care costs thus tended to be post hoc. Following their corporatist and subsidiarist traditions, the Germans fostered voluntary restraint following the guidelines of Concerted Action. As economic pressures continued or intensified, however, they have increasingly constrained the "autonomous" actors of their health care system by federal legislation through a series of cost containment acts culminating in the extensive Structural Health Care Reform Act of 1993. This led to increasingly activist regulation and controls by the federal government, with resultant dissatisfaction on the part of providers and consumers—and the economic outcome may not yet be satisfactory.

In Canada, the provinces are by constitutional right the agents of whatever cost containment efforts have been made. The federal government has done little to restrain health care costs beyond markedly reducing its proportionate contribution to the provinces. This has contributed to the high degree of tension between the national and provincial governments. The provinces have devised varyingly successful means of controlling costs, initially by imposing tight controls on capital expenditures and instituting global budgeting for hospitals and more recently through such actions as hospital consolidations and/or closures, regionalization, and kindred administrative schemes. Perhaps because, as Fooks (Chapter 8 of this volume) suggested, political will was slower to develop than recognition of the need for cost containment, the Canadian record in restraining health care cost between 1980 and 1992 was the least successful of the countries studied.

Because of the existence of a global budgetary constraint over the whole health system in Britain and Sweden, the aim of health care reforms in these countries was somewhat different from those in Canada and Germany, where overall budgetary constraints were not in place. Thus, in the latter countries, reform efforts tended to be explicitly directed toward the goal of containing health care costs. In Britain and Sweden, on the other hand, they were more often directed toward attaining greater efficiency—"value for money," as the British put it—and toward making the systems more responsive to public demands. Whereas the thrust in Germany and Canada was toward increased governmental regulation and intervention into the health care system, in Britain and Sweden, efforts were more often directed toward broadening consumer choices and to the development of an "internal market." Where cost containment was not the main priority, efforts could be directed toward making the system more flexible.

The Issue of Decentralization

When policymakers contemplate organizational reform of governments or large-scale enterprises, a common direction considered is that of "decentralization." This usually entails the downward delegation of authority and/or decision making to smaller and more locally based organizational units, and it implies greater autonomy for local units with resulting diminution of uniformity within the system. An important goal of decentralization is to attain greater responsiveness to local needs and demands, thus promoting greater efficiency. In democratic polities, decentralization is seen as a means of enhancing or protecting the "voice of the people." On the other hand, decentralization threatens the loss of possible economies of scale. It may also militate against an organization's overall ability to deal with exogenous problems, and it may risk the loss of equality among organizational units. To what extent has decentralization been a goal of the health care reforms described in this book?

The political structures of the four countries define the possibilities for centralization and decentralization in different ways. Two countries—Germany and Canada—are constitutionally decentralized, with states/provinces having major responsibilities for policy and administration in the health area. In Germany, as Altenstetter notes (Chapter 4 of this volume), in addition to the areas of competence legally reserved to them, changes in health care policy at the federal level usually require the assent of the *Länder* expressed through their representation in the *Bundesrat*. Nonetheless, in recent years, the federal government has played an increasingly active role in determining—and imposing—changes in the health care system. In Canada, regional differences and jealously guarded provincial autonomy make national policy changes difficult. Although Canadian Medicare remains a widely valued entitlement of national citizenship, it has been the subject of bitter federal/provincial dispute as the provinces have faced the constraints of the Canada Health Act while having to cope with decreasing federal contributions to health care. The national government has been able to enforce provincial adherence to the terms of the act, but such changes or reforms in the Canadian health care system as have occurred have taken place at the provincial level.

Both Sweden and Great Britain are unitary states, with power expressed on behalf of the Crown at the will of the parliament. Yet although in both nations regional and local governments are creatures of the larger state with no constitutionally guaranteed rights, the Swedes have a long-standing commitment to local autonomy, which, in the health area, is epitomized by the concentration of administrative responsibility in the hands of the county councils. If anything, the willingness of Swedes to decentralize their health care system has increased over the years, and experiments in health care organization such as the *Dalamodell* have taken place at the county level. On the other hand, the British parliament has changed the boundaries and responsibilities of counties and municipalities to suit its pleasure, and the administration of the NHS has never been made the responsibility of local government authorities.[3] Change has been dictated and monitored by the central authorities. Thus, the locus of health care reform seems not to be determined by whether a nation has a unitary or a federal structure.

In his analysis of the Swedish health care system, Professor Saltman (Chapter 11 of this volume) emphasizes the tension between policies leading to further devolution of the system to local control and those that effect integration and regionalization of services. This tension can be seen in all the study countries and has led to both "centralizing" and "decentralizing" reforms. Thus, the Swedish decision to devolve control of long-term care from county councils to municipalities and the creation of local primary care boards in Stockholm and Kopparberg County was balanced by the development of multicounty regional groupings in western and southern Sweden and by the assumption of a more activist monitoring and oversight role by the National Board of Health and Welfare.

In Great Britain, the purchaser/provider split at the heart of the internal market reforms broke up the unitary power of district health authorities (DHAs) and created complex networks of contractual obligation where there had once been clear lines of bureaucratic authority. Abolition of regional health authorities simplified and decentralized lines of authority, but this was complemented by the development of "outposts" (or, later, regional offices of the NHS Management Executive) to supervise the operations of the Service. However, the most radical "decentralizing" reform in Britain was the institution of GP fundholding—an innovation that has been somewhat misleadingly described by some American observers as the development of "mini-HMOs."[4] Fundholding not only transferred a share of purchasing responsibility from NHS administrative units (the DHAs) to practitioners but resulted in a number of geographic subunits of the districts carrying out purchasing functions independently of their district authorities (while the latter contracted for services to patients of nonfundholding GPs). This division of responsibilities quickly led to a need to amalgamate the family health service authorities (which supervised GPs) with the district health authorities, thus creating the current unified health authorities to coordinate decision making.

In Canada, most provinces have decentralized responsibility for planning and managing health services to regional or district levels. With respect to the issue of decentralization, these efforts appear to have ambiguous effects. On the one hand, they involve some devolution of provincial administrative authority over hospitals and public health services to regional boards; on the other, they involve the consolidation of management responsibilities from the hitherto autonomous institutional boards to those of the regions.

Finally, in Germany the trend has been away from the highly decentralized system of purchasing care undertaken by a multitude of *Krankenkassen*. There is a continuing trend toward consolidation of these units, which will likely be given further impetus by recent reforms designed to provide individuals with greater choice of insurer. The trend has also been toward decision making at higher levels: National negotiating committees make decisions that bind *Land* and local negotiators. Moreover, as Altenstetter (Chapter 4 of this volume) points out, the imposition, by the Structural Health Care Reform Act of 1993, of capped regional budgets for 23 regions is likely to have profound systemic effects. Traditional German mores that fostered subsidiarity and consequent decentralization have been eroded by needs for rationalization and cost containment.

Impact of the Ideology of Competition

The past 20 years have seen a vigorous assertion of the doctrines of neoclassical economics. The guiding role of markets was celebrated and the virtues of the private sector were proclaimed. Competition was seen as the key to improved efficiency and better economic performance. All of this was endorsed in the victories of conservative governments throughout the developed world and seemed to be validated by the collapse of the communist system at the end of the 1980s.

Thus, it is not surprising that the rhetoric of market-based competition has loomed large in programs for health care reform. The inspiration for many of these reforms is linked with the global influence of the United

States; the ideas of Alain Enthoven and his colleagues, who advocated a system of "managed competition," were especially influential in Europe (Enthoven, 1985, 1993). Moreover, specific American techniques, such as the use of diagnosis-related groups as a basis for determining the costs of hospital admissions, have been marketed and widely accepted in several OECD countries (Kimberly, de Pouvourville, & Associates, 1993).[5] Given the failure of the United States to contain its health care costs, there was some irony in the widespread acceptance of its procompetition ideas at the beginning of the present decade.

Procompetitive changes were important in reforms in Britain, Sweden, and Germany. They were not observed in Canada, where, within the constraints of its "single-payer" system, private fee-for-service medicine prevailed. In fact, the long-running provincial struggles to control costs have resulted in limitations on competition. Hospitals have been restrained from competing in terms of acquiring technology or providing amenities, and global hospital budgeting has removed all chance of price competition.[6] Likewise, as provinces have imposed volume controls as well as price controls on physician reimbursement, the resultant threat of "clawbacks" has turned competition among physicians from competing for more patients or referrals to avoiding being "hit" by professionwide discounts or paybacks (see Chapter 7 of this volume). It is of interest, moreover, that the Canadians have failed to emulate their neighbor to the south by developing health maintenance organizations and other organizational vehicles for managed care. They have generally reacted negatively to procompetitive innovations, fearing that their effect would be to foster a "two-tier" medical care system. Perhaps the monopsonistic power of the single payer may obviate the need for prepayment mechanisms.

The British transformation of the NHS into an "internal market" was a radical design intended to secure the benefits of competition within a nationalized health service. By making contracting between purchasers and providers central to the functioning of the system, it aimed to ensure flexibility, enhance rational decision making, and secure the dynamic benefits of competition. But, as noted by Appleby and Light (Chapters 14 and 15 of this volume), the managers of the internal market never allowed competition full play. To avoid shocks to the functioning and equity of the system, implementation of contracting was first delayed and simulated by "shadow contracting," then hedged in by a host of central directives. Failure could not be tolerated; hence, the possibility of "exit" from the market was sharply circumscribed. The long and politicized delay in reducing the hospital supply in central London is a prime example. Moreover, because contracting for medical services was scarcely extended beyond the NHS to the private sector, the possibilities for real competition among provider institutions were severely circumscribed. Yet the administrative costs of implementing the contracting system have been substantial, and since 1989 Britain has seen a major increase in the number of management personnel required for operation of the NHS.

Since the early days of the reforms, less and less has been written about the virtues of ensuring competition within the NHS. The "weaker" concept of "contestability" has been suggested as a substitute, providing an adequate stimulus to responsiveness without the caustic consequences of competition (Ham, 1996). And the new doctrine of "partnering" and "cooperation" has sought to involve providers and purchasers in cooperative rational planning and decision making, wherein the goal of attaining improved community health transcends the self-interested tactics of contracting. Though the formal structure of the internal market remains—and few suggest abandoning the purchaser/provider split—current discussion envisions a downsizing of management and more long-term contracting.

Whereas the British internal market scarcely involved the choices of patients, procompetitive overtures in Sweden aimed to broaden the range of choice for consumers. This was manifested both by experiments at the county level and by initiatives of the national government. Thus, for example, the Stockholm county initiatives allowed patients some choice about the hospital to which they wished to be admitted. At the national level, the waiting-list initiative allowed those experiencing delays in obtaining service to choose facilities that could serve them more quickly. There has also been some widening of access to private practice medicine within the system. But it was the *husläkare* reform, initiated by the Bildt government, that opened up choice of provider to the maximum degree; the abandonment of this reform after the return of the Social Democrats to power was in part dictated by an explosion in costs. As von Otter points out (Chapter 12 of this volume), the experience of cost control experiments in Sweden has been mixed, and there is little evidence that changes that might entail increased competition within the system have improved efficiency or controlled costs.

Germany has seemed ambivalent about the value of procompetitive reforms. The long series of cost containment measures detailed by Altenstetter and Kirkman-Liff (Chapters 4 and 5 of this volume) often worked to constrain competition rather than to promote it. Of special significance was the reform of the physician reimbursement system, wherein regional physician groups had to divide a pooled payment from the sick funds. Under this arrangement, undue competition for custom by physicians could only be at the expense of their colleagues, and high-charging doctors have been subjected to penalties as well. But as

Altenstetter stresses (Chapter 4 of this volume), the passage in 1993 of the Structural Health Care Reform Act and the implementation by government of its "third phase" have been accompanied by strong procompetitive rhetoric in Germany. Indeed, the fact that the *Krankenkassen* must now compete for members rather than acquiring them on the basis of members' employment status marks a major opening for competition among insurers.[7] Its effects are not yet measurable, however, and other initiatives, such as the imposition of regional budget caps, may well constrain competitive actions within the system.

On balance, it does not appear that the rhetoric of competition, widely affirmed by conservative governments, has been accompanied by aggressive procompetitive reforms in our study countries. The promise of competition as a vehicle for cost containment has not been fulfilled, perhaps because all countries have been hesitant about allowing it full play. On the other hand, some competitive reforms have indeed widened the scope of choice to consumers and, perhaps, have made providers more responsive to their needs. All countries have placed a high priority on protecting universal access within their systems and avoiding changes that might elicit dissatisfaction among the electorate. And the imperatives of cost control have repeatedly led governments to impose such "anticompetitive" measures as price controls and global budgets.

Changes in the Pattern of Medical Care Delivery

For the past generation, students of public health and medical care have warned that the way in which medical care is delivered in most countries does not have optimal effects on health outcomes. Because evidence has shown that much sickness is associated with preventable factors associated with the environment and with individual lifestyles, they have stressed the importance of prevention and of "refocusing upstream" (McKinlay, 1981) so that less emphasis would be placed on expensive—and potentially unnecessary—therapeutic interventions. They have complained that medicine has become overspecialized and has overemphasized the use of "high" technology, with the result that hospitals have become overused (e.g., Stoeckle, 1995). Therefore, at least since the Alma Ata Conference on Primary Health Care (1978),[8] there has been a worldwide effort to enhance the provision of primary care.[9] One would therefore expect the story of international health care reform to stress innovations in patterns of service delivery.

Such reforms, however, have not been a major theme of our story. The pervasive preoccupation with the issue of cost containment focused attention instead on health care financing, and this has tended to lead to changes in administrative patterns rather than in the substantive delivery of care. The vested interests of providers, sanctified by public deference to professional prerogative, may also have deflected attention away from changes in how care is actually delivered. On the other hand, it is true that the techniques of managed care, where applied, have limited professional autonomy and instituted a far-ranging revolution in patterns of health care delivery.

In more recent years, reforms have increasingly affected patterns of health care delivery "at the grass roots." Especially during the 1990s, the study countries have sought to alter the balance between hospital-based and primary care. They have also attempted to cope with the increasing burden of long-term care, dehospitalizing it and searching for ways to coordinate the multiple needs of chronically ill patients. Germany and some Canadian provinces have instituted controls on the numbers and deployment of health care personnel, and all the study countries have tried to place limits on the proliferation of "high" technology. A great deal of attention has been paid to means of improving the quality of care; thus, there has been much attention to improving and extending the collection of data on provider behavior, to instituting medical audit schemes, and to fostering the practice of "evidence-based" medicine. Finally, all countries have preached the virtues of prevention, although it may be argued that their extensive agendas for action in this area have not led to extensive investment in preventive medicine.

Hospital Medicine Versus Primary Care

Two study countries—Britain and Germany—have historically maintained sharp boundaries between hospital-based and ambulatory medicine. In both, hospital practice has been restricted to specialists whose income is largely derived from salaries. In Canada and Sweden, however, the situation is different. In Canada, as in the United States, no mandate excludes primary care physicians from hospital practice, and, especially in rural areas, GPs admit patients to hospital. In Sweden, the dominance of hospital-based medicine traditionally prevented the development of independent primary care practices, and the nation has struggled to promote primary care.

All residents of Great Britain are enrolled in the practice of an independent GP and nonemergency access to specialist and hospital care comes through the GP's referral. Although the British regard the GP as the keystone of their health care system, GPs have historically chafed under what they regarded as inferior status and working conditions. Moreover, consultants in NHS hospitals have tended to exercise major influence on British health policy, especially at the regional level. Although through the years a number of steps have been taken to improve the situation of GPs,[10] the institution of GP fundholding as part of the internal market reforms has most affected the situation of primary care in Britain.

Although begun on a small scale, by 1996, almost two thirds of British residents were enrolled in fundholding practices (see Chapters 14 and 15 of this volume). By allocating to fundholders the right to contract with providers for many services, this innovation for the first time gave GPs effective leverage over specialists. Under fundholding, specialists and trusts must compete for GPs' contracts and accordingly have become more responsive to their wishes. For the first time, the power balance between specialists and GPs shifted in favor of the latter.[11] Although studies suggest that fundholding has had some positive effects on patient care, critics argue that it may be creating a two-tier system of care in Britain; moreover, some fundholders have found the new responsibilities both difficult and irksome. At mid-1997, it is not clear what the future of this innovation will be, as the Labour Party has been among its critics (see Chapter 14 of this volume). Moreover, if GP fundholding has improved the power and status of GPs, other recent reforms have circumscribed their autonomy. Recent revisions in family practitioner contracts have subjected GPs to closer scrutiny by the management of health authorities, and controls on prescribing have been tightened by the use of indicative budgets. More recently, the historic insulation of general practice from direct ministerial control has been modified by the merger of the family health service authorities with district health authorities to form unified health authorities. Thus, although the role of general practice in the British health care system has been enlarged by recent reforms, the autonomy of practitioners may have been reduced.

In Germany, strong political and structural obstacles to changes in the separation of hospital and ambulatory care are present. There has been much criticism of the lack of coordination between ambulatory and hospital medicine.[12] It is felt that the separate treatment of these modalities leads to inefficiency and excess costs. The Structural Health Care Reform Act of 1993 attempted to address this problem by provisions aimed at fostering ambulatory surgery; however, as Altenstetter notes (see Chapter 4 of this volume), the payment schedule for ambulatory surgery remains inadequate in some cases, thus limiting its occurrence. Moreover, at the time of unification, the Germans opted for the uncoordinated West German system, allowing the well-integrated East German system to disappear. Cost containment measures, however, have had the effect of reducing the relative income of both primary care and hospital-based physicians over the years, as well as threatening their autonomy.

In Sweden, extensive efforts to promote primary care have resulted in a network of primary health centers being established throughout the country, usually under the administration of the county councils. These health centers typically have an interdisciplinary staff, including GPs, nurse practitioners, and district nurses. The centers are supported by training programs in family practice and by primary care research groups in medical school departments of community health or family medicine.[13] Such county-based reforms as *Dalamodellen* have bolstered primary care centers by establishing local boards to manage them and delegating to them the administration of the health care budget for their area. However, organizational issues such as whether primary care should be a private or a public service have been debated, and advocates of primary care still feel threatened by hospital medicine. And reforms that gave patients a wider choice of providers may have encouraged some to bypass primary health centers in favor of going directly to the hospital.

In Canada—in contrast to the situation in the neighboring United States—more than half of practicing physicians are GPs, and provincial manpower planners aim to maintain this ratio.[14] Several provinces have developed policies designed to facilitate the recruitment of family physicians, especially to rural areas; a notable example is the Quebec CLSC program (see Chapter 9 of this volume). Although throughout Canada, primary care is largely practiced by physicians in private—often solo—practice, the increasingly aggressive cost containment policies imposed by the provinces may be leading to decreased physician autonomy. Because all physicians in each province are now subject to common fiscal measures (such as clawbacks), another effect of fiscal restraint may be to reduce physicians' solidarity, pitting various specialty groups against one another. But it is the hospitals that have suffered most from cost containment policies. Throughout Canada, provinces have increasingly imposed bed closures, hospital mergers, and also hospital closures. Though Canada probably had an excess of hospital beds before 1990, this situation is quickly changing, with plans to close a third of the hospitals in metropolitan Toronto being a well-publicized example (see Chapter 7 of this volume).

The Problem of Long-Term Care[15]

Although issues of policy with respect to long-term care largely fall outside the scope of this study, a word is in order. Though at any time only a small minority of the population—around 5%—reside in nursing homes or other long-term care institutions, a much larger proportion of the aged enter them at some time in their lives. Therefore, with the aging of the population, long-term care is everywhere seen as an important policy issue. And with respect to care for the mentally ill and for the chronically disabled, the trend everywhere has been to stress deinstitution-alization and community care as a solution to the problem. By this means, it is argued, the costs of care can be reduced, and the wishes of patients to remain at home be honored.[16]

In all four of the study countries, health insurance or tax revenues provide all or most of the funding for long-term care as part of their comprehensive service packages.[17] In Canada, Germany, and Britain, much long-term care is provided by the private sector; and in Britain, recent policy has mandated that community services should, if possible, no longer be provided by the public sector. In Sweden, long-term care was delegated to the municipalities and thus removed from the control—and budgets—of the county councils.

All countries have faced problems in providing long-term care effec-tively and efficiently. In large part, this is the result of the multiple needs of disabled persons, for whom social supports often are a greater need than purely medical ones. The problem, however, is complicated by the tendency of long-term care services to be fragmented and controlled by multiple agencies.[18] The conjuncture of medical and social needs often means that administration and financing of long-term care programs may be divided between the health system and the social services system. In Britain, for example, community services are the responsibility of local authorities rather than the NHS, and financing comes from both the health and social security budgets.[19] Thus, an increasingly important aspect of health care is typically administered differently than either hospital or primary care, and multiple jurisdictions complicate the devel-opment of coordinated services. An undesirable side effect may be that from the perspective of health professionals, this situation helps to pre-serve the "separate but unequal" status of care for the chronically ill.[20]

Health Manpower Policies

In Britain and Sweden, where governmentally financed and operated health systems exist, controls over the number and placement of physicians and other health workers can easily be achieved. In Germany and Canada, on the other hand, the largely autonomous character of medical practice has rendered supply-side manpower controls more difficult to achieve. Both Canada and Germany have faced the emergence of a physician surplus,[21] and both have taken action in recent years to overcome this situation. In Canada, despite agreement by the Provincial-Territorial Conference of Ministers of Health in 1992 that there should be national strategic planning for physician manpower, policy changes have occurred at the provincial level according to local political imperatives. Though class size in many medical schools has been reduced, provinces have also imposed barriers to entry into practice, as well as imposing differential pay scales on new practitioners.[22] In Germany, the Health Care Structural Reform Act of 1993 imposed quotas on entry of physicians into practice according to whether there was a relative surplus of their specialty in a region (U.S. General Accounting Office, 1993, p. 43). Thus, the contribution of physician numbers to cost escalation has been recognized in all countries, and efforts to limit and make physician distribution more equitable have taken place. However, these policy changes have been aimed at new and future entrants into the system. Although increasing use of auxiliary workers such as community nurses has been made (especially in Sweden and Britain),[23] use of such personnel has been primarily aimed at extending services in situations of unmet need rather than substituting "less qualified" providers for physician care.

Monitoring the Content of Practice

Development of the technology of large computerized databases has made possible all kinds of administrative surveillance and controls over the health system that were unheard of 25 years ago.[24] Among these are the possibility of tracking in detail the practice behaviors of providers and, in many cases, of relating these to the outcomes of care. Though the medical profession has long engaged in audits and other self-evaluation procedures, in more recent years monitoring the conduct of practice has increasingly been mandated by governments.[25] Reforms of this sort have burgeoned in recent years.

Thus, in Britain, medical audit was mandated as part of the internal market reforms, although critics have complained that the process may have been left too much in the hands of specialist consultants. A developing professional interest in "evidence-based medicine" accords well with the drive to obtain increased "value for money," and the thrust of the joint commissioning process has been to direct funding toward "what really works" to meet population needs. The degree of adherence to the goals of the Patient's Charter is being measured, and "league tables" on the performance of NHS trusts—and other governmentally funded organizations—are being published. In Sweden, as Chapter 11 of this volume notes, the central government has in recent years increased its role of monitoring health care practice. There the National Board of Health and Welfare engages in extensive epidemiologically based evaluations drawing on its extensive system of disease registers, and it offers guidelines for practice on the basis of this research. In Germany, health reform legislation since 1986 has mandated increasingly widespread documentation and monitoring of hospital and ambulatory care practice. The Structural Health Care Reform Act of 1993 and the more recent Nursing Insurance Act both have required providers and insurers to take account of practice performance in their activities (including contracting).[26] And, of course, recent cost containment legislation has used data on the volume of procedures performed by physicians as a means of locating—and penalizing—those who engage in "overdoctoring" behaviors. In Canada, however, monitoring of practice behaviors seems not to have been so visible a part of provincial health care reforms; there, recent literature on quality assurance consists mostly of original research contributions.

Thus far, increased monitoring of practice patterns, whether voluntarily initiated by providers or mandated by governmental action, seems largely to have been carried out in a spirit of cooperation between providers and public health officials. The use of monitoring methods to sanction unwanted provider behavior is not yet widespread, and conclusions drawn from monitoring activities have been directed especially toward professional education and the development of evidence-based "guidelines" for practice. It is likely, however, that in the future monitoring activities will become more extensive and their results given wider publicity. It is possible, too, that the increased use of practice monitoring will result in further encroachment on the profession's clinical autonomy. If so, the constraints of utilization management faced by American physicians will increasingly affect their colleagues in Europe and Canada.

Emphasis on Prevention

In all four countries, there has been increased emphasis on the importance of prevention of disease. This has, of course, been justified not only as a value in and of itself but as ultimately the best way to control health care costs. So, it is argued, health policy should be directed toward greater investment in environmental and community-based activities that maintain and promote health and away from ever-increasing appropriations for curative medicine. The question, however, is the degree to which this rhetoric has been translated into meaningful action.

Canada led the way in promoting this policy reassessment, with the publication of the Lalonde Report in 1972, in which the Minister of Health argued for broadening the definition of health and for allocating resources to environmental and social activities that would promote health (Lalonde, 1974). As Béland (Chapter 9 of this volume) notes, the CLSCs were developed by the Quebec government as a venue for health promotion. Great Britain, in a manner similar to that of the United States, has developed a program of targets for achieving better health for its population (Secretaries of State for Health, 1992) and, along with Sweden and Germany,[27] has participated in prevention initiatives promoted by the World Health Organization and its European Regional Office. In Germany, the Structural Health Care Reform Act has mandated the support of prevention activities as a responsibility under statutory health insurance. Though progress has been made in the development of screening programs, smoking cessation, and environmental protection, the commitment to an emphasis on preventive medicine has not yet resulted in a major diversion of funds from curative medicine. The tempo of change in this area may only be beginning—and its effectiveness can only be established in the future.

Conclusion

It is clear that the principal motor driving change in the health care systems of our study countries is the need for cost containment. Though the countries have varied in the degree to which budget deficits and poor economic outlook have forced action on them, all have taken action aimed at moderating the costs of medical care. The main factors contributing to increased costs—the aging of populations, technological innovation leading to more intensive care and increased capital and recurrent costs, and heightened demands for better and more responsive care—either are uncontrollable or have been politically unassailable. Although since 1980 the rate of growth in medical care expenses has been successfully reduced in all OECD countries, policymakers continue to feel a pressing need for restraint even in the face of an "underfunding crisis" as in Britain or of inability to maintain historic entitlements to comprehensive and "free" care for all. Indeed, during the 1990s, the frequency and scope of reforms aimed at cost containment seem to have increased.

The reforms analyzed in this book have largely been administrative or fiscal: for example, imposition of global budgets on hospitals, modifications in the mechanisms by which physicians are paid, and creation of an "internal market" by means of a payer/provider split. In Britain and Sweden, where health services are largely provided by government, administrative innovation could be easily implemented. However, policymakers in both countries, desirous of quick results and fearful of adverse public reactions to change, have tended repeatedly to modify their reforms. In Germany and Canada, on the other hand, reforms have mostly involved successively rigorous regulation of the health care industry and have at times involved strenuous political struggle. In these countries, providers have been a force to reckon with as they have fought a rearguard action against erosion of their perquisites.

Yet in many cases, health care reform has resulted in threats to or diminutions in the autonomy of providers. Laws and regulations restricting the adoption of new technology[28] as well as consolidations or closures of facilities reduce the opportunities available to providers. So, more directly, do limits on the entry and placement of physicians into practice. Governmental imposition of fee schedules and expenditure caps—even over the objections of professional societies in some cases—and controls on volume of services provided are further constraints. An important effect of internal market reforms, clearly observed in Britain, is to modify the historic balance of power among professionals and provider institutions. Demands for increased accountability, enforced through mandates for medical audit or other quality assurance mechanisms, also restrict provider freedoms while underlining their responsibilities.

The effects of such measures go beyond constraining providers' unlimited freedom of action. They may result in overt hostility toward health policy makers on the part of the provider community and, as in several Canadian provinces and in Germany, to doctors' strikes and kindred actions. As Charles and Badgley (Chapter 7 of this volume) suggest, they may also pit elements of the provider community against one another. And they certainly underline the fact that the mandate of health care providers is not an entitlement but rather a grant dispensed by society and subject to its pleasure.

In this respect, hospitals have been the "big losers." Subject in all countries to increasingly tight budgetary constraints, they have also seen many of their erstwhile therapeutic functions transferred "beyond the walls." It is likely that bed reductions and hospital consolidations or closures will continue. The dominance of hospital specialists within the health care community has been seriously challenged.

In addition to omnipresent economic pressures, these changes reflect the increasing grasp of managerial techniques over the health care system.

Modern information systems make it possible for distant "managers" to monitor and control the activities hitherto conducted in the privacy of the consulting room. The guidelines and protocols of "evidence-based" medicine may well improve the quality of care. But they may also be seen as part of a trend toward increasing standardization and control over the health care system.

All of the study countries have long committed themselves to ensuring comprehensive and accessible care to their populations. All agree on the importance of the value of health care as a basic human right and on the importance of equity in their health care systems. But all find the economic pressure of the costs of modern health care to be suffocating. And all are engaged in a struggle to somehow continue to ensure good health care for their populations at a price that they can afford. In the process, they have moved increasingly toward reforms that affect the historical autonomy of the medical profession and its associated provider community. The evidence seems to suggest that the responsibility and authority of providers must be brought into a new relationship of dialogue and cooperation with the larger community if that autonomy is to survive. Health care reform at the end of the 20th century may be seen as a search for the institutional framework that will best facilitate this realignment.

We have sought to associate variations in the process of health system change with structural differences among our study countries. Despite important differences in political structure, in control of the health care system, in patterns of remuneration of providers, and in political values and ideology, the patterns of reform seem not to be clearly differentiated by these structural factors.[29] Rather, the common effects of demographic changes and technological advances seem in large part to overwhelm unique historical and structural patterns. The changing global economy and the progressive ability of rational management to direct and control heterogeneous systems lend credence to the convergence hypothesis (see Chapter 3 of this volume). If health care reform in international perspective may be seen as a set of variations on a theme, it is certain that the theme itself will dominate the counterpoint.

Notes

1. Though we consider only provisions for health care, it is important to realize that modern health care systems developed within a larger social movement that culminated in the modern "welfare state." Thus, in addition to health insurance or governmentally provided health care, citizens of developed countries saw the development of systems providing old-age

pensions, unemployment insurance, cash payments in case of sickness or disability, family support payments, provision of free education, housing subsidies, and so forth. This panoply of programs in most countries had attained its basic shape and extent by the 1970s. For histories of the welfare state, see de Swaan (1988), Flora and Heidenheimer (1981), and Hage, Hanneman, and Gargan (1989).

2. Thus, per capita health care expenditures increased between 1970 and 1992 from $146 to $1,151 in Britain, which spends relatively the least on health care; from $274 to $1,317 in Sweden; from $199 to $1,775 in Germany; from $274 to $1,949 in Canada; and from $346 to $3,094 in the United States. These data were abstracted from Schieber, Poullier, and Greenwald (1994, Exhibit 2, p. 102) and from Schieber and Poullier (1991, Exhibit 5, p. 113). With respect to Germany, it should be pointed out that health care costs for that country include expenses not usually reported under this rubric by other Organization for Economic Cooperation and Development (OECD) countries, such as sickness/disability pay and maternity benefits. See U.S. General Accounting Office (1993).

3. It is true, however, that the "internal market" reforms of the NHS involved giving greater autonomy to units of the NHS such as district health authorities and trusts.

4. In further extension of this decentralizing trend, eligibility criteria for fundholding practices were progressively relaxed to allow smaller and smaller practice units to participate in the fundholding process.

5. It should also be noted that this innovation, along with many possibilities for market-based reforms, depends on the availability of modern technology for the collection, management, and analysis of health care data. Much of this technology has been developed and marketed by American firms.

6. A few institutions, especially in Alberta, have attempted to compete by offering extra services or amenities for an extra charge, but this has put them into possible violation of the regulations of the Canada Health Act (see Chapter 7 of this volume).

7. The U.S. General Accounting Office (1993, p. 49) reported that before the passage of the Health Care Structural Reform Act, about 50% of the insured could choose their insurer. After 1996, this choice was expected to be available to 80% of the insured.

8. For a summary of the World Health Organization's program aimed at "Health for All by the Year 2000" and of the controversy over its concept of primary health care, see Basch (1990, Chapter 7). The text of the Alma Ata declaration is reprinted at pp. 226-230.

9. It has also been claimed by many that most primary care can be adequately provided by appropriately trained nonphysicians (given proper supervision and access to channels of referral).

10. Thus, improved postgraduate training programs for GPs were instituted, and pay and allowances increased on several occasions, most notably in 1966 with the institution of the Family Doctor Charter. The NHS also has encouraged the formation of GP practice groups and has underwritten much of the costs of facilities and of community and ancillary personnel associated with the practices.

11. With the abolition of the regions, in which they had had a powerful voice, and with the increased assertiveness of general management within the trusts, specialists found their status and power challenged in other ways. On the other hand, the institution of contracting often involved specialists in direct participation in that process.

12. In Germany, the nonhospital physician sector includes many specialists—about 60%—as well as GPs. The 1993 reforms attempted to enhance primary care by creating a new category of MD—"family physician"—to which practitioners might affiliate. This category was to be given a special place in the payment schedule, thus providing an incentive to primary care. See U.S. General Accounting Office (1993, pp. 41-43).

13. That research on problems of primary care in Sweden is active is shown by the existence of some 200 citations on "primary health care and Sweden" in Medline since 1992.

14. Whitcomb (1996) claimed that on a per-population basis, Canada has twice as many generalists as does the United Kingdom, with Germany and the United States falling between the two. He concluded that the United States does not need to increase its supply of generalists.

15. See Mechanic's discussion of the importance of this problem in Chapter 2 of this volume.

16. The savings in costs, however, may be overstated. The costs of informal home care to patients' families are considerable, and the opportunity costs to them are even larger. Yet payers often have resisted the establishment of new funding for community-based services on the grounds that new expenditures are certain, whereas presumed savings from the institutional care budget may not immediately appear.

17. Germany was the last country to do so, introducing statutory nursing care insurance as recently as in 1995 (see Chapter 4 of this volume).

18. For example, Williams (1996) reported that in Ontario there are no fewer than nine separate provincially sponsored home care programs—leaving aside the many providers of institutional care. Hence the need to establish "all-inclusive" multiservice agencies throughout the province.

19. This entails the further complication that whereas health services are in principle free to all at the point of service, social security funding may be means tested.

20. In our study countries, care for the mentally ill also tends to be offered and administered under somewhat different arrangements than medical care and to suffer from relative deprivation of funding and attention.

21. In Canada, this surplus largely resulted from a major expansion in medical school places in the 1960s and 1970s (see Chapter 7 of this volume), whereas in Germany the surplus is linked to the historic policy of keeping medical school admissions open to all qualified secondary school graduates. In Germany, the surplus has resulted in noticeable levels of unemployment among physicians.

22. See Chapter 7 of this volume. In Ontario, for example, regulations were proposed to limit entry into practice by physicians from outside the province.

23. Whitcomb (1996) reported that auxiliary medical practitioners have been used sparingly in Canada and Germany and much more heavily in Britain.

24. This change was symbolically acknowledged when Germany substituted a "smart card" for its century-old system of vouchers that allowed patients to use their health insurance benefits. (See Chapter 4 of this volume.)

25. An early example was the establishment in the United States of the Professional Standards Review Organizations under the Social Security Amendments of 1972.

26. See U.S. General Accounting Office (1993, p. 44). This has led to widespread research and publication on the subject of quality assurance in Germany; since 1992, Medline has cited 463 articles on this subject in Germany, more than twice the number that appeared in Britain, Sweden, or Canada. This literature includes formal statements by various professional organizations on their legal responsibilities. The areas of ambulatory surgery, radiology, and psychiatry have been especially represented in the German literature.

27. In Germany, the Health Care Structural Reform Act made a modest new appropriation to cover some preventive services, such as periodic physical examinations (U.S. General Accounting Office, 1993).

28. Procedures for assessment of new technology, often aimed at inhibiting its premature acquisition as well as limiting its distribution among providers, exist in all the study countries.

For example, recent legislation in Germany is discussed in U.S. General Accounting Office (1993, p. 34).

29. Of course, the study deals with a sample of only four countries. Extension of the analysis to a large sample of health care systems might allow us to establish the effects of structural differences more clearly.

References

Abel-Smith, B. (1992). Cost containment and new priorities in the European Community. *Milbank Quarterly, 70,* 393-411.

Basch, P. (1990). *Textbook of international health.* New York: Oxford University Press.

Culyer, A. (1989). Cost containment in Europe. *Health Care Financing Review, 21* (Suppl.).

de Swaan, A. (1988). *In care of the state: Health care, education, and welfare in Europe and the USA in the modern era.* New York: Oxford University Press.

Enthoven, A. (1985). *Reflections on the management of the National Health Service: An American looks at incentives to efficiency in health services management in the UK.* London: Nuffield Provincial Hospitals Trust.

Enthoven, A. (1993). The history and principles of managed competition. *Health Affairs, 12* (Suppl.), 24-48.

Flora, P., & Heidenheimer, A. (1981). *The development of welfare states in Europe and America.* New Brunswick, NJ: Transaction.

Hage, J., Hanneman, R., & Gargan, E. J. (1989). *State responsiveness and state activism.* Boston: Unwin Hyman.

Ham, C. (1996). Contestability: A middle path for health care. *British Medical Journal, 312,* 70-71.

Kimberly, J., de Pouvourville, G., & Associates. (1993). *The migration of managerial innovation: Diagnosis related groups and health care administration in western Europe.* San Francisco: Jossey-Bass.

Lalonde, M. (1974). *A new perspective on the health of Canadians: A working document.* Ottawa: Government of Canada.

McKinlay, J. (1981). A case for refocusing upstream: The political economy of illness. In P. Conrad & R. Kern (Eds.), *The sociology of health and illness* (pp. 613-636). New York: St. Martin's.

Newhouse, J. (1977). Medical care expenditures: A cross-national survey. *Journal of Human Resources, 12,* 115-124.

Organization for Economic Cooperation and Development. (1987). *Financing and delivering health: A comparative analysis of OECD countries.* Paris: Author.

Reinhardt, U. (1993). Reforming the health care system: The universal dilemma. *American Journal of Law and Medicine, 19,* 21-36.

Schieber, G., & Poullier, J. (1991). International health spending: Issues and trends. *Health Affairs, 10* (1), 106-116.

Schieber, G., Poullier, J., & Greenwald, L. (1994). Health system performance in OECD countries, 1980-1992. *Health Affairs, 13* (4), 100-112.

Secretaries of State for Health. (1992). *The health of the nation: A strategy for health for England.* London: HMSO, Command No. 1986.

Stoeckle, J. (1995). The citadel cannot hold: Technologies go outside the hospital, patients and doctors too. *Milbank Quarterly, 73,* 3-17.

U.S. General Accounting Office. (1993). *1993 German health reforms: New cost control initiatives* (GAO/HRD-93-103). Washington, DC: Government Printing Office.

Whitcomb, M. (1996). A cross-national comparison of generalist physician workforce data. *Journal of the American Medical Association, 274,* 692-696.

Williams, A. (1996). The development of Ontario's home care program: A critical geographical analysis. *Social Science and Medicine, 42,* 937-948.

CHAPTER 17

Patterns of Health Care System Change

Francis D. Powell

The sociopolitical structure is a factor in the various types of change that occur in national health care systems. In Western countries, the structure of the central government alone seldom determines the type of change that takes place in the health care system. More frequently in Western countries, change in the health services is influenced by specific but varying relationships between the central government and other constitutionally established institutions within the society.

Within the four health systems discussed in the preceding chapter, only in that of Great Britain does the type of change in health services derive solely from the structure of the central government. Thus, in the British case, the unitary structure of the central government is not counterbalanced by any separate effective institutionalized structure. Other than the elective process itself, no officially established constitutional obstacle stands in the way of ruling-party parliamentary programs initiated by the ministerial government in London. This lack of countervailing power in a unitary political structure is a dominant factor in the "directive" (goal- and means-setting) change that occurs in the British health system.[1]

Although Sweden has a somewhat similar type of unitary central government, the authority of the government in Stockholm is counterbalanced by politically organized community structures and a national commitment to decentralization. With regard to health services, the

393

county councils are responsible for the administration of local facilities. They are elective political bodies, owing their allegiance primarily to their local community. Moreover, an unelected body, the Federation of County Councils in Stockholm, functions as an advisory "corporatist" body in health policy formation. This diffusion of policy-making and administrative power is a key factor determining the "adaptive" change that occurs in Swedish health services. Adaptive change is change that is responsive to the needs of local communities.

In the case of Canada, the sociopolitical structure involves special relationships between the central government and the 10 provinces. These special relationships are based on the high degree of autonomy that is accorded to the provincial governments by the Canadian constitution. In recent years, these relationships have been complicated by the tightened economic conditions existing in Canada, which have compelled the central government to cut back on its contributions to the provinces for health services. As a result, the latter have sought ways of sustaining services with reduced finances while retaining a commitment to universal access as guaranteed by Canadian Medicare. A number of provincial governments have, therefore, maintained their systems in a "static" manner by pursuing policies of consolidation featuring mergers and the elimination of services judged to be unnecessary. The province of Quebec has met this financial constriction by expanding services to underserved populations through organizations constructed to provide these services without increasing the costs of care. The ability of Quebec to increase services while not expanding costs is an innovative instance of "dynamic system maintenance" change. Such change aims to institute a more efficient means of sustaining fundamental but seriously threatened goals.

Like those of Sweden and Canada, the health system of Germany is embedded in a sociopolitical structure that is complicated by relationships other than those within the central government. This sociopolitical structure includes relationships between central and state governments as well as with nongovernmental corporatist bodies. These corporatist bodies are officially recognized organizations having the legal right to represent the interests of consumers or providers of health services. Policies regarding health affairs are regularly arrived at through negotiations between governmental and corporatist bodies. This structure of negotiated compromise between major interest groups with governmental participation produces "integrative" changes in the health system. Integrative changes involve negotiated compromise between major opposing group interests. The autonomous basis of these sociopolitically structured negotiations, however, has been severely circumscribed recently through governmental decisions necessitated by restrictive economic conditions.[2]

The present chapter will consider whether the types of change that have occurred in the health systems of these four Western countries have also taken place in certain jurisdictions in the United States. A broad and impressive array of health "reforms" have been initiated in a number of states in recent years. These state-level initiatives contrast with the general condition of gridlock that has blocked such efforts at health system reform at the federal level as the Clinton plan.[3]

Certain specific innovative state-level programs have been selected for comparison with the reforms in the health systems of the four countries analyzed in this book. These local programs have been chosen for analysis because of the presence of a distinct sociopolitical structure in a particular state that is analogous to that of a corresponding specific Western country. We suggest that the existence of a comparable prevailing sociopolitical structure is a determining factor of the *type* of change that occurs in both contexts.

In the health systems of each of the four countries, the sociopolitical structures determining change in the health care system are the result of legally and formally established institutional arrangements.[4] In the U.S. context, the structures that give rise to these reform programs are the result of a constellation of economic, demographic, and historic-political factors that are specific to a particular state. The specific pattern of the sociopolitical structure constituted by these factors produces the types of change that differentiate these local reform programs.

In the U.S. context, a given sociopolitical structure consists of a specific constellation of factors in the social fabric of a state (or region of a state). This sociopolitical structure determines the ways in which political activities are organized regarding health care reform and how state health service reforms are carried out. The political, economic, and demographic factors constituting the sociopolitical structure of each of the four states analyzed form patterns that stress either an "integrative," an "adaptive," a "directive," or a "system maintenance" configuration. Such configurations are thought to determine the nature of health care reform in a particular state. The configurations of the sociopolitical structure of the states selected for analysis in this chapter are parallel to those of the political structure and thus to the types of change occurring in the countries discussed in this volume.

The purpose of making these comparisons is to demonstrate that different paths that specific states have taken are similar to those adopted by specific Western countries. The comparisons also indicate basic alternative patterns of change that may be manifested by health care systems.

Integrative Change in the German Health Care System Compared to Innovations in the State of Oregon

The German political system is described by Altenstetter in Chapter 4 of this volume as based on a democratic parliamentary system and on a corporatist institutional structure. The administration of health services is carried out by officially recognized corporatist institutions representing the interests of consumers and providers of health services. Negotiated decisions of these corporatist bodies are often subject to official approval and review by governmental authorities. The sickness funds and the provider associations are representative of two basic complementary functions—namely, the consumption and provision of health services. These complementary functions of the corporatist bodies provide the basis for their status as the principal responsible parts of the health system as a whole. The inclusive character of the corporatist bodies is a necessary condition for maintaining an effective part-whole relationship because only an inclusive body can speak for all consumers or providers of health services. Any competitive breakup of the monopoly position of the corporatist bodies might introduce fragmentation of the system and loss of effective orientation of the parts to the whole. This functional type of organization is the basis for the structural "integration" of the German health system.

The reliance of the German health system on the functionally complementary corporatist bodies is consistent with the use of negotiations as a means of organizing relationships between these institutions. Negotiations maintain the autonomous position of these organizations as responsible complementary parts of the health system as a whole.[5] However, this autonomy is not absolute.[6]

The German health system has been regulated through "integrative" change negotiated among corporatist bodies and, since 1977, within the "umbrella" corporatist body that is Concerted Action (see Chapter 4 of this volume). Through negotiation, a balance was achieved that "integrated" the interests of consumers and providers under a common commitment to control costs. Attainment of the policy goal of effective cost containment was based on recognition of the obligation of the health care system to the society as a whole.[7] Since the reunification of the country in 1989, the sickness funds have continued to successfully defend the interests of consumers in negotiations. A smaller body, the Federal Committee of Sickness Funds and Sickness Fund Physician Association (BAA/K), continues to maintain an "integrative" balance between the interests of consumers and providers. Through this "integrative" balance of negotiated change, the holistic goal of effective cost containment is achieved in Germany.

In the state of Oregon, a combination of sociopolitical factors makes possible changes that are parallel to those that have occurred in the German health system. For example, in Oregon, a process of change has taken place in the care of the elderly poor that departs substantially from the purely market-oriented conditions prevalent in many areas of the United States.[8] The Oregon approach to change is the result of a relationship between voluntary nongovernmental organizations and the state government that parallels in some ways conditions existing in Germany. Voluntary group involvement in the Oregon program is exemplified by the United Seniors, which has been a dominant force in changes in the care of the poor among elderly Oregonians.

Under the leadership of the United Seniors, a "negotiated investment strategy" has been instituted on behalf of elderly Medicaid recipients in need of subsidized community-based health care services. The strategy involves planning meetings between the United Seniors and representatives of community-based providers of care for the elderly. At the meetings, providers and United Seniors representatives prepare their demands as circumscribed by restraints of costs and resources available. Because the negotiating parties believed that nursing home providers offered inferior care, they were not included in the meetings (Falcone et al., 1992). With a prepared agenda, the United Seniors and the providers negotiated with state agencies an improved program of community-based health and home care services that covers approximately 20,000 of 27,000 aged Medicaid recipients (as estimated by the Oregon Senior and Disabled Services Division).

The type of voluntary social action manifested by the United Seniors was influenced by the specific sociopolitical structure of the state of Oregon. This sociopolitical structure is the result of political, economic, and demographic factors that have shaped the way in which politics is conducted in the state. Among these factors are historical effects of the populist and progressive movements within the state of Oregon, which led to direct participation by the citizenry and focused on general economic and social issues that transcend the interests of any particular group

(Dodds, 1986). This orientation constitutes an "integrative" factor in the sociopolitical life of Oregon. The relatively autonomous and uncomplicated structure of the economy is a factor fostering a sense of broader community among Oregonians. Principal segments of the economy, such as the timber and wood product industries, fisheries and canning, electric power, and agriculture, all involve processing of local or regional resources. Though some analysts have judged that the locally autonomous and relatively less complex structure of the economy is a factor in a weak Oregon political party system,[9] an emphasis on social issues characterizes Oregon politics. With its emphasis on issues rather than party affiliation, Oregon tends to elect candidates whose views are consistent with those of the general electorate. The tendency toward consensus through voting based on social issues constitutes an "integrative" factor in Oregon political life. The relatively uncomplicated economy, which discourages the formation of enduring and opposed constituency groups, is a factor in the tendency toward political consensus and "integration" in Oregon.

This tendency toward political consensus and integration, supported by a relatively noncomplex economy, is invigorated by the proliferation of voluntary advocacy groups. A prominent example of these advocacy groups is Oregon Health Decisions (OHD), which played a major role in the controversial "rationing" proposal for Medicaid.[10] The proposed "rationing" program advocated by OHD, though initially applied only to Medicaid beneficiaries, had implications for the health system as a whole. The proposal transcended the interests of any social segment and posed possibilities of change for the health care received by the entire society. This feature of presenting new alternatives that have implications for the society as a whole marks the behavior of Oregonian advocacy groups.

The relatively homogeneous and assimilated composition of the population has facilitated the ability of voluntary groups to form and to develop effective coordinated efforts. Oregonians have learned through long experience ways of joining in effective constructive social action through such voluntary groups as the United Seniors. By facilitating responsible unified action, the homogeneity of the population constitutes an "integrative" sociopolitical factor in the Oregonian political system.

A definite structural similarity exists between the Oregon program for the elderly poor and the German health care system. Both Germany and the Oregon program have representation by major health-related interest groups along with participation by state authorities. In both instances, consumer and provider groups engage in consensual negotiations to reach mutual agreement. In both cases, these mutual agreements gain binding force with the approval of the appropriate state authority. The presence in the negotiations of the key interest groups along with the state agencies gives the Oregon aging program much in common with the corporatist sociopolitical structure of the German system.

However, the Oregon program described here has a number of elements that are not corporatist. Negotiations between the United Seniors and the providers of community health services for the elderly poor take place in accordance with pluralistic assumptions of health services in the United States. Individuals entering into these voluntary groups, and the groups forming these negotiating relationships, do so without legal compulsion. The parties to these negotiations are not legally bound to continue in these relationships, nor must the state recognize health service negotiations for the elderly poor as the exclusive responsibility of these two organizations. Moreover, the exclusion of the nursing home industry from the negotiated investment strategy is inconsistent with corporatist standards. In Germany, the nursing home operators, as legitimately licensed providers of housing for the elderly, would not be legally excluded from the negotiations.

Nevertheless, within a pluralistic market-oriented context, the Oregon program has important corporatist components. The interest of the United Seniors is in quality health services for the elderly poor. The interest of the providers is in profitable business conditions. The interest of the state agency is in keeping costs within Medicaid allotments. Despite these differences in interests, all three parties agreed on a commitment to community-based care for the elderly poor. In fact, given the pluralistic setting, the exclusion of the nursing home industry permitted the three interest groups to find a common ground for the negotiated investment strategy. Because the three negotiating parties had this common commitment, compromises were possible short of state regulation or market outcomes that might be inimical to the interests of the elderly poor.

The capacity of the Oregon program for the elderly poor to produce integrative change derives from its "quasi-corporatist" sociopolitical structure. Consumer and provider interest groups participating in negotiations with the authorizing state agencies are essential corporatist elements. The program displays a "solidarity" commitment to community-based health care as serving best the needs of the elderly poor. This commitment binds the differing tripartite group interests under a common social service understanding. Though operating within a pluralistic market context, the Oregon aging program presents significant components of a "quasi-corporatist" sociopolitical structure capable of integrative system change parallel to that existing in the German health system.

System Maintenance Change in Quebec Compared to Innovations in Tennessee

An innovative example of distinct provincial health reform is the CLSC program described by Béland in Chapter 9 of this volume. This new style of clinic introduced an approach to primary care combining traditional medical services with a strong emphasis on prevention and health teaching. Stress is also placed on the social dimensions of health, with physicians working on a team basis with nonphysicians, including nurses, paramedics, social workers, and community organization personnel. In contrast with the episodic focus of most traditional medical practice, the CLSCs are particularly dedicated to health promotion, prevention, and health teaching.

The CLSCs are well adapted to remote rural conditions. The sparsely settled remote regions of Quebec present powerful deterrents to private practitioners. Under a tax-supported fee-for-service system, private practices prosper best in urban settings with large populations. Physicians in the CLSCs are either on salary or paid on a session basis, with reimbursement offered for each day or half-day of service. More importantly, CLSC physicians have a commitment to the social dimensions of health, which inclines them to offer services in remote areas where the population suffers from a severe shortage of health care. The provincial ministry of health has also provided special financial support for the new clinics in the remote regions.

The CLSCs represent a creative program launched by the provincial ministry of health. It was developed in the context of a financial squeeze occasioned by reduced contributions from the central government. Rather than cut back services as other provinces have done, Quebec expanded care in the underserved northern regions. It succeeded in this policy by introducing more economical means of reimbursement and by offering institutional support for the CLSCs in the remote regions. Through its CLSC program, the province has "maintained the system" by keeping costs within straitened budgetary limits. It has also maintained the system goal of universal access as the basic commitment of Canadian Medicare.

A specific sociopolitical structure in the state of Tennessee produced a situation regarding health care reform that was parallel to the situation faced by the government of Quebec. But in Tennessee, unlike the Canadian province, many of the problems in the administration of health affairs are attributable to conservative policies that have been pursued by the state government, including low taxation and relatively small allocations for education and social welfare. Thus, Tennessee has failed to attract suffi-cient numbers of white-collar and professional workers needed to operate high-wage industries such as electronics, finance, and specialized machin-ery manufacturing. A significant portion of the state's economy involves low-paying industries such as textile, clothing, and furniture manufactur-ing. These industries are unstable and often buffeted by severe competi-tion. Tennessee, in consequence, has been marked by high levels of unemployment and by low levels of income.[11] Moreover, a conservative electorate, divided by enduring regional ecological and economic interests and distrustful of government, tends to discourage political action on issues until a crisis has arisen.[12]

The sociopolitical structure of the state involves a combination of "system maintenance" factors that help to determine Tennessee's approach to health care policy. Its conservative tax and low expenditure policies have prevented the state government from taking an anticipatory approach in regard to health policy issues. In particular, distrust of government by the electorate has forced the administration in Nashville to react to crises as they arise rather than to act on the basis of long-range planning. Funds and political resources have not been available to prepare and educate the public for proposed health care reforms. Given these sociopolitical factors, the reforms undertaken were designed to "maintain the system" in circum-stances that might have threatened its existence as previously constituted.

These "system maintenance" factors in its sociopolitical structure help to account for Tennessee's response to a recent crisis in the Medicaid program. Faced with surging and uncontrollable Medicaid costs, a con-servative Democratic governor with little advance notice unveiled the new TennCare program in April 1993. The proposal included the simultaneous repeal of the hospital tax (to cover uncompensated care), the broadening of Medicaid to cover most of the state's uninsured, and a decision to enroll the entire existing Medicaid population in capitated managed-care net-works. As a result, the current enrollment in TennCare amounts to over 1,180,000, of which about 842,000 are Medicaid eligibles and approxi-mately 346,000 are categorized as either uninsured or uninsurable.[13]

Consistent with the restrictive economic conditions facing the state government, the TennCare program came into being under the heading of "stealth reform" (Bonnyman, 1996). This expression aptly describes the political maneuvers employed by the governor's office in getting the program under way. The program as initially proposed in the spring of 1993 received reluctant approval by the legislature in November. How-ever, this tentative support began to erode rapidly under unfavorable comment from the media and through efforts to block the program by the state medical association. With support slipping away, at the stroke of midnight on January 1, 1994, Tennessee moved all 800,000 Medicaid beneficiaries into capitated managed-care networks and began to accept applications from persons who were newly eligible. As of June 1997, TennCare has been able to enroll 400,000 previously uninsured and uninsurable Tennesseans. At the same time, by shifting over 1 million recipients from fee-for-service treatment to capitated managed care, TennCare has held costs of the program to a minimum.

Both the TennCare program and Quebec's CLSCs developed within an economically restricted political structure. In both cases, the political authorities faced a situation in which a significant portion of the population had inadequate access to health services. In both instances, the governments could not afford to provide appropriate services for these underserved groups while retaining existing reimbursement policies. In Quebec, as in Tennessee, the decision was to increase care for inadequately served groups by switching from costly fee-for-service reimbursement to a more economical payment system.[14] In contrast with the static approaches of a number of Canadian provinces, both of these programs are examples of "dynamic system maintenance" change.[15] For the health services to be "dynamically maintained" as a viable system, the governments had to increase access to care without causing new budgetary strains. The Quebec and Tennessee programs have generated "dynamic system maintenance" changes in the context of economically restricted political structure.

Comparison of Adaptive Changes in Sweden to Innovations Sponsored by Minnesota Institutions

The Swedes have a long tradition of decentralization of power and a commitment to local autonomy. This commitment has been realized in the health care system through the county councils. In recent years, this decentralization has been highlighted by the introduction of a number of local programs designed to meet rising demands for a health service that is more sensitive to community needs.

Among these programs is the *Dalamodell* plan of the Dalarna region. The plan features local health centers in which general practice physicians, nurse practitioners, and district nurses constitute the main providers of care. These centers arose in response to local community complaints regarding lack of continuity and quality of care. In line with Swedish decentralization policy, the county council also delegated the coordination of primary care and hospital services to subareas of the Dalarna region. This delegated authority, however, is subject to review by the county council, as indicated by Saltman in Chapter 11 of this volume.

Several important structural components of the Swedish system facilitate "adaptive" changes that are responsive to the needs of local communities. The national government, though establishing a common framework for the health services, has delegated its administration to county councils. As elected local bodies, the county councils are in a position to be sensitive to the wishes of community residents. The Federation of County Councils is available as a communication link to the central government and as an advisory body.[16] Moreover, county council members in the *Riksdag* are in position to formulate local views for possible legislative action. These features of the political structure have enabled the Swedes to introduce "adaptive" changes that are sensitive to local community needs.

In the state of Minnesota, a number of demographic, economic, and political forces have fostered the capacity of local communities to assume an active role in dealing with their problems. Their New England roots and the strong influence of their Scandinavian immigrant stock have given local communities the sociopolitical "adaptive" capacity to act on local issues as they arise. Historic economic struggles, many of which were carried out in local settings, have reinforced the "adaptability" of communities in meeting challenges to jobs and livelihood.[17] The Democratic Farmer Labor Party, which grew out of these economic struggles, has often been linked with these local issues and operates politically to facilitate the "adaptive" capacity of local communities to deal with problems as they arise.

Although a sociopolitical structure of "adaptive" local activism characterizes Minnesota as a whole, this pattern is even further emphasized by the institutions located in the northeastern and Duluth region of the state. A common experience of difficult economic times, perhaps seasoned by a rather bitter climate, has produced a sense of solidarity embraced by the institutions in this section of Minnesota.[18] Community attention has focused on the health area because of the problems of an aging and at-risk population with incomes well below state and national levels.

A project based in the Duluth area is an expression of this sociopolitical local activism. The Health Quest Program involves collaboration among 70 health care institutions serving the region of northeastern Minnesota and northwestern Wisconsin. The initial phase of the project was a jointly developed study of the health status and health behavior of residents of these 16 Minnesota and Wisconsin counties. This "Bridge to Health Survey" was constructed and designed through close collaboration by representatives of many of the 70 provider organizations. From the very beginning of the project, officials from the Minnesota Department of Health and academics from Duluth and the Twin Cities played key advisory roles in the preparation of the survey. They also provided continuous support in carrying out goals of the project.

The principal results of the survey are twofold. First, the survey provides information not previously available on the health status and health behavior of residents of the two-state region. In particular, reliable data for the first time are now in existence for rural areas of the region. A second area of interest has emerged from the survey. This involves proposed programs of preventive intervention by the providers. Issues that have been highlighted for these interventions include smoking behavior and cancer screening. Priority attention is being given to a proposed joint program focusing on control of smoking.[19]

In both the Dalarna plan and the Duluth area project, the local community and government constitute a joint sociopolitical structure for instituting change. In both cases, the initiative for change came from the local community. In Sweden, the link between the local community and the government is institutionally established through the role of the county councils. In Duluth, the link between the local community and the state government is achieved through informal institutional commitment to social democratic localism.

In Sweden, the county council exercises administrative control over the facilities involved in the Dalarna plan. Because these facilities are publicly owned, the competition between separate units is minimized.[20] The Dalarna plan operates under fixed budget limits set by the government that are not existent in the Duluth area. The competitive conditions and lack of control over provider behavior in the Minnesota-Wisconsin region contrast with the highly regulated pattern in Sweden. However, the Health Quest Program has a number of similarities with the Dalarna region plan. In both contexts, institutions in the local community have constituted the driving force that initiated the reforms. Because of a common commitment to social democratic localism, the reforms were "adapted" to the needs of the local community. Moreover, in both contexts, expert consultation has played an important part in the development of the reforms. The use of expert consultation to achieve greater "adaptation" to local needs is important in both cases. "Adaptive" change is the result of a sociopolitical structure that is attuned to local needs.

Directive Change in the Health Care Systems of Britain and Hawaii

The state of Hawaii stands in sharp contrast with the United Kingdom with respect to size of population, ethnic composition, degree of industrial development, and political history. However, with regard to one dimension that is important for health policy determination, these two political systems have much in common. Thus, over the last three decades or so, Hawaii, like Great Britain, has had a political structure in which the executive and legislature have been under unified party control. In the British case, this is the result of the parliamentary system, in which the victorious party in an election controls both executive and legislative decisions. The Hawaiian unity of political structure resulted from dominance of government by the same party. Since not long after the establishment of statehood in 1959, the Democratic Party has regularly controlled the governorship and the state legislature and has also dominated the Hawaiian congressional delegation in Washington. In both systems, there exists an extraordinary potential for the exercise of power in regard to change in the health system. The decision to exert this power for health system change requires a commitment to an agenda on the part of the ruling administration. In recent years, the willingness to use this available power has been displayed in both Britain and Hawaii.

Certain specific "directive" factors have contributed to the type of health care policies initiated by the Hawaiian Democratic Party. These consist of economic, demographic, and political forces that encourage active long-term policies on the part of the state government. The economic landscape of Hawaii has been fundamentally altered since the advent of statehood in 1959. A rural economy has been supplanted by a more modern economy increasingly oriented to tourism. A plantation system of agriculture, marked by low wages and paternalistic practices, has been restructured by vigorous union organization of sugar cane and pineapple growers. In particular, an active government employee union leadership has assumed an important role in the politics of the state.[21] The unions have regularly called on the aid of the government in Honolulu for assistance. Thus, they have been a sociopolitical factor encouraging "directive" and activist policies in the governing of the state. Since achieving statehood, Hawaii has also acquired an articulate academic community that has made itself felt in political life on the islands.

The continued dominance of state politics by the Democratic Party also derives from the heavily ethnic character of the population and its identification with statehood as a cause espoused by the Democrats. Thus, Japanese, Filipino, Chinese, and native Hawaiian residents all saw in the goal of statehood an opportunity for social and economic advancement. After admission to the union in 1959, the Democratic administration fostered a generous program of public education that solidified the allegiance of all of these groups to the party. The support of these ethnic communities has been a "directive" sociopolitical factor encouraging an active and long-term commitment by the state government to policies favoring the interests of these constituencies.[22]

With this social base offered by union and ethnic community support, the leadership of the party gravitated in the direction of the liberal wing of national Democratic politics. This liberal orientation of the Hawaiian Democratic Party constitutes a third sociopolitical "directive" factor conducive to long-term, active policy planning on the part of the state government.

With the support of this sociopolitical structure, and under vigorous Democratic executive department direction, Hawaii has embarked on an ambitious program of reform of the health services. Support for these programs was ensured by party control of the state legislature. The goal of these reforms was to achieve fully insured health care access and coverage for all Hawaiians. An incentive for reaching this objective entailed the desire to be the first state in the nation to achieve universal insured health service access.

The first step toward this policy goal was the passage of the Prepaid Health Care Act of 1974. This legislation mandates health insurance coverage for all employees who are not insured under collective bargaining agreements. Financing for the plan is provided by equal payments from employers and employees. Subsidies are offered for smaller companies not able to meet the financial burdens of coverage.

At the time of its passage, it was thought that the Prepaid Health Care Act would be a step toward universal health insurance in Hawaii. This expectation derived from the anticipated adoption of a program of national health insurance. The failure of such a nationwide initiative led to development of the State Health Insurance Plan (SHIP) for the state of Hawaii, which was passed in 1989. SHIP was designed to cover all residents of the islands that were not embraced by the Prepaid Health Care Act or who were not beneficiaries of private insurance plans or public programs such as Medicaid and Medicare. The SHIP program sought to provide insurance for all those falling between cracks in the system. In

1989, persons served by the plan numbered around 35,000, consisting mainly of the unemployed, dependents of low-income workers, part-time employees, immigrants, the seasonally employed, and students. This program still left small segments of the Hawaiian population that did not have access to insured health services. However, the state progressed very far toward achieving its goal of a universal system of insured care as set forth in its original initiative of 1974.[23]

The institutional conditions and the legislative processes that have taken place in Hawaii may be compared with changes initiated under the "internal market reforms" in Great Britain. In making this comparison, it is necessary to note that the issues dealt with in the two contexts differ widely in scope. The NHS had long since established universal health care coverage for all residents of the United Kingdom. This policy goal having been long realized, the Thatcher government set for itself the objective of achieving greater "value for money" on the part of health care providers. This objective was sought by giving greater autonomy to providers in managing budgetary allotments. A key element in the development of this autonomy is the separation of the provider function from the purchasing function.[24] Through a process of trial and error, movement toward the goal of greater efficiency was implemented through adoption of "community needs assessment" and "joint commissioning."[25] This entire process was carried out by the central administration in London, with little need to consult with countervailing forces. The ability of the Thatcher government to complete this entire process without significant input from other institutional structures represents an example of "directive" health system change.

This "directive" pattern of change was, of course, achieved over the opposition of the Labour Party and various sectors of public opinion. Notable among social forces often opposing the internal market reforms were elements of the medical profession, due to chariness in accepting the power being given to business managers in the health system. The recent defeat of the Conservative government is an adequate indication of the political limits of British constitutional power. The extent to which the new Labour government may modify the "internal market" changes introduced under the Conservative regime is a matter of considerable conjecture (as suggested by Appleby in Chapter 14 of this volume).

Despite vast differences in constitutional and health services conditions, clear parallels exist between the changes that have occurred in Britain and in Hawaii. There existed a de facto similarity between the political situations in Hawaii and Great Britain. In both instances, no effective countervailing officially established institutional forces were available to block or modify "directive" health system change initiated by the ruling administration. In the absence of such countervailing forces, both the Thatcher administration and the Democratic leadership in Hawaii were free to set their respective objectives for health system reform.[26]

Although their objectives differed and although the constitutional conditions varied greatly, the Thatcher "internal market reforms" in the NHS and the Hawaiian health insurance programs of 1974 and 1989 both exemplify "directive" change. In both instances, the political administration achieved realization of its health policy goal through means selected by itself, without effective interference from countervailing institutional forces.

Conclusion

According to the analysis presented in this chapter, patterns of change in health care systems are derived from the overall sociopolitical structure in which the reform programs are embedded. The sociopolitical structure determining the pattern of health care change is in each case organized primarily with respect to a specified system problem. This approach to analysis of health care change makes possible the comparison of reforms occurring in large national systems with those taking place in smaller local systems. This approach also makes possible the examination of reforms in local systems through the analysis of sociopolitical factors that are similar in type to those found in large national health systems.

The system problem approach to health system reform facilitates an understanding of the functioning of a system as a whole. For example, the joint action of union and employer sickness fund representatives in achieving negotiated compromise between consumers and providers of services brought about integrative change in German cost containment reforms. It exemplifies the negotiating pattern that is common to other parts of the German social structure. This type of integrative approach to reform in a mature national health system helps us understand changes of a similar type in smaller, less developed systems.[27] Thus, the small and incipient health care reform program for the elderly poor in Oregon is of interest because of its structure and its approach to change. The "negotiated investment strategy" between opposing interest groups representing consumers and providers parallels the structure of German cost containment negotiations. The involvement of the state agencies completes a tripartite negotiating structure similar to that in Germany.

Using the system problem conceptual approach, four overall value patterns have been identified—namely, "integrative," "adaptive," "directive," and "system maintenance" configurations. Factors associated with each of these patterns present in the state social fabric are determinants of the structure and type of change that accompanies each local health service reform. Further investigation of these sociopolitical factors should bring to light the structures and processes by which incipient health service reforms evolve from the social matrix with which they are articulated.

There are indeed important potential fallacies and pitfalls in the way of this system problem approach to health care reform. The approach makes the assumption that a given health care system tends to give special attention to a particular type of system problem. On theoretical grounds, one must assume that other system problems are also given some attention by each health system. The initial identification of the system problem emphases presented in this chapter is a topic worthy of further investigation. Other health systems may well be not as readily classified in this manner. Some systems may give equal emphasis to several system problems. However, the comparison of reforms in these four national systems with corresponding local state reform programs suggests the possible usefulness of a system problem approach to comparative analysis of health system change.

Notes

1. The types of change discussed in this chapter involve behavior designed to deal with the functional problems of a system identified by Parsons and Shils (1951) and by Parsons, Bales, and Shils (1953), as applied to the health system context. Each health care system tends to give special attention to one system problem in particular. In the case of the British system, the term *directive change* is used to indicate the means-ends, self-contained, "goal attainment" behavior of the National Health Service. The terms *adaptation, system maintenance,* and *integration* are retained from Parsons's structural-functional analysis.

2. This description is generally consistent with the analysis of Cawson (1986) and that of Schmitter and Lehmbruch (1979).

3. A careful analysis of the approach to changes introduced by the United Seniors in Oregon is presented by Falcone, Ensley, and Moore (1992). This approach contrasts with the establishment of commissions, which involves early intervention by government.

4. An account of the historical factors that led to the structuring of the health care systems of the four Western countries is beyond the scope of the present chapter. However, an analysis of some of the historical forces that led to the formation of the German health system is presented by Altenstetter in Chapter 4 of this volume. Major steps in the establishment of the Canadian health system are described by Charles and Badgley in Chapter 7, and key elements in the development of Swedish health services are presented by Immergut in Chapter 10. For analysis of events before and after the foundation of the NHS, see Webster (1988).

5. Altenstetter in Chapter 4 of this volume stresses the centrality of functional organization in the German health system. The corporatist approach does not accept the mechanistic solution of the pure market and its assumption of preestablished harmony. The corporatist system relies on negotiations rather than on the market to achieve effective part-whole relationships. See Glaser (1991) for discussion of the role of negotiations in the German health system.

6. The Structural Health Care Reform Act of 1993 has reduced the scope of corporatist negotiations in Germany, owing to the tightened economic conditions following on the reunification of the country. Since passage of the reform of 1993, although the size of the health care budget has been closely controlled through federal and state action, prices and volume of services continue to be negotiated by the corporatist bodies, as indicated by Altenstetter in Chapter 4 of this volume.

7. See Kirkman-Liff (1990) for a discussion of the role of Concerted Action in cost containment policy.

8. As noted by Anderson (1989), the reliance on market-oriented forces with regard to distribution of health care services is more extreme in the United States than in any other Western country.

9. Morehouse (1983) and Hendrick and Ziegler (1987) maintained that the relative simplicity of the economy is a factor in a weak Oregon political party structure. These authors conceived the capacity of a majority party to obtain the election of their own gubernatorial candidates as an indicator of the strength of a state party system.

10. Leichter (1992, pp. 117-146) compared the behavior of Oregon Health Decisions in the Medicaid "rationing" proposal with that of the United Seniors in the aging program as examples of the "moralistic political subculture" of Oregonians. This moralistic subcultural pattern was also attributed to Oregon by Elazar (1988) and by Mahood (1990), who emphasized commitment to issues relating to society as a whole.

11. This description is based in part on data on rankings of the 12 southeastern states regarding employment and income rates and on rankings as to levels of state taxes and expenditures for such areas as education, highways, and police, as presented in the *Tennessee Statistical Abstract, 1996-1997* (1997). See Luebke (1990) for a related analysis of core and peripheral industries.

12. Grantham (1995) pointed out the role of regional differences in Tennessee state politics during the present century. See also Lamis (1990) and Corlew (1990) for analysis of political and social conditions in Tennessee.

13. The foregoing description and the following summary of the TennCare program are based on the report of Bonnyman (1996). Later figures for June 1997 are from the TennCare Fact Sheet as provided through the TennCare web site, http://170.142.16.205/health/tenncare/pdffiles.htm.

14. The savings achieved by TennCare and the CLSCs are also related to the extensive employment of nonphysician professionals in both programs.

15. Other Canadian provinces have dealt with restricted economic conditions by cutting back or consolidating services while retaining the fee payment system. As pointed out by Fooks in Chapter 8 of this volume, the fee-for-service system is a factor in the inability of Canada to effectively control costs. Through the CLSCs, Quebec employs an alternative less costly reimbursement system as a "dynamic" means of dealing with the common "system maintenance" problem facing many of the Canadian provinces.

16. The Federation of County Councils is not elected by popular vote but represents the councils in their administrative duties throughout the country. In this exclusive nationwide capacity, the federation exemplifies "administrative corporatism," consistently with von Otter's designation of the Swedish health system in Chapter 12 of this volume.

17. See Lass (1977) for an account of some of these local economic struggles. See also related articles in Clark (1989).

18. Elazar (1970) remarked that "the Scandinavian influence so prevalent in Minnesota is almost undiluted in Duluth" (p. 273). It should be noted that allegiance to the Democratic Farmer Labor Party with its commitment to local activism is particularly strong in the Duluth area. Because of common problems embracing the entire region, 16 adjacent Minnesota and Wisconsin counties have been involved in the project described below.

19. This description of the Health Quest Program is based on the *Bridge to Health Survey: Summary Report* (St. Mary's Medical Center, 1996), supplemented by telephone interviews with the steering committee, and with data and communication team members advising on the project.

20. According to officials at SPRI, a research organization affiliated with the Federation of County Councils in Stockholm, some offers of choices for users between alternative providers have been recently withdrawn for reasons of cost.

21. The role performed by the unions in the evolution of the Hawaiian economy from a rural system to that of a modern industrial society is presented by Aller (1957), by Beechart (1985), and by Lee (1987).

22. The central role played by these ethnic groups in the changed political landscape of Hawaii is documented by Mondragon and Schweig (1995) and by Neubauer (1997).

23. Neubauer (1997) detailed the steps by which the Prepaid Health Act of 1974 and the SHIP program were enacted. The analysis also discussed recent trends in Hawaiian health policies that suggest some retreat from the earlier commitment to universal insured access for all Hawaiians. From the present comparative perspective, these recent trends do not call into question the dominant role of a unitary political structure in fostering "directive" health system change.

24. The importance of the separation of these functions in the internal market reforms is stressed by Ham (1994). Since the introduction of internal market reforms, providers have been able to manage allocated budgets without the need for continuous approval by the local funding authority. For a related analysis of "planned markets," see Saltman and von Otter (1995).

25. As indicated by Light in Chapter 15 of this book, "community needs assessment" involves a planning process that "reconceptualizes" purchasing as "joint commissioning" and as "creative rethinking . . . of what kinds of services will best maximize the health of a population or a community."

26. The British health system's capacity for "directive" change is enhanced by the centrally controlled bureaucracy of the NHS and by a unified budgetary system under central government administration.

27. For this reason, various local reform programs in the United States can be seen as laboratories of change, in the sense of being useful foci for comparative international analysis. From this perspective, these local reform programs are of interest not so much for their accomplishments in the way of reform as for their similarities in structure and approach to reform.

References

Aller, C. (1957). *Labor relations in the Hawaiian sugar industry.* Berkeley, CA: Institute of Industrial Relations.

Anderson, O. (1989). *The health services continuum in democratic states.* Ann Arbor, MI: Health Administration Press.

Beechart, E. (1985). *Working in Hawaii: A labor history.* Honolulu: University of Hawaii Press.

Bonnyman, G. (1996). Stealth reform: Market-based Medicaid in Tennessee. *Health Affairs, 15*(2), 306-314.

Cawson, A. (1986). *Corporatism and political theory.* Oxford, UK: Basil Blackwell.

Clark, C. (1989). *Minnesota in an era of change: The state and its people since 1900.* St. Paul: Minnesota Historical Society Press.

Corlew, R. (1990). *Tennessee: A short history.* Knoxville: University of Tennessee Press.

Dodds, G. (1986). *The American Northwest: A history of Oregon and Washington.* Arlington Heights, IL: Forum.

Elazar, D. (1970). *Cities of the prairie: The metropolitan frontier and American politics.* New York: Basic Books.

Elazar, D. (1988). *The American constitutional tradition.* Lincoln: University of Nebraska Press.

Falcone, D., Ensley, D., & Moore, C. (1992). Political culture, political leadership, sustained advocacy and aging reform: The Oregon and North Carolina experience. In H. Leichter (Ed.), *Health policy reform in America: Innovations from the states* (pp. 73-101). Armonk, NY: M. E. Sharpe.

Glaser, W. (1991). *Health insurance in practice.* San Francisco: Jossey-Bass.

Grantham, D. (1995). Tennessee and twentieth century American politics. *Tennessee Historical Quarterly, 54,* 210-229.

Ham, C. (1994). *Management and competition in the new NHS.* Oxford, UK: Radcliffe Medical Press.

Hedrick, W., & Ziegler, L. (1987). Oregon on the politics of power. In R. Hrebenar & C. Thomas (Eds.), *Interest group politics in the American West* (pp. 105-112). Salt Lake City: University of Utah Press.

Kirkman-Liff, B. (1990). Physician payment and cost containment in West Germany: Suggestions for Medicare reform. *Journal of Health Politics, Policy and Law, 15,* 69-99.

Lamis, A. (1990). *The two party South* (2nd expanded ed., pp. 163-178). New York: Oxford University Press.

Lass, W. (1977). *Minnesota: A bicentennial history.* New York: Norton.

Lee, A. (1987). Planters, public employees and public interest. In R. Hrebenar & C. Thomas (Eds.), *Interest group politics in the American West* (pp. 59-66). Salt Lake City: University of Utah Press.

Leichter, H. (1997). *Health policy reform in America: Innovations from the states* (2nd ed.). Armonk, NY: M. E. Sharpe.

Luebke, P. (1990). *Tarheel politics: Myths and realities.* Chapel Hill: University of North Carolina Press.

Mahood, H. (1990). *Interest group politics in America: A new intensity.* Englewood Cliffs, NJ: Prentice Hall.

Mondragon, D., & Schweig, B. (1995). Enactment of mandated health insurance in Hawaii. *Review of Social Economy, 53,* 243-259.

Morehouse, S. (1983). *State politics, parties and policies.* New York: Holt, Rinehart & Winston.

Neubauer, D. (1997). Hawaii: The health state revisited. In H. Leichter (Ed.), *Health policy reform in America* (2nd ed., pp. 163-188). Armonk, NY: M. E. Sharpe.

Parsons, T., Bales, R., & Shils, E. (1953). *Working papers in the theory of action.* Glencoe, IL: Free Press.

Parsons, T., & Shils, E. (1951). *Toward a general theory of action*. Cambridge, MA: Harvard University Press.

Prepaid Health Care Act of 1974, Hawaii Revised Statutes, Chapter 393.

Saltman, R., & von Otter, C. (1995). *Implementing planned markets: Balancing social and economic responsibilities*. Philadelphia: Open University Press.

Schmitter, P., & Lehmbruch, G. (1979). *Trends toward corporatist intermediation*. Beverly Hills, CA: Sage.

St. Mary's Medical Center, Health Quest Program. (1996). *Bridge to Health Survey: Summary report. Northeastern Minnesota and Northwestern Wisconsin Regional Health Status Survey* (2nd ed.). Duluth, MN: Author.

Tennessee Statistical Abstract, 1996-1997. (1997). Knoxville: University of Tennessee, College of Business Administration, Center for Business and Economic Research.

Webster, C. (1988). *The health services since the war: Vol. 1. Problems of health care: The National Health Service since 1957*. London: HMSO.

Index

About the Editors

Francis D. Powell received his PhD from Georgetown University and did postdoctoral work in sociology at Harvard. He has held research appointments at the Tavistock Institute of Human Relations in England and the Mediziniches Hochschule in Hannover, Germany. He is currently an adjunct faculty member at the Massachusetts Institute for Social and Economic Research at the University of Massachusetts-Amherst. Among his publications is *Theory of Coping Systems: Change in Supportive Health Organizations*.

Albert F. Wessen received his PhD from Yale University. He is Professor of Medical Science and Sociology at Brown University. Formerly the Chief of the Behavioral Science Unit of the World Health Organization, he has specialized in social epidemiology and the comparative study of health care organizations. His most recent book is *Migration and Health in a Small Society*.

About the Contributors

Christa Altenstetter received her PhD from the University of Heidelberg. She is currently Professor of Political Science at Queens College and the Graduate School of the City University of New York and is a member of the research staff of the GSF-MEDIS Institute of the National Research Center for Environment and Health, Neuherberg, Germany. She has served as an adviser to the Regional Office for Europe of the World Health Organization and as Chair of the Study Group on Comparative Health Policy of the International Political Science Association. Her research interests in the area of comparative health policy concern evolving policies in the European Union and its member nations, with special reference to Germany. Among her many publications are *Comparative Health Policy and the New Right* (with Stuart Haywood), *Health Policy Reform: National Variations, and Globalization* (with J. W. Björkman), and *Health Policy-Making and Administration in West Germany and the United States*.

John Appleby joined the King's Fund in London as Director of the Health Systems Program at the end of 1998. Currently, he is Senior Lecturer in Health Economics at the University of East Anglia, Norwich, England. He received his MSc in Health Economics from the University of York and has held appointments with the National Health Service, the National Association of Health Authorities and Trusts, and at the Health Services Management Center, University of Birmingham. He has published numerous papers on health economics, with special reference to the

424

recent reforms of the National Health Service, and he is also the author of *Financing Health Care in the 1990s*.

Robin F. Badgley received his PhD from Yale University and for many years has been a member of the Faculty of Medicine of the University of Toronto, where he was Chair of the Department of Behavioral Science and of the Graduate Department of Community Health. He has been active in health policy research in Canada, having chaired or been a member of several national inquiry commissions. His special research interest is the problem of attaining equity in health care. He has published widely in medical sociology and on Canadian health care. Among his publications are *Doctors' Strike: Medical Care and Conflict in Saskatchewan* and *The Family Doctor* (with Samuel Wolfe).

François Béland received his PhD in sociology from Laval University. He is Professor in the Department of Health Administration at the Faculty of Medicine of the University of Montreal. He is also a researcher in the Interdisciplinary Health Research Group. His interests include the study of health, aging, and long-term care in Quebec, Canada, and Spain. He has published over 100 scholarly articles.

Catherine A. Charles received her PhD from Columbia University. She is currently Associate Professor in the Department of Clinical Epidemiology and Biostatistics and a member of the Centre for Health Economics and Policy Analysis at McMaster University in Hamilton, Ontario. Her research interests include: public and patient participation in health care decision-making, the health professions and public policy, and the use of research evidence to improve decision-making regarding the organization and delivery of health care.

Patricia Day received a degree in sociology from the University of London. She is Senior Research Fellow at the Center for the Analysis of Social Policy, University of Bath. Her research interests include hospital organization and public housing as well as the study of the National Health Service.

Mark G. Field, who received his PhD in Social Relations from Harvard University, is an Associate of the Davis Center for Russian Studies and

Adjunct Professor, School of Public Health, Harvard University. He is also Professor of Socilogy Emeritus at Boston University. A specialist in health care in the Former Soviet Union, his books include *Doctor and Patient in Soviet Russia* and *Soviet Socialized Medicine: An Introduction.* He has written widely on issues of comparative health care systems, including *Success and Crisis in National Health Systems: A Comparative Approach.* He is a former Chairman, Committee on the Sociology of Health, International Sociological Association.

Catherine Fooks received a graduate degree in political science from Queen's University. Her research interests include quality assurance activities, methods of physician payment, and issues of health and child development. Formerly a Senior Policy Advisor to the Ontario Minister of Health, she is now Director of Policy and Research at the College of Physicians and Surgeons of Ontario.

Ellen Immergut is Professor in the Faculty of Political Science at the University of Konstanz. She was formerly on the faculty of the Massachusetts Institute of Technology. Her interests in health policy led to the publication of *Health Politics: Interests and Institutions in Western Europe,* a comparative study of developments in France, Sweden, and Switzerland.

Bradford Kirkman-Liff is Professor of Health Administration and Policy at the Arizona State University School of Business. He received a doctor's degree in public health from the University of North Carolina. He has published widely in the areas of quality assessment, managed care, and medical practice organization, as well as in the field of comparative health policy. His research on health care systems has focused on the Netherlands, Germany, and England as well as on the United States.

Rudolf Klein, who received his graduate degree in history from Oxford University, is Professor of Social Policy and Director of the Center for the Analysis of Social Policy at the University of Bath. A leading analyst of health and social services in the United Kingdom, he has published many articles and monographs on the National Health Service, including the very influential *Politics of the National Health Service.*

Donald W. Light is currently Professor and Director of the Division of Behavioral and Social Medicine at the University of Medicine and Dentistry of New Jersey and has been Senior Fellow at the Leonard Davis Institute of Health Economics at the University of Pennsylvania. He received his PhD from Brandeis University. He has published widely in sociology and is a specialist on comparative health care systems. Among his books are *Becoming Psychiatrists: The Professional Transformation of Self*, *Benchmarks of Fairness for Health Care Reform* (with Norman Daniels and Ronald Caplan), *Political Values and Health Care: The German Experience* (with Alexander Schuller), and *Britain's Health System: From Welfare State to Managed Markets* (with Annabelle May).

David Mechanic, a leader in medical sociology, was formerly a faculty member at the University of Wisconsin. Since 1979, he has been at Rutgers University, where he served as Dean of the Faculty of Arts and Sciences. He is the founder and Director of the Rutgers Institute for Health Policy and Aging Research and is the Rene Dubos Professor of Behavioral Sciences. He has received numerous awards for distinction in research and is a member of the Commission on Behavioral and Social Sciences and Education of the National Research Council. In addition to his wide-ranging research on health care in the United States, he has been especially interested in the British health care system. Among his books are *Mental Health and Social Policy, From Advocacy to Allocation: The Evolving American Health Care System, Handbook of Health, Health Care and the Health Professions,* and *Inescapable Decisions: The Imperatives of Health Reform.*

Richard B. Saltman is currently Professor of Social Policy and Management at the Emory University School of Public Health. A political scientist, he has specialized in the comparative analysis of recent trends in the health systems of Western nations. He is the author of *The International Handbook of Health-Care Systems, Fixing Health Budgets: Experience From Europe and North America* (with Friedrich Wilhelm Schwartz and Howard Glennerster), and *Planned Markets and Public Competition: Strategic Reform in Northern European Health Systems* (with Casten von Otter).

Bradley Scharf is Professor in the Department of Political Science at Seattle University. He has specialized in analyzing Soviet politics and the affairs of the German Democratic Republic. Among his publications is *Politics and Change in East Germany: An Evaluation of Socialist Democracy.*

Casten von Otter, a sociologist, specializes in the analysis of issues of social and health policy in Sweden. He is currently a Senior Researcher at the Arbeitslivcentrum (Center for the Study of Workers' Life) at the University of Stockholm. Among his monographic publications are *Public Sector Transformation: Rethinking Markets and Hierarchies in Government* (with Frieder Naschold) and *Implementing Planned Markets in Health Care: Balancing Social and Economic Responsibility* (with Richard Saltman).